Comments from readers on Ragnar Hanas's book, **Type 1 Di[...]
Children, Adolescents and Young Adults**

'I have no hesitation in thoroughly recommending this book to
adolescents and young people with Type 1 diabetes, their families,
and also to all healthcare professionals involved in their care.'

PROFESSOR MARTIN SILINK
in *Diabetologia*

'The information is clear, concise and extremely readable. All imaginable
topics are covered from hypoglycaemia, through pregnancy and on to
psychological issues! It is difficult to imagine anyone, including
healthcare professionals, teachers and grandparents, not learning
something helpful.'

Practical Diabetes International

'This is far and away the best diabetes resource I have ever come across.
It has information you will not find anywhere else and is well presented
and indexed. If you are serious about managing your child's diabetes
to the best of your ability, you cannot afford to do without this book.'

Reader from London,
featured on the Amazon website

Comments from readers on Charles Fox's book, **Type 2 Diabetes:
Answers at your Fingertips**

'I can pass on much more information now after this marathon read!
I'll be the first to purchase the new edition when it's published.'

CLARE MEHMET,
Diabetes UK Newham Voluntary Group

'I have no hesitation in recommending this book.'

SIR STEVE REDGRAVE,
Vice President, Diabetes UK

'It is an invaluable guide to the subject: authoritative, nicely written and
packed with facts.'

P L, Acton

Type 2 Diabetes in Adults of All Ages

How to become an expert on your own diabetes

Dr Charles Fox BM, FRCP
*Consultant Physician with Special Interest in Diabetes,
Northampton General Hospital, UK*

Dr Ragnar Hanas MD, PhD
*Consultant Paediatrician, specialising in diabetes,
Uddevalla Hospital, Sweden*

CLASS PUBLISHING · LONDON

NOTICE
For dosages and applications mentioned in this book, the reader can
be assured that the authors have gone to great lengths to ensure that
the indications reflect the standard of knowledge at the time this work
was completed. However, diabetes treatment must be individually
tailored for each and every person with diabetes. Treatment methods
and dosages may change. Advice and recommendations in this book
cannot be expected to be generally applicable in all situations and
always need to be supplemented with individual assessment by a
diabetes team. The author and the publishers do not accept any legal
responsibility or liability for any errors or omissions, or the use of the
material contained herein and the decisions based on such use.
Neither the authors nor the publishers will be liable for direct, indirect
or consequential damages arising out of the use, or inability to use,
the contents of this book.

Printing history
First published 2008

The authors and publishers welcome feedback from the users
of this book. Please contact the publishers.

Class Publishing, Barb House, Barb Mews, London W6 7PA, UK
Telephone: 020 7371 2119
Fax: 020 7371 2878 [International +4420]
email: post@class.co.uk
Website: www.class.co.uk

A CIP catalogue for this book is available from the British Library

ISBN 978 1 85959 166 6

10 9 8 7 6 5 4 3 2 1

Edited by Richenda Milton-Thompson

Typeset by Martin Bristow

Printed and bound in Finland by WS Bookwell, Juva

Contents

Preface

This book on Type 2 diabetes was inspired by Dr Ragnar Hanas's book on *Type 1 Diabetes in Children, Adolescents and Young Adults,* which contains a wealth of detail and wisdom. The aim, in both the Type 1 book and this book, is to enable readers to become *the* experts on their own diabetes.

Diabetes is a condition which forces people to make unwelcome changes in their lives. This is true of both Type 1 and Type 2 diabetes. The more information available to you, the more motivated you are likely to be when it comes to making choices.

There is no such thing as 'mild diabetes', but that it is not to say it needs to rule your life. Type 2 diabetes is a progressive condition and people move inevitably through different stages of treatment starting with diet, through increasing numbers of tablets and eventually to insulin. Each new stage leads to anxiety and a feeling of failure and loss of control. This book aims to provide you with the information you need to understand what it happening to you at each stage, and why. Once you are armed with this information, you will begin to be able to take back control of your life.

We hope this book will become a valuable source of information for people with Type 2 diabetes, and for everyone with whom they share their lives. The style is informal and friendly and we have tried to avoid jargon. More detailed information about physiology or research findings can be found in boxes so it is readily available for reference but does not interfere with the readability of the text itself. We write for the reader who wants to be fully informed so that they can make the choices necessary for staying healthy. Wherever possible, we provide evidence to support our views.

We want this book to be as good as it can be, and to remain so. In order to achieve this, we welcome feedback from our readers. If you feel there are errors or gaps, please contact Class Publishing at Barb House, Barb Mews, London W6 7PA, or via info@class.co.uk.

Enjoy the book, explore the information, and live your life to the full!

Dr Charles Fox, Northampton, UK
Dr Ragnar Hanas, Uddevalla, Sweden

Acknowledgments

Many people have contributed to this book, but particular thanks are due to Dr Phil Ambery and Dr Anne Kilvert for their detailed comments on the whole manuscript. Without their input, this would be a lesser book.

Dr Peter Swift and Dr Stuart Brink advised on the preparation of sections of the book, and the dietitians Ellen Aslander, Carmel Smart and Sheridan Waldron gave invaluable comments on drafts of the Nutrition chapter.

We would like to thank our editor, Richenda Milton-Thompson, for steering this project to completion.

A large number of cartoons were commissioned especially for this book and drawn by David Woodroffe who seemed to know exactly what we wanted to portray. The cartoon on the front cover is by Randy Glasbergen.

Finally, we would like to thank our patients – the people for whom this book has been written. We hope it will prove useful and inspire confidence.

Charles Fox and Ragnar Hanas

Introduction

If you want something done properly, do it yourself. This is all very well, but of course you need to know how to do it first. If you are to manage your diabetes, you will need a thorough understanding of the disease and how it affects you. As anyone living with diabetes knows, it is a condition that is with you 24 hours of every day.

This book helps you take control of your own life with Type 2 diabetes. The only person you can rely upon to be there 24 hours a day is yourself. So after a while you will become the best authority on your own diabetes. Learning to care for your diabetes from scratch, like learning anything else, is a matter of trial and error. During the process you are bound to make some mistakes – but you can learn from each one of these. Indeed you will learn more from your own mistakes than from the mistakes other people have made. Taking an active part in lifestyle

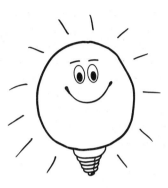

The diabetes clinic will often function as an information centre where we pass on good ideas from one person to another.

management and having an understanding of your drug treatments and why they are important is crucial to preserving your health over the longer term. It is rapidly becoming clear that clinics where treatment is truly a partnership between doctor and patients achieve far better long-term results.

Once you have come to terms with your diagnosis of diabetes, you will probably find it takes about a year to experience most of the day-to-day situations that are likely to be affected. These may include holidays, birthdays, parties, heavy exercise and periods of sickness. As you become more confident, you will begin to draw upon your own experiences and discover things about your condition that your diabetes team will find it helpful to know about. This sort of free exchange of information not only helps us to help you. It also enables the clinic to function as an information centre, passing on suggestions and knowledge from one person to another. You are not alone, and you can be sure that whatever problem you've had, someone attending your clinic will already have encountered it.

Knowledge changes over time. What was advisable 10 or 15 years ago may not necessarily apply today. At one time, health professionals

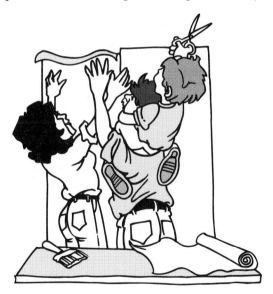

The underlying theme of this book is: 'If you want something done properly, do it yourself'. You are the only person who will be involved with your diabetes 24 hours every day so it won't be long before you are the greatest expert on it.

would tell a person about some new development, only to hear, 'Actually, I have been doing it that way for years, I just didn't dare tell anyone'. Nowadays we share knowledge and learning with each other instead. Ask your practice nurse or doctor about your local Diabetes UK group. Regular meetings allow for sharing of experiences and quite often have a speaker who may be your local diabetologist, a dietitian or an exercise coach. Even if you can't attend the meetings, you may at least be able to acquire some telephone numbers so you can 'phone a friend' for advice.

This book deals with Type 2 diabetes in adults of all ages, including the specific problems of Type 2 diabetes encountered by older people. It does not address the treatment of Type 1 diabetes, except in the briefest of ways. This is dealt with in the companion book *Type 1 Diabetes in Children, Adolescents and Young Adults,* by Dr Ragnar Hanas. This book describes methods of treating diabetes that are common in much of Europe as well as in North America and elsewhere in the world. However, the methods used may vary from one centre to another. The goal is to find a way of managing your diabetes effectively, and there may be more than one way of reaching this goal.

Don't try to read the book from cover to cover or memorize it. Rather, use it as a reference book. A number of medical jargon terms are included, but their meaning should be obvious from the context so you don't necessarily need to learn them. If you find some parts of the book difficult to understand, especially on the first reading, please don't be discouraged. When you come back and read it a second time, and when you have more experience of living with diabetes, it will all begin to fit together. More detailed information, aimed at those who want to learn a little bit more, can be found in the boxes in the text. Key references that have been used in the writing of each chapter can be found at the back of the book.

Remember that you can learn things in many different ways. Many education programmes involved lessons arranged around one aspect of diabetes at a time. You will be encouraged to

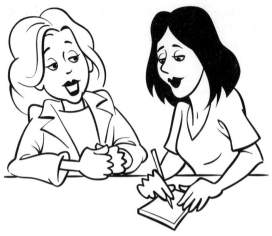

Body language can make more impact than words, and many people find that if it comes to a choice between remembering official information or informal information, they usually find it easier to remember informal information.

attend with a partner or friend who will help you to take in everything you're told. Generally, people learn better in a relaxed atmosphere where they are encouraged to participate. However, you may also learn a great deal from an unplanned conversation with a nurse, for example. The nurse's intonation, body language and expression may give you as much information as the spoken words. So, while you will be given official information during a formal consultation, you will also hear unofficial views and additional information from health professionals, other people with diabetes and their family members. It is also helpful if you can be aware of their body language, what they say and how they say it, as well as what they do *not* say. This type of information is also available from every day contact with doctors and nurses.

Your previous experience of diabetes from a relative or colleague may give you a false picture of what living with diabetes will be like for you. In particular, perhaps, your treatment regime immediately after diagnosis is likely to be very different from the regime followed by someone who has been living with diabetes for a number of years.

It will be quite natural after diagnosis to be preoccupied by concerns about your future and the difficulties that may lie ahead. Your diabetes team will give you straightforward information about possible complications, and how to avoid or reduce the risks. Many doctors, including the authors of this book, will tell you all there is to tell, not leaving out any information. Sometimes there is no straight answer to a question, but we will tell you as much as we know.

During the first few weeks, you will need to get to know yourself all over again. You now know you have diabetes. To begin with, having to take this knowledge on board may make you scared about various aspects of your life. You may feel anxious and insecure, since you don't yet know how to tackle the different situations that daily life throws at you, but gradually you will feel more confident about getting on with your life. Alternatively, you may feel relieved that you now have an explanation for feeling unwell (particularly if this has gone on for a considerable time) and be glad that you are going to have treatment to make you feel better.

Getting to grips with diabetes

Managing Type 2 diabetes involves a journey of therapy, which begins with changes to your diet and pattern of exercise. This continues as a way of life. As time goes by, you will probably start taking tablets, need to combine treatments, and eventually start taking insulin injections. Good diabetes care includes both medical treatment and education. We want everyone with Type 2 diabetes, and their relatives, to feel that they can assume responsibility for their own treatment and take charge of their own life. You can control your diabetes rather than let your diabetes control you. Once your diabetes has become manageable, so other aspects of your life will fall into place.

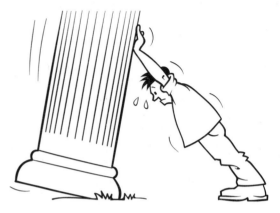

When a problem is too large and seems unsolvable, don't feel you have to cope with it all at once, all by yourself.

When you first find out you have diabetes

In the UK and many other countries, newly diagnosed Type 2 diabetes is usually looked after in general practice, where patients have an initial consultation with their GP, and later with the practice nurse. It is usual if you have Type 2 diabetes to receive advice about changes to your diet and lifestyle at the time of diagnosis, but this should be reinforced a few days later by a longer consultation with the practice nurse. A few months after this, you should have a follow-up appointment to look at whether the changes you have made to your lifestyle have brought your blood glucose levels under control. Long-term glucose control is measured by a test called

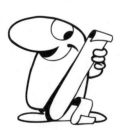

Keep a list of your questions so you can remember to ask them at your next diabetes review.

HbA_{1c} which gives you an estimate of how much sugar is being carried in your red blood cells. This can improve substantially in people who are able to change the way they eat and the amount of exercise they take. It is essential to ask questions about your diet in the early stages and you should try to work out the best way of changing your pattern of eating. Changes made early on can set you up for better glucose control throughout your life with Type 2 diabetes.

What happens next?

The first week will seem chaotic. You may well have had no symptoms of diabetes, but suddenly you find yourself being given a number of depressing facts about long-term problems associated with diabetes. You may also be given a number of new drugs to keep you well. By the second week, things will seem much more routine and you will find yourself beginning to understand a lot more about Type 2 diabetes and how it may affect your life.

During the first few days, many people may experience a feeling of resentment, disappointment and thoughts of 'Why me?'. If you are in this situation, you may have difficulty taking in the fact that you actually have diabetes. You will need time to examine your feelings and adjust gradually to this strange new situation that now faces you and the rest of your family. Most things will be new and you may find them difficult to understand at first but, bit by bit, the different pieces of information should fall into place. By the end of the second week, you will begin to understand how taking care with food and drink choices can be really helpful in lowering your blood sugar and improving your symptoms. You may end up with a wholesale clearance of your fridge and food cupboard!

If you succeed in taking control of your diabetes early, you can be the one in charge of the situation, rather than your diabetes taking charge of you.

Most people find that managing diabetes is easier than they had anticipated. To feel confident caring for yourself at home, you should revise what to do if you become unwell (see Chapter 21).

In the first few months, you should expect to meet a specialist dietitian. There is only so much that you can learn about healthy eating for

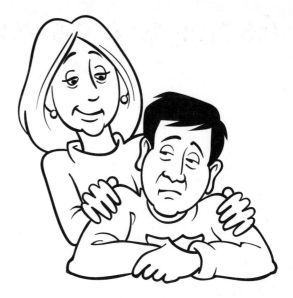

After a few days, as you begin to come to terms with your diagnosis, it's worth broaching your diagnosis with close colleagues and friends. They are much more likely to be sympathetic to a change of lifestyle if you briefly explain why.

diabetes from books; a face-to-face meeting helps to put many of the changes you need to make into context. Some of the necessary changes to your eating pattern might seem really difficult to make, but if you take them one step at a time, and have the right amount of support, you will find they are achievable.

Older people

Older people are being diagnosed with Type 2 diabetes in ever greater numbers as GPs take increasing opportunities for screening. Unfortunately, as you get older it may be more difficult to make the necessary lifestyle changes. With help and support from relatives and carers, people often find the motivation to accept the diagnosis and alter their eating habits and take the medication. Even if you're on your own, there will be a skilled practice nurse to offer advice and support.

More information about diabetes and older people can be found in Chapter 34.

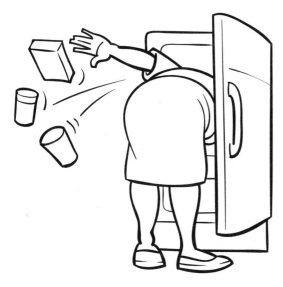

As you discover how taking control of what you eat can help your symptoms, you may find yourself clearing out most of the contents of your fridge!

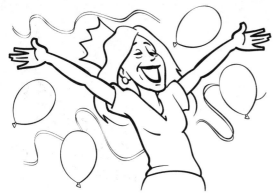

Whether it is a birthday, an anniversary or a new job, some days call for celebration. Once in a while, you can be a bit more relaxed about routines and rules.

Teenagers and young adults

Unfortunately, more and more young people are now being affected by Type 2 diabetes. This is due, in part, to the increasing burden of weight gain affecting our society in general. If you are in your teens or 20s and have just been diagnosed with Type 2 diabetes, it can feel as though the world is falling in. But rest assured, you will get the help and support you need. Specific strategies around weight loss and the management of Type 2 diabetes in teenagers and young adults will will be discussed in Chapter 22.

Self-help groups

Knowledge and self-confidence are your best armour when you are confronted with other people's opinions about diabetes. They will help you to recognize and deal with the prejudice and out-of-date views that, unfortunately, you are likely to meet. It is important for patients and health professionals to help each other spread better knowledge and understanding about diabetes.

Our goal is for everyone with Type 2 diabetes, however young or old, to do something proactive in the management of their condition. You don't suddenly have to get up every morning and run a marathon. Simple changes like getting off the bus one stop early, or forgoing that mid-morning snack, can make all the difference to your long-term health with diabetes.

Routine check-ups

After the initial phase, you are likely to see the nurse or doctor at the surgery for a check-up every third month or so. At these check-ups, you can discuss your health over the last few months, and the nurse or doctor will measure your long-term blood sugar control using an HbA_{1c} measurement. You will also be weighed, and the healthcare professional leading the clinic will ask about changes to your diet or routine. You may not achieve perfect results straight away, but as long as there is a steady improvement, that in itself is enough. Because raised blood pressure and cholesterol go hand in hand with Type 2 diabetes, you will also have your blood pressure and cholesterol checked at regular intervals. There is good evidence that keeping these other risk factors under control has a positive effect on your health in the long term.

If you are in a steady relationship, it is very important that your partner comes with you when you visit your diabetes healthcare team.

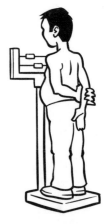

It is important that you continue to maintain a healthy weight. We check your weight at every visit to monitor and encourage your efforts with respect to weight loss. If your weight is stuck, this can be a cue for more encouragement and specific advice from the dietitian.

Once a year, you will usually have a more thorough check-up, including a full physical examination. Several additional tests (mainly blood tests) may be included in your annual check-up.

Living the life you choose

Diabetes is a long-term condition that will affect you every day for the rest of your life. Try to accept your diabetes (or at least not to see it as an enemy) since you can't escape it and there is currently no known cure. Although it is important to make changes to your lifestyle to support your treatment goals, you can still be very flexible in your day-to-day activities involving work and leisure time.

It is essential, however, that from the very beginning you plan how to carry on with your life in a manner that suits you. Don't let your diabetes dictate the type of life you should live. A lot of people find themselves thinking: 'I can't do such and such any more, now that I have diabetes . . . but I used to enjoy it so much before my diagnosis'. However, most activities are not only allowed, but you can do them perfectly well. Nothing is absolutely forbidden, but you would be wise to think things through more carefully than you used to, in all sorts of situa-

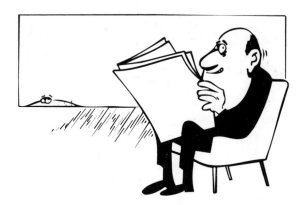

It is much easier to have a strong opinion if you don't know all the facts involved. You and your family will find that many people you come in contact with think they know a great deal about diabetes. Often their knowledge about diabetes treatment is far from up to date. Be sceptical when you hear generalized statements about diabetes, especially early on before you have your own knowledge and experience to rely upon.

tions. It is important to experiment and learn by trial and error. You should try to work with your practice nurse and doctor to agree a treatment regime which fits in with your lifestyle. If, as your diabetes progresses with time, you need insulin, this will have an impact on certain occupations (Chapter 27 on Social and employment issues).

Caring for your own diabetes

Goals for managing diabetes

A number of international authorities have put together recommended guidelines for the treatment of diabetes. The International Diabetes Federation has recently launched guidelines specifically for the management of Type 2 diabetes. A summary of the recommendations for management of blood glucose can be found on page2 88–9, and the full guidelines can be downloaded from their website (www.idf.org). Other organizations that have produced guidelines include the Canadian Diabetes Association and the English National Institute for Health and Clinical Excellence (NICE) which is currently preparing updated guidance. The latest updates on progress can be found on the NICE website (www.nice.org.uk).

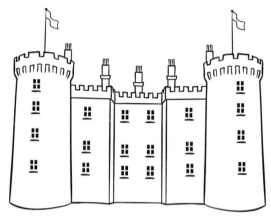

My home is my castle, as the saying goes. Build yourself a castle of knowledge and motivation so you can feel safe and comfortable while dealing with your diabetes.

Diabetes should not disrupt your work patterns. It is difficult to apply yourself if your blood glucose is too high or too low, as this disturbs concentration. During times of stress, there may be a temptation to relax your pattern of eating. But of course, it may be even more important to keep yourself feeling well when there are extra pressures in your life. Many people with Type 2 diabetes lead enjoyable and full lives but maintain good control in order to reduce the long term risks of diabetes.

> ### Goals of treatment
>
> - No symptoms or discomfort in everyday life.
> - Good general health and wellbeing.
> - Normal social relationships.
> - Normal professional life.
> - Normal family life including the possibility of pregnancy.
> - Prevention of long-term complications.

An important goal of diabetes management is to reduce the number and severity of the symptoms and side effects you may experience. Particularly during the early stages after diagnosis you may suffer tiredness, frequency of passing urine and thirst. It is important for your own personal wellbeing to avoid these as much as possible. For this reason we regularly review control of blood sugar and ensure it is the best it can possibly be.

How can you achieve these goals?

Traditionally, exercise and lifestyle changes have been the cornerstone of good Type 2 diabetes management – and this is still the case. Lifestyle changes underpin the way most of our treatments for diabetes work and improve their effectiveness. In the past, clinicians have started one treatment for blood sugar but not started a second one until the first is at maximum dose, a stepwise approach. Many doctors and health professionals are starting to question this now, and believe that earlier combination of two drugs may be more effective at lowering blood sugar, with fewer side effects. Managing Type 2 diabetes isn't just about blood sugar though: studies have shown that changing what you eat in order to reduce your fat intake can be combined with drugs to reduce fats in the blood. Along with exercise and tablets to help reduce your blood pressure, these can be important in helping you avoid problems later. See also Chapter 8 on Nutrition, and Chapter 9 on Weight reduction.

Traditional approach

- Diet and exercise.
- Stepwise addition of tablets to control blood sugar.
- Insulin – eventually.

Doctors' understanding of Type 2 diabetes, and the armoury of treatments they can prescribe to help you manage it, have both increased with time. Unfortunately those aspects of your lifestyle that put you at risk of developing Type 2 diabetes tend to be with you for a very long time. So health professionals have learned that they must work with people to help them change habits and behaviour patterns which are particularly damaging. Drug combinations, not just

for sugar but for blood pressure and blood fats as well, allow us to avoid or reduce the chance of complications later in life. But the key factor in all of this is you, and your own level of motivation. If you have the knowledge to be fully involved in managing your own diabetes care, this will be enormously helpful both for you yourself and for your medical team.

Diabetes today – cornerstones of management

- Diet and exercise.
- Earlier combinations of drugs to lower sugar to improve effectiveness and reduce side effects.
- Avoidance of complications by managing a range of problems, not just sugar.
- Knowledge.

Motivation of your own → Self-care

If you want to manage well with diabetes you must:

1 Become your own expert on diabetes.

2 Have more knowledge about diabetes than the average doctor.

3 Accept your diabetes and learn to live with it.

'It is no fun getting diabetes, but you must be able to have fun even if you have diabetes.'

Professor JOHNNY LUDVIGSSON, Sweden

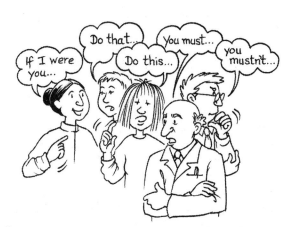

The key factor in managing your diabetes is you.

Becoming your own expert

The more motivated you are, the better you will be able to manage your own diabetes. It is important you realize the treatment is for your own sake, not your family's, and certainly not to benefit your doctor or nurse. Your motivation for the best possible self treatment might be:

- to be as good (or better . . .) at coaching your son's football team as you were before;

- to achieve a good performance at work while keeping good control of your blood sugar levels;

- to be able to enjoy an active retirement and look after your grandchildren.

If you have diabetes, you must become your own expert, learning to handle whatever life may throw at you in a satisfactory way.

The treatment of diabetes has changed a great deal in recent years, but public awareness has not necessarily caught up. So you are likely to come across a lot of people with out-of-date or fixed ideas, who think they know a great deal more than they actually do. You need to be able to rely on your own knowledge. Indeed, in order to live your life in the way you want without too many unpleasant symptoms, you will actually need to know even more about diabetes than the average doctor! To gain this knowledge you will have to ask questions and clarify your own thoughts about diabetes. Be sure to contact a member of your diabetes team whenever you have questions about your medication or anything else. If you save the question until your next visit, which might be 3 months away, you may simply forget all about it.

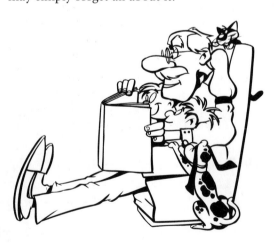

No matter how good our health or our fortune, we all need to feel loved and needed.

Becoming fully engaged with your diabetes and your own care is vitally important. Because you have to live with diabetes 24 hours a day, it is crucial that you decide as early as possible whether you are going to adjust your life around your diabetes, or whether you prefer to decide on a particular lifestyle and then adjust your diabetes treatment to enable you to achieve it. We encourage all people both young and old to be as active as possible in the management of their own diabetes from the start.

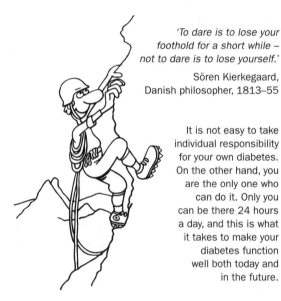

'To dare is to lose your foothold for a short while – not to dare is to lose yourself.'

Sören Kierkegaard, Danish philosopher, 1813–55

It is not easy to take individual responsibility for your own diabetes. On the other hand, you are the only one who can do it. Only you can be there 24 hours a day, and this is what it takes to make your diabetes function well both today and in the future.

Can you take time off from diabetes?

This really isn't possible since your diabetes is with you 24 hours a day. But you can make a distinction between everyday life and having a good time on special occasions. Most people (with or without diabetes) will allow themselves something extra once in a while, even if they know that this little extra is not necessarily terribly healthy. If your usual lifestyle is appropriate for diabetes, you too can allow yourself to be a bit more relaxed with food, if you are celebrating for example (see also 'Party-time' on page 48).

If you go on holiday or a business trip, your routine is bound to differ from the one you have at home. The goal on these occasions should not be to have perfect control over your blood glucose. The important thing is that you feel well enough to participate in all activities. This may mean you have to accept having a slightly higher than usual blood glucose level, but of course you shouldn't let it get so high that it affects your wellbeing.

It is better to have 15 rough days when your control is not what it should be, and 350 days when your diabetes is well controlled, and feel happy about life, than 75 'so-so' days and 290 when your diabetes is under strict control, but you feel miserable all the time. Many people with diabetes choose to have a slightly higher blood glucose level when they are about to do something important, such as an interview for a new job. And there are good reasons for this. In certain situations, it is much more important to avoid hypoglycaemia than to have a perfect blood glucose level.

Alternative and complementary therapies

Sometimes we encounter questions about complementary or alternative treatment methods. Unfortunately some stories from the world of Type 1 diabetes, where insulin is required in all patients, make disturbing reading – particularly where choosing an 'alternative' has resulted in the death of a child. This does still happen occasionally.

In Type 2 diabetes, many herbalists claim to have products which promote weight loss or improve blood glucose levels. Although some may be genuine and well-meaning practitioners, others may prey on vulnerable individuals who have had trouble losing weight or maintaining a diet in times gone by.

Unlike an alternative therapy, which is used instead of a conventional one, complementary therapy means exactly what its name implies. It should be used in addition to medical treatment, to complement rather than replace it. So, while

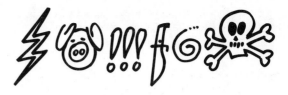

Sometimes you may feel like this when everything you have planned goes wrong and your blood glucose level ends up much too high or too low. At a time like this, it might be a good idea to put your monitoring and adjustments on hold for a week and just take time off. Then, you can start afresh with renewed enthusiasm. Check your blood glucose only to avoid hypoglycaemia. Most things in life are learned this way, in waves. As you become more familiar with your diabetes, these moments of exasperation will occur less and less often.

a complementary therapy cannot be a substitute for prescription medicines, you may benefit from it in other ways. For example, an aromatherapy massage may help you to relax, or a reflexology treatment may make it easier for you to cope with the anger you feel at having to organize your life rather differently from the way you did before.

Three issues are especially important when thinking about complementary or alternative treatments:

1 We must talk frankly with each other about this subject. If you want to try an alternative or complementary treatment for your diabetes despite recommendations not to, it is better that you do this openly so that your doctor and diabetes nurse know about it.

2 Adolescents and adults with diabetes must continue taking their medical treatments as prescribed by the doctor, otherwise their health may be in serious danger.

3 The alternative or complementary treatment must not be in any way dangerous or harmful to the person with diabetes.

Diabetes: some background

Diabetes mellitus, usually referred to simply as 'diabetes', has been known to mankind since ancient times. Diabetes means 'flowing through' and mellitus means 'sweet as honey', referring of course to the high volume of urine laden with sugar found in uncontrolled diabetes. Diabetes used to be described as either 'insulin-dependent' (IDDM) or 'non-insulin dependent' (NIDDM). Nowadays, you are more likely to hear the terms '*Type 1 diabetes*' and '*Type 2 diabetes*'.

Egyptian hieroglyphic findings from 1550 BC illustrate the symptoms of diabetes. Some people believe that the type of diabetes depicted was Type 2 and that Type 1 diabetes is a relatively new disease, appearing within the last two centuries.

In the past, diabetes was diagnosed by tasting the urine. No effective treatment was available. Before insulin was discovered, Type 1 diabetes always resulted in death, usually quite quickly.

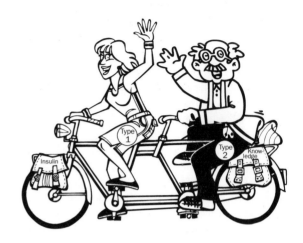

Insulin history

- The first human to be treated with insulin was a 14-year-old boy, Leonard Thomson, in Canada in the year 1922.
- James Havens was the first American to be treated with insulin, in 1922.
- In the UK, insulin was first given as part of a research trial later the same year.
- In Sweden, the first insulin injections were given in 1923 to, among others, a 5-year-old boy who subsequently lived almost 70 years with his diabetes.
- In the early days, insulin was distributed as a powder or tablets which were mixed with water before being injected.

Type 1 diabetes

If you are going to get Type 1 diabetes, you will probably know before your 40th birthday. Most people whose diabetes is diagnosed in childhood or the teenage years used to have Type 1 diabetes, but now there is an alarming increase in Type 2 diabetes in young people.

Type 1 diabetes is insulin-dependent, meaning that treatment with insulin is necessary from the time the disease is first diagnosed. In Type 1 diabetes, the insulin-producing cells of the pancreas are destroyed by a process in the body known as 'autoimmunity' (i.e. in which the body's cells attack each other). This leads eventually to a total loss of insulin production. In the absence of insulin, the blood glucose level rises inexorably and without insulin, the person will die.

Type 2 diabetes

Type 2 diabetes is also called adult-onset diabetes as the onset usually used to take place after the age of 40. Unfortunately, due to lifestyle changes over the last few decades, many more people are developing Type 2 diabetes at a younger age. There always were some people presenting with Type 2 diabetes early in adulthood, but these were the exception rather than the norm. Many years before the development of Type 2 diabetes, individuals usually become overweight. This leads to insulin becoming less effective ('insulin resistance') meaning that people with this condition have to produce more and more insulin to control their blood sugar. Eventually, the pancreas can no longer produce enough insulin and blood sugars begin to rise. This is the point at which Type 2 diabetes occurs. The best way to improve blood sugar levels in the early stages is by diet and exercise, though there is a trend for people to be treated with tablets straight after diagnosis. After 5–10 years, the body's ability to produce insulin will tail off so that insulin injections are required.

> ### Risk factors for Type 2 diabetes
>
> ● Overweight, particularly around the middle: (a waist measurement of 37 inches in men and 33 inches in women puts you at greater risk).
> ● Genetics (i.e. having a parent or other close relative with Type 2 diabetes).
> ● Poor nutrition.
> ● A history of high levels of cholesterol and other fats in your blood.
> ● A history of heart problems.

Tablets for Type 2 diabetes

The mainstay of Type 2 diabetes drug treatment in patients both young and old is metformin. This drug reduces the amount of glucose produced by the liver in the period between meals and has been shown in a very large study called the United Kingdom Prospective Diabetes Study (UKPDS) to reduce the risk of heart attacks and strokes in people with Type 2 diabetes.

Since the year 2000, a new class of drugs, the glitazones or insulin sensitizers have been available. These drugs act by improving the action of insulin on tissues like muscle and fat, improving the way in which these parts of the body take up and use the sugar from the bloodstream. The glitazones cause fluid retention and should not be used in people with heart failure. It has also been suggested that rosiglitazone may lead to a small increased risk of heart attacks. On the other hand, in many people, the glitazones have a powerful lowering effect on lowering blood glucose and most doctors feel that the benefits outweigh the drawbacks.

Another type of drug, the sulphonylureas, act by increasing the amount of insulin released by the beta cells in the pancreas. They are good at bringing blood sugars down quickly and are useful in thinner patients with Type 2 diabetes or those with many symptoms of high blood sugar. Patients taking sulphonylureas must be careful about their blood sugars falling too low (hypoglycaemia)

More information about tablets for lowering blood sugar is given in Chapter 13.

Young people with Type 2 diabetes

An increasing number of reports from North America, Japan, the UK and other parts of the industrialized world indicate that overweight teenagers are now beginning to develop Type 2 diabetes. This appears to be more common in

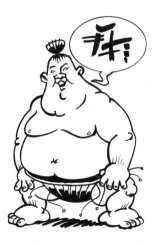

Being overweight will make you more vulnerable to Type 2 diabetes as, in the long run, your body will not be able to produce the large amounts of insulin necessary to keep your blood sugar normal. Japanese sumo wrestlers with a body weight of 200–260 kg have an increased risk of Type 2 diabetes when they stop their intensive training.

> ### Principles of treatment for Type 2 diabetes
>
> ➤ Change what you eat to include smaller portions with less fat and carbohydrate.
>
> ➤ Take up a form of regular exercise that involves your friends too. Walking, jogging or team sports can all be fun in groups.
>
> ➤ If you are a teenager or still at school, then get your school on board. Changing the type of food offered in the school canteen and ensuring regular physical exercise on the school timetable will help.
>
> ➤ Metformin can generally be used across all age groups, young and old, as long as they don't have kidney trouble. It is the mainstay of drug treatment for high blood sugar levels in Type 2 diabetes, and other drugs are added around it.
>
> ➤ Newer drugs such as the glitazones can't be used in children but offer promise for the future.

girls than in boys. In North America, Type 2 diabetes and heart disease among young and middle-aged members of the native American population is reaching epidemic proportions.

In certain groups, the number of cases of Type 2 diabetes as a proportion of the total number of newly diagnosed diabetes among children is extremely high. This proportion is nearly 100% in native Americans, 31% in Mexican Americans, and 70–75% in African Americans. Type 2 diabetes is often diagnosed in African Americans after they become ill with the symptoms of ketoacidosis (see page 33).

Other risk factors for Type 2 diabetes in children and young people are low birth weight, Type 2 diabetes in the family, ethnic origin (Canadian and American First Nation's people, Hispanic, African American, Japanese, Pacific Islander, Asian and Middle Eastern), high-fat and low-fibre diet, lack of exercise, and signs of insulin resistance such as high blood pressure and dark velvety discolouration of the skin (known as acanthosis nigricans).

A possible reason for the increase in Type 2 diabetes in young people may be that some people were 'programmed' thousands of years ago to survive famine by conserving energy compared with periods when there was better access to food. Today, when we have easy access to food, these 'survival capacities' may lead to obesity. For example, the number of young people with Type 2 diabetes is much higher in African Americans than among Africans still living in their home continent, although the genetic make-up of these two groups is very similar. This suggests that lifestyle and diet may be particularly important.

Maturity-onset diabetes of the young (MODY)

Some young adults, and even adolescents and children, have a rare form of genetic diabetes (MODY, maturity onset diabetes of the young). This is associated with a definite family history of diabetes, and people with this condition are usually slim at time of diagnosis.

More information about MODY can be found in Chapter 22 on Type 2 diabetes and young people.

Latent autoimmune diabetes in the adult (LADA)

This is a form of Type 1 diabetes that appears in adults and is caused by the body's own immune mechanisms. People with LADA are relatively thin and are very insulin-sensitive. They usually produce insulin of their own for many years, much longer than the typical remission or 'honeymoon' period seen in most young people with Type 1 diabetes. Because of their age on presentation, many people with LADA are initially diagnosed wrongly as having Type 2 diabetes, but this can be determined by measuring the level of certain antibodies that attach to the insulin producing cells in the pancreas.

How common is diabetes?

The number of individuals with diabetes varies enormously from country to country. In Europe and the US it is estimated that 50 million people have Type 1 or Type 2 diabetes. In the UK alone it is estimated that 1.5 million people have diagnosed Type 2 diabetes, with a further 1 million undiagnosed cases. In Europe as a whole, it is estimated that around 90% of the total number of diabetes cases are due to Type 2 diabetes.

Can you catch diabetes?

Diabetes is not infectious. This may be obvious to adults but young children may be less confident. It is very important to get the message across to all friends – and children and grandchildren – that they cannot 'catch' diabetes off you or anyone else.

Does eating too much sweet food cause diabetes?

Eating sweet food will not influence your risk of getting Type 1 diabetes at any stage of life. You can fall into the trap of thinking: 'If only I had done this or that differently, perhaps I wouldn't have diabetes'. Generally speaking, there is nothing you can do to change your chance of getting Type 1 diabetes.

Type 2 diabetes is rather different, however. While sweet foods do not in themselves cause Type 2 diabetes, excess calories of any kind (sweets, cake, potatoes, sugary drinks, alcohol), or just insufficient physical exercise coupled with eating too much, is clearly related to obesity. And if you have a genetic susceptibility to Type 2 diabetes, obesity will make you much more likely to develop it. Nutritional issues relating to diabetes are discussed more fully in Chapter 8.

How your body works

It is important to understand how the body works in order to understand what goes wrong when you have diabetes. If you are not familiar with medical terms, or not interested in learning them, you can skip the terms in brackets. You do not need to know them to understand what is being said.

The three most important components of the food we eat are sugar or starch (carbohydrates), fat and protein. When we eat, the digestion of starch (long chains of sugar; see page 38) begins immediately in the mouth with the help of a special enzyme (salivary amylase). An enzyme is a protein compound that breaks the bonds holding chemicals together. The food collects in the stomach, where it is mixed and broken down by the acidic gastric juice. The stomach then empties this mixture, a little at a time, into the small

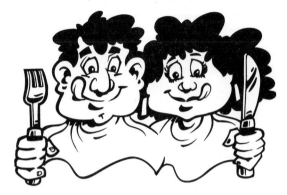

As soon as you see food your mouth will water and your body will begin to prepare to digest it.

intestine through the lower opening of the stomach (pylorus; see illustration on page 20).

Once the food is in the small intestine, it will be broken down further by digestive enzymes from the pancreas and suspended in bile produced by the liver. Sugar cannot be absorbed directly from the mouth or stomach and can only reach the bloodstream once it has passed through the stomach into the small intestine. The emptying rate of the stomach for different foods is variable and has an impact on the rate at which glucose is absorbed into the blood. Thus if you have a hypo (see Chapter 18) and need to increase your` blood glucose as quickly as possible, fluids containing concentrated glucose (e.g. Lucozade™, orange juice) are most effective as they pass through the stomach rapidly.

The carbohydrates we eat are broken down into the simple sugars (mono-saccharides), glucose (dextrose, grape-sugar), fructose (fruit sugar) and galactose. Fructose must first be transformed into glucose in the liver before it can affect your blood glucose level. Food proteins are broken down into amino acids, and fat into very tiny droplets (known as chylomicrons, and composed mainly of triglycerides). Simple sugars and amino acids or very small proteins are

Phases in glucose metabolism

1 Storing at meals:
During a meal and for the following 2–3 hours, glucose from the meal will be used as fuel by the cells. At the same time the stores of glycogen (glucose in long chains; see illustration on page 38), fat and protein are rebuilt.

2 Fasting between meals:
After 3–5 hours, the carbohydrate content of the meal is used up and the blood glucose level starts to decrease. The glycogen stores in the liver will then be broken down to maintain a constant blood glucose level. The glucose produced in this way will be used by the brain while the body uses free fatty acids from fat tissue for its fuel.

absorbed directly into the blood while the fat droplets are absorbed into the lymph system and enter the bloodstream through the lymph vessels.

The venous blood draining the stomach and intestines passes through the liver before reaching the rest of the body. A large amount of glucose will be absorbed by the liver with the help of insulin, and then stored as a reservoir as glycogen (see illustration overleaf). These stores can be used between meals, during the night, and when a person is starving. Glucose can only reach the bloodstream and circulate throughout the body if it is either *not* stored, or if it is released from glycogen stores in the liver. This glucose can be measured by a finger prick or a blood test from the vein.

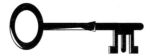

How insulin works

1 Insulin switches off glucose production by the liver.

2 It stimulates the storage of glucose as glycogen.

3 It opens the door for glucose to enter the cells.

4 It stimulates the development of fat from excess carbohydrates.

5 And it stimulates the production of protein compounds in the body.

Muscles can also store a certain amount of glucose as glycogen. Whereas the glycogen store in the liver can be used to raise the blood glucose level, the store in the muscles can only be used by the muscles themselves as fuel during exercise. The body's ability to store glucose is very limited. The glycogen stores are only sufficient for 24 hours without food for an adult and 12 hours for a child.

The glucose content of the blood remains surprisingly constant during both day and night in a person without diabetes (approximately

4–7 mmol/L, 70–120 mg/dl). In adults, this blood glucose level corresponds to only about two lumps of sugar. If you think about it this way, you won't find it surprising that even a small amount of sugar, a few sweets for example, can disturb the balance of glucose in the body of a person with diabetes.

The smallest building blocks in your body are called cells. All the cells in your body need glucose to function well. With the help of oxygen, glucose is broken down into carbon dioxide, water and the vital energy to make cells work throughout the body (see 'A healthy cell' on page 22).

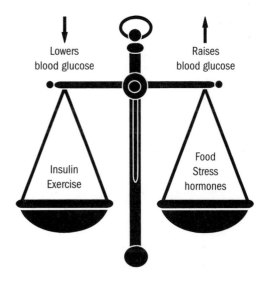

The blood glucose in your body is controlled by many different actions that balance each other to achieve as even a level as possible throughout the day.

Insulin

Many of the different things your body does are controlled by hormones. Hormones act through the blood and work like keys, 'opening doors' to different functions in the body. Insulin is a hormone that is produced in the pancreas in special types of cells called beta cells. The beta cells are found in a part of the pancreas known as 'the islets of Langerhans' which also contain alpha cells producing the hormone glucagon (see illustration on page 20). Other hormones are

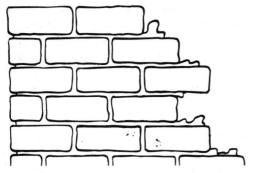

All the organs in the body are built of cells, which are like the bricks in a house. Each organ contains specialized cells to enable it to perform its function, so there are identifiable kidney cells, liver cells and muscle cells.

also produced by the islets, and help the islet cells to communicate with each other. The pancreas has another very important function. It produces enzymes to help you digest your food. In someone with diabetes, this part generally works normally.

The reason that insulin is so important is that it acts as the key that 'opens the door' for glucose to enter the cells. As soon as you see or smell food, signals are delivered to the beta cells to increase insulin production. Once the food has gone into your stomach and intestine, other special hormones send more signals to the beta cells to continue increasing their insulin production.

What happens to the carbohydrates in the food?

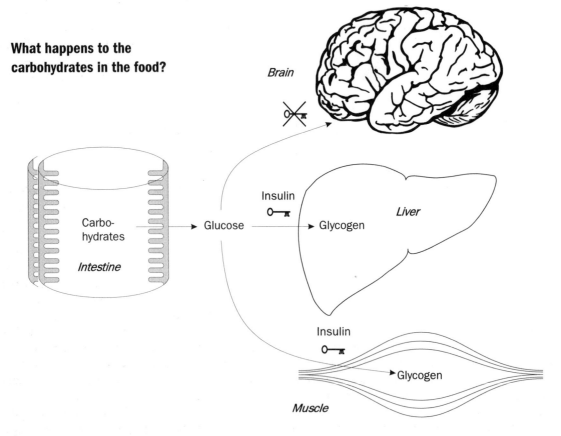

The complex carbohydrates in food are broken down to simple sugars in the intestine. Glucose is absorbed into the bloodstream and stored as glycogen in the liver and muscles. The key hormone insulin is needed to transport glucose into the cells of these organs. The brain cannot store glucose, so it has to depend upon a regular supply if it is to function well. The nervous system and some other cells (for example, those in the eyes and kidneys) can take up glucose without the help of insulin. There are advantages to this in the short term as the nervous system will not experience a lack of glucose, even if no insulin is present. However, in the long term, there are disadvantages for a person with diabetes, as the nervous system will be exposed to high levels of glucose inside the cells when the blood glucose level is high.

The beta cells contain an inbuilt 'blood glucose meter' that registers when the level of glucose in your blood goes up and responds by sending the correct amount of insulin into your bloodstream. When a person without diabetes eats food, the insulin concentration in their blood increases rapidly (see illustration on page 23) to take care of the glucose coming from the food, transporting it into the cells. This person's blood glucose level will normally not rise more than 1–2 mmol/L (20–25 mg/dl) after a meal.

Insulin travels in the bloodstream to the different cells of the body, where it sticks onto special insulin receptors on the surface of the cell. The receptors allow the glucose to pass through the cell wall into the cell. Insulin causes certain proteins inside the cell to come to the cell surface, collect glucose from the blood and then release it inside the cell. In this way, the blood glucose level is kept at a constant level.

Not all cells require insulin to transport glucose into their interior. Some cells are 'insulin-independent' and these absorb glucose in direct proportion to the blood glucose level. Such cells are found in the brain, nerve fibres, retina, kidneys and adrenal glands, as well as in blood vessels and red blood cells. These cells probably behave differently because they make up the most essential parts of the body. So if the glucose level starts to fall, insulin will be switched off and other cells will be unable to take up glucose, leaving it available for the essential body organs.

Certain cells can absorb glucose without insulin. However, in a situation where there is not enough glucose in the body, the insulin production will be stopped, thus keeping the glucose in reserve for the most important organs. If you have diabetes and your blood glucose level is high, the cells that can absorb glucose without the need for insulin will absorb large amounts of glucose. In the long run, this will poison the cells, putting those organs at risk of long-term damage.

The body needs a small amount of insulin, even between meals and during the night, to prevent the liver from breaking down glycogen stores to form glucose. This is often referred to as 'background' or 'basal' insulin to distinguish it from the "boluses" of insulin needed to control the blood glucose any time we eat. Around 40–50% of the total amount of insulin produced by a person without diabetes, over any 24-hour period, will be secreted as basal insulin between meals.

A large amount of carbohydrate from a meal will be stored in the liver (as glycogen, see previous page). If you eat more than you need, the excess carbohydrate is transformed into fat and stored in the fat tissue. The human body has an almost unlimited ability to store fat, so fat left over from a meal is stored in the same way. Proteins (amino acids) from the meal can be used by different body tissues and the liver can convert them into glucose, in particular when fasting and insulin levels are low. However, there is no mechanism for storing amino acids, and if insulin is deficient in the long term, body proteins are broken down.

Your body doesn't realize it has diabetes

When you read about how your body functions if you have diabetes, remember that it always 'thinks' and reacts as if it does not have diabetes, that is to say, as if insulin were being produced and working normally. Your body doesn't understand why things go wrong when you become insulin deficient, because it doesn't realize what has happened. On the other hand, your brain can help you by thinking through what will happen when your insulin production stops working. It is very important therefore that you remember to stop and think about how your body reacts in particular situations, why it reacts like this, and how you can influence these reactions.

If you are taking insulin, the doses will vary as a result of changes in your lifestyle. If you did not have diabetes, your beta cells would adjust to any changes automatically. It is now up to you to notice how your body reacts on different days, and how much insulin you need in different situations.

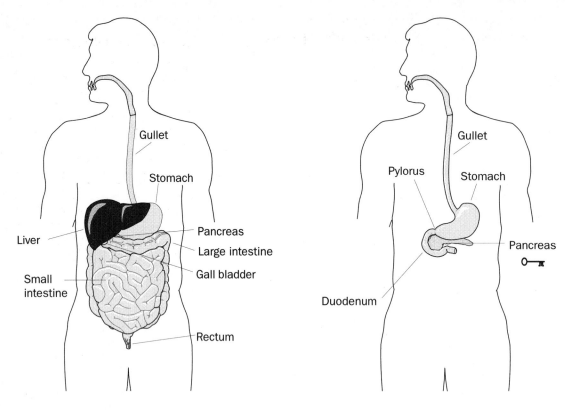

Your body's anatomy

When you eat, the food passes from your mouth through your gullet (oesophagus) and into your stomach. Sugar can not be absorbed into your blood until the food has passed through the lower opening of your stomach (pylorus) and entered the intestine. In the intestine, it will be digested by enzymes from your pancreas and intestinal lining.

The small intestine is very long (3–5 metres or 9–15 feet in an adult) and is folded or coiled in order to fit comfortably inside your abdominal cavity or tummy. The first part of the small intes-

Pancreas

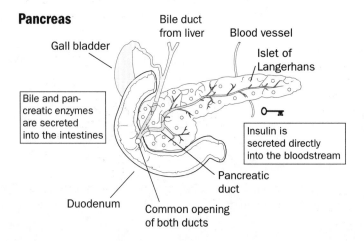

'I am now your pancreas but one day, when you are older and learn to take care of yourself, your brain will become your pancreas.'

The mother of Maria de Alva, former president of the International Diabetes Federation

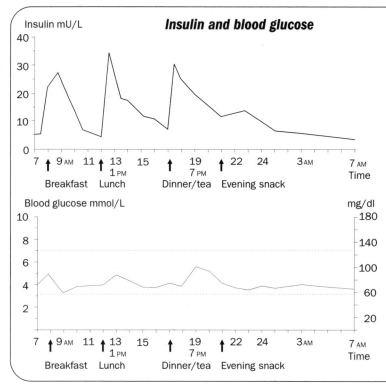

Insulin and blood glucose

Insulin mU/L

40
30
20
10
0

7 | 9 AM | 11 | 13 | 15 | | 19 | 22 | 24 | 3 AM | 7 AM
 | | | 1 PM | | | 7 PM | | | | Time

Breakfast Lunch   Dinner/tea Evening snack

Blood glucose mmol/L   mg/dl

10   180
8   140
6   100
4   60
2   20

7 | 9 AM | 11 | 13 | 15 | | 19 | 22 | 24 | 3 AM | 7 AM
 | | | 1 PM | | | 7 PM | | | | Time

Breakfast Lunch   Dinner/tea Evening snack

A person without diabetes

If an individual doesn't have diabetes, the insulin concentration in the blood will increase rapidly after a meal. When the glucose in the food is absorbed from the intestine, and the blood glucose has returned to normal levels, the insulin level will drop back to baseline once again. However, the insulin level will never go right down to zero, as a low level of basal insulin is needed to take account of the gluose coming from the reserve stores in the liver between meals and during the night.

The resulting blood glucose level will be very stable in a person without diabetes as this graph illustrates. The normal blood glucose level is between about 4 and 7 mmol/L (70–120 mg/dl).

tine, the duodenum, is 25–30 cm (10–12 inches) long.

After leaving the small intestine, the food passes into the large intestine (or colon) which is approximately 1½ metres (4–5 feet) long. The large intestine passes around the abdominal cavity before entering the rectum.

Pancreas

Your pancreas is about the size of the palm of your hand. It is positioned under the left rib cage in the back of the abdominal cavity, close to the stomach. The pancreas has two main functions: it produces enzymes which help you digest food, and it produces insulin which helps control blood sugar. The digestive enzymes from the pancreas reach the intestine through the pancreatic duct. This drains into the duodenum together with the duct from the liver and the gallbladder. The cells in the pancreas that produce insulin are called islets of Langerhans

and there are about one million of these. Insulin produced in the beta cells of the islets is secreted directly into the small blood vessels passing through the pancreas.

The islets of Langerhans

If you look at an islet of Langerhans through a microscope, you will find it contains beta cells,

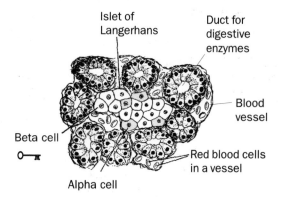

Islet of Langerhans

Duct for digestive enzymes

Blood vessel

Red blood cells in a vessel

Beta cell

Alpha cell

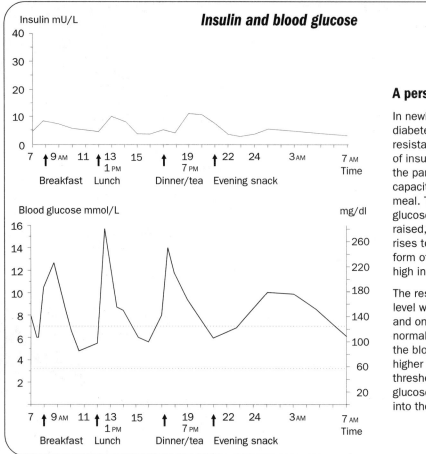

A person with diabetes

In newly diagnosed Type 2 diabetes, because of insulin resistance, the basal levels of insulin may be high, but the pancreas loses the capacity to respond to a meal. Thus, fasting blood glucose may be only slightly raised, but the blood sugar rises to high levels after any form of food, particularly if high in carbohydrate.

The resulting blood glucose level will be very unstable and only occasionally within normal levels. Every time the blood glucose level is higher than the renal threshold (see page 244), glucose will be passed out into the urine.

which produce insulin, and alpha cells, which produce glucagon. Both of these hormones are secreted directly into the blood. The beta cells contain a sort of 'built-in' blood glucose meter. If the blood glucose level is raised, insulin will be secreted. If it is lowered, the secretion of insulin stops. If it falls below the normal level, glucagon is secreted.

The islets of Langerhans are very small, only 0.1 mm (four thousands of an inch) in diameter. All the islets together contain approximately 200 units of insulin in an adult. The volume of them all combined is no larger than a fingertip.

Cellular metabolism

A healthy cell

Sugar in the food is absorbed from the intestine into the blood in the form of glucose (dextrose) and fructose. Glucose must enter the cells before it can be used for producing energy or for other metabolic processes. The hormone insulin is needed to 'open the door', i.e. make it possible for glucose to penetrate the wall of the cell. Once it is inside the cell, glucose is metabolized with the help of oxygen into carbon dioxide, water and energy. The carbon dioxide travels to the lungs, where it is exchanged for oxygen.

Energy is vitally important to the cell if it is to function properly. In addition, glucose is stored

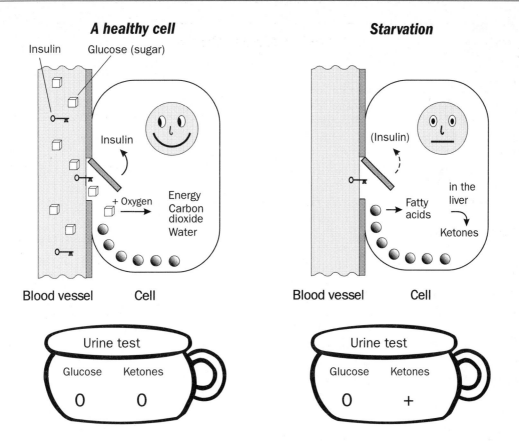

(in the form of glycogen) in liver and muscle cells for future use. The brain, however, is not capable of storing glucose as glycogen. It is therefore dependent on an even and continuous supply of glucose from the blood.

Starvation

When no food is available, there is a shortage of glucose in the blood. In this case, opening the 'cell door' with the help of insulin will not do any good. In a person who does not have diabetes, the production of insulin will be stopped almost completely when the blood glucose level goes down. The alpha cells in the pancreas recognize the lowered blood glucose level and secrete the hormone glucagon into the bloodstream. Glucagon acts as a signal for the liver cells to release glucose from the reserve supply of glycogen. Adrenaline, cortisol and growth hormone are other hormones that

are produced when the body is starving (see Chapter 6 on Regulation of blood glucose).

If starvation continues, the body will use the next reserve system for glucose supply. Fat is broken down into fatty acids and glycerol with the help of the stress hormone adrenaline. The fatty acids are transformed into ketones in the liver (these are known as 'starvation ketones') and glycerol is changed into glucose. These reactions will take place if you are fasting or if you are too ill to eat, for example if you have gastroenteritis.

All the cells of the body (except the brain) can use fatty acids as fuel. Only the muscles, the heart, the kidneys and the brain, however, can use ketones as fuel. The cells will retrieve some energy from this but less than when glucose is available. If the body is without food for too long, proteins from muscle tissue will start to break down too so that they can be converted into glucose.

Diabetes, insulin deficiency and insulin resistance

Type 2 diabetes is a condition which results from increased requirements of insulin at a time when the beta cells are no longer able to produce adequate supplies of this hormone. Thus, Type 2 diabetes is caused by insulin deficiency in the face of insulin resistance. This makes the insulin that is available less effective, and puts extra demands on the pancreas at a time when it is failing. This lack of insulin leads to an increase in the fasting glucose. However, the insulin resistance is usually more obvious when the beta cells are really stretched to produce enough insulin to cover a meal. Thus blood glucose levels rise high after food and take many hours to return to baseline levels.

So, while Type 1 diabetes is a 'deficiency disease' in which the hormone insulin is missing, people with Type 2 diabetes often have reasonable levels of insulin, but not enough to overcome the insulin resistance. So the blood sugar may be slightly high when fasting but tends to rise higher after food.

In Type 1 diabetes, there is complete lack of insulin which promotes the formation of ketone bodies, similar to those seen in starvation. In Type 2 diabetes, however, complete insulin lack is very rare and so ketone bodies never appear in large amounts. This is only seen when Type 1 diabetes is completely out of control, and in some people with Type 2, at the onset of their diabetes. This is not uncommon in teenagers.

Diabetes and insulin deficiency

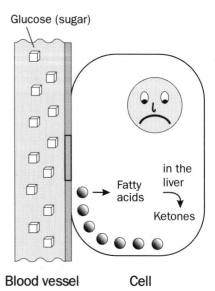

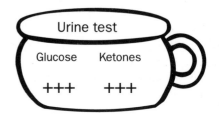

Regulation of blood glucose

Someone who does not have diabetes has a very small amount of glucose in their blood. The glucose content of their entire bloodstream in the fasting state amounts to only 5 g (⅕ ounce) of glucose – barely two lumps of sugar. However, the liver, which produces glucose, needs to provide 10 g of glucose every hour as fuel to the organs of the body. Thus if the supply of glucose dries up, the level of blood glucose will fall rapidly.

In someone who does not have diabetes, the body is able to regulate its own blood glucose levels within narrow boundaries, normally between 4 and 7 mmol/L (70–120 mg/dl). When your blood glucose falls below 3.5–4.0 mmol/L (65–70 mg/dl) you will feel unwell. A reduction in blood glucose level affects all bodily reactions, as the body struggles to channel all remaining glucose to the brain, which in general terms can only operate when enough glucose is available as fuel. Cells outside the brain attempt to use as little glucose as possible. The brain is unable to store glucose, so it depends on an uninterrupted supply of glucose from the blood. However, if no food has been eaten for several days, the brain can adapt to use other types of fuel, such as ketones.

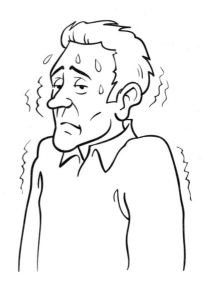

While the hormone insulin lowers your blood glucose level, there are a number of hormones in your body which can raise it. The body reacts to low blood glucose with a defensive reaction known as counter-regulation. In this process, the brain and nerves work with a number of different hormones to raise the blood glucose level. This defence against hypoglycaemia is extremely important. The symptoms associated with hypoglycaemia are caused by the brain's response to a lack of glucose as well as by the direct effects of the counter-regulatory hormones.

In Type 2 diabetes, insulin is less effective due to insulin resistance, in particular with respect to

---

Where does the glucose in your blood come from?

1 From your food, via the liver.
2 From the breakdown of glucose stored as glycogen in the liver (called glycogenolysis).
3 From protein and fat, converted in the liver to form glucose (called gluconeogenesis).

Counter-regulatory hormones that increase blood glucose levels

1 Adrenaline.
2 Glucagon.
3 Cortisol.
4 Growth hormone.

Effects of insulin

⇒ Insulin is produced in the beta cells of the pancreas.

1 Insulin decreases blood glucose by:

⇒ Decreasing the production of glucose from the liver.

⇒ Increasing the uptake of glucose into the cells.

⇒ Increasing the body's ability to store glucose as glycogen in the liver and muscle.

2 Insulin prevents the production of ketones from the liver. It stimulates utilization of ketones in the cells.

3 Insulin also increases the production of muscle protein.

4 It increases the production and decreases the breakdown of body fat.

Body reserves during fasting and hypoglycaemia

⇒ The store of glycogen in the liver is broken down to glucose.

⇒ Fat is broken down to free fatty acids that can be used as fuel. Fatty acids can be transformed into ketones in the liver. Ketones can also be used as fuel, mainly by the brain.

⇒ Proteins from the muscles are broken down to be used in the liver in order to produce glucose.

---

blood glucose and blood fats. This leads to increased glucose production in the liver, and reduced uptake of glucose into the cells. The level of fats in the blood is also increased.

The liver

The liver functions as a bank for glucose. When times are good (after feeding) glucose is laid down in the liver and when times are bad (starvation) glucose is released. Excess glucose following a meal is stored in the 'reservoir' of the liver and muscle cells in the form of glycogen (see illustration on page 18). Insulin is needed to transport the glucose into both liver and muscle cells.

The liver can also produce glucose from fat and proteins to raise the blood glucose level (by a process called gluconeogenesis). The adult liver produces about 6 g (⅕ ounce) of glucose per hour in between meals. The majority of this glucose will be consumed by the brain which can make use of glucose without the help of insulin. After a longer period without food, the kidneys can produce glucose in the same way as the liver does. Recent research suggests that the kidneys can contribute as much as 20% of the body's total glucose production after a night without food.

People with diabetes can also use the stores of glycogen when their blood glucose is low. If you have emptied your stores of glycogen, for example during a game of football when the body needs a lot of extra glucose, you will have smaller reserves for dealing with any hypoglycaemic episode that might occur later, including during the night. This leads to an increased risk of hypoglycaemia several hours after physical exercise (see page 60).

A healthy pancreas produces insulin. Since the blood from the pancreas goes directly to the liver, this organ will be the first in line to receive a high concentration of insulin. When people with diabetes inject insulin subcutaneously, it has to pass through the general circulation and the heart before it reaches the liver. Because the insulin has been diluted on its passage through the circulation, the concentration in the liver is much lower than in the non-diabetic situation where insulin passes directly from pancreas to liver.

Liver and muscle stores

- Liver cells can release glucose into the blood from the store of glycogen.

- Muscle cells can only use the glucose released from the glycogen stores as fuel inside the cell.

- An adult has about 100–120 g (3.5–4.2 ounces) of glucose stored in the liver.

- The glycogen store can be broken down to glucose when the blood glucose is low (glycogenolysis) and can compensate for about 24 hours without food in an adult.

- Children have smaller glycogen stores and can compensate for a shorter time without food.

- A pre-school child has enough glucose for about 12 hours without food, a smaller child even less.

- A child will use up glucose faster than an adult will, even when not very active. This is because a child's brain is larger in relation to body mass than an adult's brain.

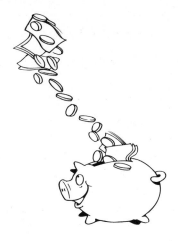

The liver acts like a bank for glucose in your body. When times are good, i.e. during the hours after a meal, glucose is deposited in the 'liver bank' to be stored as glycogen.

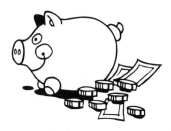

When times are bad, i.e. a couple of hours after the meal and during the night, glucose is withdrawn from the 'liver bank' to keep the blood glucose level adequate.

Glucagon

During the day you tend to feel hungry at intervals of about 4 hours, whereas during the night you can do without food for up to 8 or even 10 hours. This is because glycogen from the liver is broken down into glucose during the night, with the help of the hormones glucagon and adrenaline.

Glucagon is produced by the alpha cells in the pancreas and has the opposite effect to insulin, namely it leads to glucose production by the liver. In Type 1 diabetes, glucagon production is normal at the time of diagnosis but becomes blunted after about a year and by 5 years is absent. The cause for this failure of alpha cells is

not well understood but may be related to the nervous system control of glucagon release. People with Type 2 diabetes do not lose the ability to produce glucagon as long as they are able to produce some insulin themselves. However once they reach the stage of being completely devoid of their own insulin, they also lose the ability to produce glucagon. Up till this point severe hypos leading to dangerous mental confusion are rare in insulin-treated Type 2 diabetes.

Glucagon injections

If a person with diabetes is unconscious or unable to eat or drink, an injection of glucagon

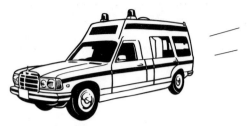

Give a glucagon injection if a person with diabetes develops severe hypoglycaemia and becomes unconscious or has a seizure. If the person has not woken up within 10–15 minutes, call an ambulance. However, if the individual has woken up and has a normal blood glucose level by the time the ambulance arrives, it won't be necessary for him or her to go to hospital.

will stimulate the breakdown of glycogen in the liver and raise the blood glucose level. Glucagon injections are not difficult to administer. If you take insulin and are prone to hypos, it would be a good idea to encourage a partner or family member to learn how to give glucagon so they are able to help in the unlikely event of you being unable to deal with a hypo yourself. The most common cause of severe hypoglycaemia is unaccustomed activity such as a long walk or a sight-seeing holiday, and it would be a good idea to take a pack of glucagon with you if you expect to be unusually active or are going somewhere where food may not be immediately available.

Glucagon can be given as a subcutaneous injection in the same way as insulin. It is packaged as 1 mg of powder, which has to be dissolved in the water provided before injection. A syringe is included in the pack and the standard dose is to give half the total volume in the syringe, i.e. 0.5 mg of glucagon. Wait about 5 minutes to assess the response and, if there has been no improvement, give the rest of the dose, making a total of 1 mg. The higher dose is more likely to cause the common side effects of headache, nausea and sometimes even vomiting. Giving only half the full dose will reduce the risk of these side effects. Whenever possible, some carbohydrate should be given as soon as the person has recovered sufficiently to eat and drink, but if they feel sick, wait until they are feeling better.

If you have to give glucagon, wait 10–15 minutes for the person to wake up. If they are still unconscious after this time, call an ambulance. However, if the person has revived, is feeling well and has a normal blood glucose when the ambulance arrives, it may not be necessary for them to go to hospital. It goes without saying that if someone has a severe hypo and glucagon is not available, an ambulance should be called immediately.

If you have a glucagon pack, keep an eye on the expiry date and ask for a replacement when it becomes out of date. Your partner can use the old kit to practise how to dissolve the powder and draw it up. It is never easy to do this in the real life situation when you have to deal with a confused person.

Some people with diabetes feel sick after a difficult hypoglycaemic episode, even if glucagon has not been injected. One explanation is that the production of glucagon from their own pancreas also can result in nausea as a side effect. At present, glucagon can only be given as an injection.

This all sounds very complicated and worrying but, in practice, very few people with Type 2 diabetes have hypos which are serious enough to need glucagon.

Adrenaline

Adrenaline is a stress hormone secreted by the adrenal glands. It raises the blood glucose primarily by breaking down the glycogen stores in the liver. The concentration of adrenaline rises when the body is exposed to any stress, such as fever or danger. One of the greatest stresses the body can experience is a low blood glucose, which immediately puts the brain at risk. For

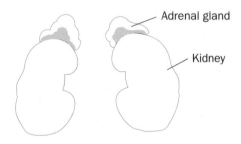

Adrenaline and cortisol are produced in the adrenal glands.

Glucagon

➤ Every individual with Type 2 diabetes treated with insulin who has had problems with hypoglycaemia should have a glucagon kit and know how to use it.

➤ Give glucagon if a person with diabetes is unconscious, has seizures or cannot eat or drink.

➤ Dose: 0.5 mg (half the volume provided). Give the remainder if no improvement after 5 minutes. Glucagon is not dangerous if you accidentally overdose.

➤ Glucagon takes effect within 10–15 minutes.

➤ The effect lasts for up to 60 minutes.
Eat something when you are feeling better to keep your blood glucose level up until the next meal.

➤ Nausea is a common side effect.

➤ Do not repeat the dose! One full injection (1 mg) gives a sufficient level of glucagon in the blood.

➤ Loss of effect can be caused by:

Store of glycogen depleted by:	Glucagon counteracted by:
1 Exercise	1 Alcohol
2 Recent hypoglycaemia	2 High dose of insulin

➤ If you have a tendency to become hypoglycaemic during exercise, take glucagon with you, e.g. when going on a picnic, hiking trip, sailing trip or holiday abroad.

➤ Teach people close to you how to administer glucagon!

➤ Glucagon has the same effect whether injected into subcutaneous tissue or into the muscle.

this reason, hypoglycaemia causes a brisk release of adrenaline.

Adrenaline also reduces the amount of glucose taken up by the cells of the body. This is in order to allow as much glucose as possible to go to the brain, which can only operate if glucose is available.

The human body was originally designed for living in the Stone Age. If a person ran into a polar bear or a mammoth, the only alternatives were to fight or take flight. In both situations extra fuel, in the form of glucose, was needed by the body. The problem with our present way of life is that adrenaline is still secreted when we get excited or fearful, though this is more likely to be caused by a frightening TV programme than by an activity which actually calls for extra

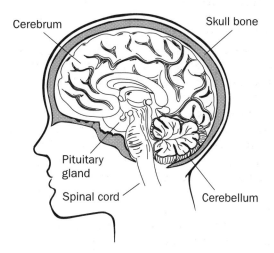

Cross-section of the brain. Growth hormone is produced in the pituitary gland.

Effects of adrenaline

⟹ Adrenaline is produced in the adrenal glands.

1 Adrenaline raises blood glucose by:

⟹ Releasing glucose from the glycogen stores in the liver.

⟹ Activating the production of glucose from proteins.

⟹ Reducing the uptake of glucose into the cells.

⟹ Reducing insulin production in people who don't have diabetes.

2 Adrenaline causes symptoms of hypoglycaemia, such as shakiness, rapid heartbeat and sweating.

3 It also stimulates the breakdown of body fat.

Effects of cortisol

⟹ Cortisol is produced in the adrenal glands.

1 Cortisol raises blood glucose by:

⟹ Reducing the cellular uptake of glucose.

⟹ Breaking down proteins that can be used to produce glucose in the liver.

2 It also stimulates the breakdown of body fat.

---

strength. A healthy person, whose insulin production is working as it should, will not find this causes a problem. However, a person with diabetes will find that their blood glucose level rises (see Chapter 20 on Stress).

When a person with diabetes becomes hypoglycaemic, secretion of adrenaline can raise the blood glucose by stimulating the breakdown of the glycogen stores in the liver and at the same time causing shakiness, anxiety, and a pounding heart. Adrenaline also stimulates the breakdown of body fat to fatty acids which can be converted into ketones in the liver.

Cortisol

Cortisol is another important hormone which is secreted by the adrenal glands in response to stress and affects the body metabolism in many ways. It increases the amount of glucose in the blood by producing glucose from proteins (called gluconeogenesis) and by decreasing the amount of glucose that is absorbed and used by the cells. Cortisol also promotes the breakdown of body fat into fatty acids that can be converted into ketones.

Growth hormone

Growth hormone is produced in the pituitary gland, which is found just below the brain. Some of the body's most important hormones are produced in this gland. The most important effect of growth hormone is to stimulate growth. It has the effect of raising blood glucose by counteracting insulin on the cell surface, thereby reducing the uptake of glucose into the cells. Growth hormone not only stimulates growth during childhood and adolescence; it also increases muscle tissue and stimulates the breakdown of body fat.

The effects of growth hormone

⟹ Growth hormone is produced in the pituitary gland:

1 It stimulates growth.

2 It raises blood glucose by reducing the cellular uptake of glucose.

3 Growth hormone breaks down body fat.

4 It increases muscular mass.

High blood glucose levels

When your blood glucose level is high, the only way the body can eliminate the excess sugar is via the urine. Because there are large amounts of glucose to be removed, the body has to provide a lot of fluid to dilute the glucose. Thus anyone with a high glucose level and normal kidneys will pass a copious volume of sugary urine. This in turn leads to dehydration, a potentially serious condition. In order to correct this problem, you will become very thirsty and will need to drink abnormally large quantities of fluid. If you choose to slake your thirst with high sugar drinks, such as CocaCola or lemonade, you will add fuel to the flames and cause a further rise in your blood glucose level. This then leads to the vicious circle of even greater thirst and urine output. When your sugars are high, your skin and mucous membranes can become dry and uncomfortable as a result of dehydration. High blood glucose levels also leave you prone to infection, particularly with *Candida*, which in

Infection can often precipitate an increase in symptoms of Type 2 diabetes and may be associated with a rapid loss of control over blood sugar levels.

men may cause balanitis (infection of the penis), or in women, vulvo-vaginitis (infection, inflammation and itching around the vagina). In addition, your immune system is less effective at fighting off infections once your blood sugar goes above 14 mmol/L (250 mg/dl).

What happens in the body when there is not enough insulin?

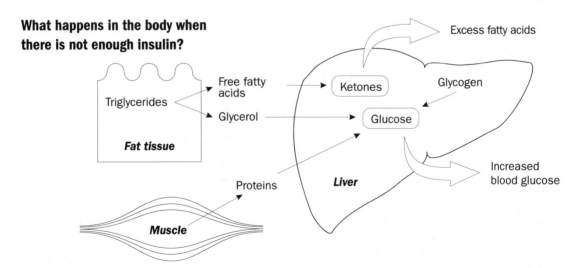

The reaction of a person's body without diabetes to shortage of insulin is quite logical if you remember that, in a healthy person, levels of insulin are low when the blood glucose is low too. In Type 2 diabetes, insulin resistance and a relative lack of insulin stops glucose being taken up as fuel into the muscle or fat and encourages the liver to release more glucose. In addition, large amounts of fats usually used as fuel circulate in the blood.

If your blood glucose level rises temporarily (e.g. following a large meal), you may not even notice. Many people feel fine, even with a blood glucose level of 16–18 mmol/L (290–325 mg/dl). You may be a bit more tired and thirsty than usual, but the symptoms are not nearly as obvious as when your blood glucose level is low. One study of adults found no difference in neuro-psychological function (simple motor abilities, attention, reaction time, learning and memory) when comparing blood glucose levels of 8.9 and 21.1 mmol/L (160 and 380 mg/dl).

Insulin resistance – not enough insulin to do the job?

In Type 2 diabetes, insulin being unable to do its job properly (insulin resistance), along with a relative lack of insulin, results in a lack of glucose inside the cells (see illustrations on pages 23 and 24), and a rise in blood sugar levels. A moderate increase will cause the usual symptoms of thirst, tiredness and frequent visits to the bathroom. However if there is another medical problem, such as a chest infection or even a heart attack, blood sugar levels may rise above 25 mmol/L (450 mg/dl). This can also result from trying to quench the thirst with sugary drinks such as lemonade or cola. Confusion, profound drowsiness and lethargy will follow, and patients can rapidly become very unwell. This condition is called HONK (hyperosmolar non-ketotic) coma, and more information about this is given below. The coma is 'non-ketotic' because people with Type 2 diabetes have enough residual insulin to stop the formation of ketones.

(See Chapter 21, Coping with sickness, for further information about what to do in an acute illness.)

Remember that your blood glucose level may rise during an acute illness even if you don't eat anything. This is caused by an increased level of hormones stimulating the liver to release more glucose (see Chapter 6, Regulation of blood glucose).

Early need for insulin in Type 2 diabetes

Some people who apparently have Type 2 diabetes do not respond to the normal early treatment with diet and tablets. They continue to have the symptoms of thirst and especially weight loss despite large doses of tablets and careful diet. In such cases, the only treatment is insulin. It is hard to know whether such people actually have Type 1 diabetes at an older age, or whether they simply progress rapidly through the stages of Type 2 diabetes.

What to do with a high blood glucose level

If your blood glucose levels are high for more than a few days, you will have to take action. If you think you may have an infection, you should contact your doctor, who may prescribe antibiotics. However, your response will depend on the treatment you normally have for your diabetes.

Diet alone

If there is no obvious reason for the high glucose levels, it is likely that your diabetes has just moved into a different phase – this often happens quite suddenly. If so, you will need tablets and metformin is the usual first-line treatment.

Anti-diabetes tablets

If you take metformin and your sugars are high, you could try taking an extra one or two tablets each day. Unfortunately higher doses of metformin are more likely to cause the recognized side effects of nausea and diarrhoea.

If you take a sulphonylurea (such as gliclazide or glimepiride), you could try increasing the dose. These drugs normally have a fairly fast response but if you are already taking 4 of these tablets a day, increasing the dose will not have any effect.

Rosiglitazone and pioglitazone are very slow-acting drugs so increasing the dose in the short term will not have an effect on the blood sugar levels for several weeks.

Sometimes the rise in blood glucose may be caused by your diabetes reaching the stage where you either need more tablets or insulin should be considered. Your diabetes specialist will be able to advise you about this.

Insulin treatment

This is the only heading in this section where the advice is simple. If you are taking insulin and, for whatever reason, your glucose levels suddenly run high, you need to increase the dose of insulin. If your morning blood glucose is high, an increase in bedtime/basal insulin should help. If, on the other hand, your sugar level rises during the day, you should take larger doses of mealtime insulin. If your initial increase in dose fails to correct your sugars, you will have to get help from your specialist nurse or doctor.

Ketoacidosis

In Type 1 diabetes, a common result of low insulin levels is ketoacidosis. This is a serious condition which usually develops over the space of several hours or even days. Because of insulin lack, the body produces ketones as an alternative fuel to glucose. Since ketones too can only be utilized if insulin is present, they accumulate in the bloodstream. Because they are very acidic, they unbalance the body chemistry and lead to vomiting. At this stage people are already dehydrated from the raised glucose levels, and vomiting tips the balance into an emergency situation. Ketoacidosis requires urgent admission to hospital for therapy with fluids and insulin.

People with Type 2 diabetes can usually produce enough insulin to avoid ketoacidosis becoming established. They still have an excess of the hormones which make more energy available (i.e. adrenaline, cortisol, glucagon and growth hormone). Acute infections or stresses such as a heart attack can lead to a rise in blood

---

Symptoms of persistently high blood glucose

1 Glucose in the urine:
- Needing to go to the toilet more frequently, including at night.
- Passing a lot of urine at a time.
- Fluid loss:
  Very thirsty, dry mouth.
  Dry skin, dry mucous membranes.
- Lack of energy.

2 Weight loss, weakness.

3 Blurred eyesight.

4 Difficulty in concentrating, irritable behaviour.

---

sugar without the production of excess ketones. High blood sugar levels may cause severe dehydration, and people may not feel well enough to replace all the fluid they have lost in the form of urine. They may then end up being admitted to hospital as an 'emergency' in a very unwell state. This is particularly likely to affect teenagers.

Hyperosmolar non-ketotic coma (HONK)

Hyperosmolar non-ketotic coma may also be referred to as 'hyperosmolar hyperglycaemic non-ketotic coma' or 'HHNC'.

The onset of HONK often occurs slowly with several days of ill health and severe dehydration before people ask for medical help. Unfortunately the dehydration (which may amount to 9–10 litres of fluid) leads to confusion, which may prevent people from realizing how unwell they are, especially if they live alone. Eventually, drowsiness, coma and, sometimes, even fits occur.

People with HONK still have enough residual insulin to inhibit the formation of ketones but not enough to prevent high blood glucose levels, which may reach 30–60 mmol/L (540–1000 mg/dl). and consequent dehydration.

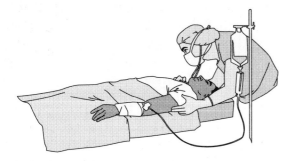

Hyperosmolar non-ketotic coma (HONK) can rapidly develop into a life-threatening condition. This must be treated adequately in hospital with intravenous fluid and insulin.

The loss of fluid, combined with high blood glucose levels, also causes increased thickness (viscosity) of the blood in people with HONK. This can lead to other problems such as an increased risk of heart attack or stroke.

Up to two thirds of cases of HONK occur in people who have not previously been known to have Type 2 diabetes. It is important to start treatment as soon as possible with fluids and insulin. Unfortunately, because patients with HONK may often have problems with other systems in the body, an episode such as this can be very dangerous and lead to serious consequences.

If you are admitted to hospital with HONK, you will receive fluid replacement therapy and insulin to lower your blood sugar, although you may only need this for a few days or weeks. Once your condition is stable, you will probably be able to control your blood glucose with tablets. You will also be given heparin to thin the blood to prevent the formation of clots.

If you have already experienced HONK, the best way to avoid problems in the future is to be aware of the symptoms of high blood glucose and dehydration, to recognize early when things are running out of control, and to consult your doctor or diabetes nurse at an early stage.

Blurred eyesight and diabetes

Blurred eyesight can be a symptom of a high blood glucose level. This is caused by a mismatch between the glucose content of the lens and that of the blood. The lens contains no blood vessels (if it did, they would block the passage of light into the eye). Glucose from the blood must therefore be transported into the lens through the surrounding fluid (aqueous humour; see illustration on page 199). So when the glucose content of the blood is changing rapidly, the glucose content of the lens is bound to be different. If the glucose content of the lens is higher than that of the blood, the lens will try to absorb water, and this will make it swell. The lens will then refract the light differently, causing temporary shortsightedness. It affects your vision in very much the same way as if you borrow someone else's glasses.

The eye itself will not be damaged by short-term high blood sugar levels, and vision often returns to normal within a few hours. It is like borrowing somebody else's glasses – you can still focus, but it is tiresome for your eyes. This type of visual disturbance is common at the onset of diabetes and usually happens when the glucose level is changing rapidly. It has nothing to do with the eye complications that can occur after many years of diabetes. See also page 199.

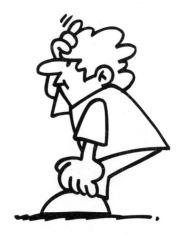

Symptoms of a low blood glucose level are usually fairly easy to recognize. However, when the blood glucose level is high many people won't have any symptoms at all. Thirst and the need to pass a lot of urine both occur when your blood glucose level goes above the renal threshold, but remember that this level can vary from one person to another. Other common symptoms are apathy and a sense that everything is 'slowing down'. What signs can you see to indicate your own blood glucose level is high?

Nutrition

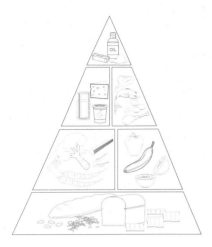

From a historical perspective, dietary advice for people with diabetes has been very restrictive when it comes to carbohydrate intake. This has generally encouraged people to believe that once someone has been diagnosed as having Type 2 diabetes, they will no longer be able to take any carbohydrate in their diet. However, although it is important to make significant reductions in the amount of refined carbohydrate (sugar) you eat, it is not essential to stop eating this altogether.

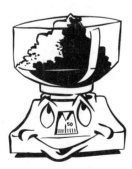

Kitchen scales can be useful for weighing food. Reducing portion size is difficult, and actually being able to visualize the weight of food being eaten is important. If you are estimating calories, then weighing portions of foods like meat or cheese can also help make your estimates more accurate.

Sticking to a rigid pattern of mealtimes and selected food is not necessary because of Type 2 diabetes alone, especially if you are taking metformin, rosiglitazone or pioglitazone, which are less likely to cause hypoglycaemia than sulphonylureas or insulin. If you are on multiple injections of insulin or insulin pump therapy, you should tailor your insulin to the size or type of meal that you are eating. Most people with diabetes live full and varied lives, enjoy an interesting diet, and still manage to control their blood glucose levels effectively. The more knowledge you have about diet, the more control you will have over your diabetes. This chapter will give you many details about blood glucose and different foods, but you will learn the general aspects of healthy eating from your dietitian.

It is important to be careful about what you eat, even if you don't have diabetes. But remember that food should not be looked upon as medicine. Food should look and taste good. Meals are meant to be pleasurable: we should enjoy food and feel satisfied afterwards. You should be able to discuss what you can eat with a dietitian who will help you draw up a meal plan based on the mealtimes, routines and preferences that are important to your family. To quote the British dietitian Sheridan Waldron, 'You should never eat what you don't like'.

'What can I eat?', 'What should I avoid?' Such questions are commonly asked by people who have only recently discovered they have diabetes. Usually, the comment after the first consultation with a dietitian will be: 'I am glad to discover I can eat most of the things as I used to before getting diabetes; I just need to learn to avoid more of the bad choices'. Dietary advice should be directed towards the whole family from the very beginning. If your wife, husband or children aren't bought in to the concept of making better dietary choices, you won't be able to stick to them.

Absorption of carbohydrates

Glucose from food can only be absorbed into the bloodstream after it has passed into the intestines. It cannot be absorbed through the lining of the mouth, as used to be believed. To reach the intestines, the food must first pass through the lower opening of the stomach (pylorus; see illustration on page 20) where a special muscle, the pyloric sphincter, acts as a 'gateway' to the intestine below. The sphincter will only allow very small pieces to pass through.

Complex carbohydrates in the food must first be broken down to simple sugars before they can be absorbed into the bloodstream. The length of the carbohydrate chain does not seem to affect absorption as much as was once believed since 'cleavage' (breaking) is a fairly rapid process. Simple carbohydrates are broken down by enzymes in the intestinal lining while more complex carbohydrates and starch are first prepared for digestion by amylase, an enzyme found in the saliva and pancreas. Starch fibre cannot be broken down into carbohydrates in the intestine.

At one time, carbohydrates were divided into quick-acting and slow-acting, mainly depending on the size of the molecules. It is more accurate to speak of quick-acting and long-acting foods and to evaluate the composition, fibre content and preparation in order to determine the effect on the blood glucose level, rather than simply its content of pure sugar. The term 'glycaemic index' (GI) is used to describe how the blood glucose level is affected by different food. More detailed information about the GI can be found later in this chapter (see pages 42–43).

Dietary fibre content and particle size seem to be particularly important, according to recent studies. The starch in vegetables is broken down more slowly than the starch in bread. The starch in potatoes is quick to break down to glucose. The starch from pasta products is broken down much more slowly, even though it is made from white flour, which is low in fibre.

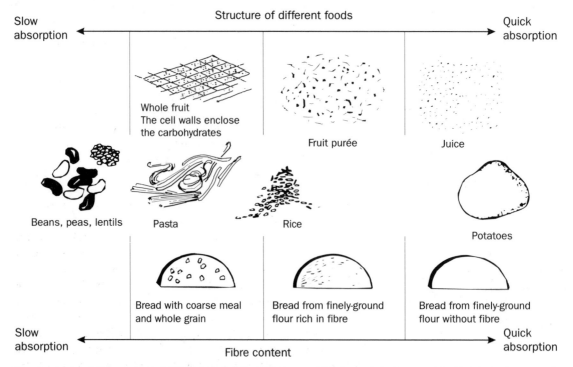

The structure and fibre content of different foodstuffs affect how quickly the carbohydrate content is absorbed.
The illustration is from the book *Food and Diabetes* by the Swedish Diabetes Association, printed with permission.

Factors that raise the blood glucose level more quickly
(*increase the glycaemic index*)

1 Cooking:
Boiling and other types of cooking will break down the starch in food.

2 Preparing food:
Prepared food, e.g. polished rice, will give a quicker rise in blood glucose than unpolished, mashed potatoes quicker than whole potatoes and grated carrots quicker than sliced. Wheat flour gives a higher blood glucose response when baked in bread than when used for pasta.

3 Fluids with food:
Drinking fluids with a meal causes the stomach to empty more quickly.

4 Glucose content:
Extra sugar as part of a meal can cause the blood glucose level to rise, but not by as much as was once believed. Particle size and cell structure in different food compounds give them different blood glucose responses in spite of their containing the same amount of carbohydrate.

5 Salt content:
Salt in the food increases the absorption of glucose into the bloodstream.

Factors that raise the blood glucose level more slowly
(*decrease the glycaemic index*)

1 Starch structure:
Boiled and mashed potatoes give a quicker blood glucose response (as fast as ordinary sugar) while rice and pasta give a slower blood glucose response.

2 Gel-forming dietary fibre:
A high fibre content (as in rye bread) gives a slower rise in blood glucose by slowing down the emptying rate of the stomach and binding glucose in the intestine.

3 Fat content:
Fat in the food will delay the emptying of the stomach.

4 Cell structure:
Beans, peas and lentils retain their cell structure even after cooking. Whole fruits affect the blood glucose level more slowly than peeled fruits and juice.

5 Size of bites:
Larger pieces of food take longer to digest in the stomach and intestine. Larger pieces also cause the stomach to empty more slowly.

How much you chew the food and the size of the food particles swallowed also influences the blood glucose response. Industrially manufactured mashed potatoes contain a fine powder that is mixed with fluid. The glucose in mashed potatoes is absorbed just as quickly as a glucose solution. Pasta and rice are swallowed in larger bites and must be digested before they can be absorbed. Likewise, a whole apple will give a slower rise in blood glucose than apple juice which contains smaller particles and is in a liquid form.

Heating decomposes starch, making sugar more accessible and faster to digest. Industrial food processing usually involves higher temperatures, which give food a quicker blood glucose raising effect compared with home-cooked meals.

Indigestible carbohydrates (dietary fibre) cannot be broken down in the intestines and will therefore not give a blood glucose response. The amount of carbohydrate listed on a food label can be misleading as no distinction is made between digestible and indigestible carbo-hydrates. Do ask your dietitian for more infor-mation about this.

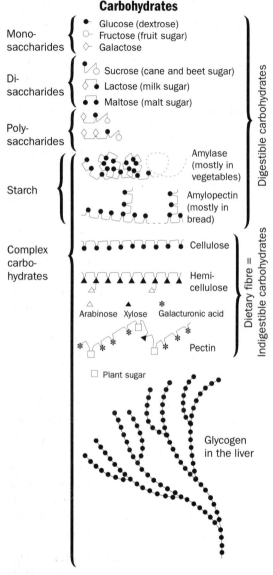

Carbohydrates

Carbohydrates are important for metabolism in the body. Only mono-saccharides can be absorbed from the intestine. Di-saccharides and starch must first be broken down by digestive enzymes. Dietary fibre cannot be broken down to saccharides in the intestines. The glycogen store in the liver is composed of very long chains of glucose.

This illustration is modified from the article by Anderssen, Asp and Hallmans in the *Scandinavian Journal of Nutrition*, 1986.

Emptying the stomach

Everything that causes the stomach to release food more slowly into the intestines will also result in a slower increase of the blood glucose level (see illustration on page 36). From this, it follows that the composition of the meal will be important, and not only the amount of carbo-hydrates it contains. Fat and fibre cause the stomach to empty more slowly, while a drink with the meal will make it empty more quickly. A meal containing solid food (such as pasta) is emptied more slowly than liquid food like soup. Swallowing without chewing also causes a slower rise in blood glucose. Extremely cold (4°C, 39°F) or hot (50°C, 122°F) food will also slow down stomach emptying.

The emptying of the stomach is also affected by the blood glucose level. The stomach empties more quickly if the blood glucose is low and more slowly if it is high. Both solid and liquid food are emptied from the stomach twice as fast when the blood glucose drops from a normal level (4–7 mmol/L, 72–126 mg/dl) to a hypo-glycaemic level (1.6–2.2 mmol/L, 29–40 mg/dl). If your blood glucose level has been lowered by a large dose of insulin, for example, you want your stomach to empty as quickly as possible so that the glucose can be absorbed into the blood. In this situation, you should take something with a high glucose content, such as glucose tablets, glucose gel, fruit juice or a sports drink.

A high insulin level in the blood (for instance if you have taken too large a dose of insulin) does not affect the emptying of the stomach in itself. It is the high blood glucose level that causes a slower emptying. Even small changes in blood glucose level, well within the normal ranges for individuals without diabetes, seem to affect the rate of stomach emptying. One study of people without diabetes showed a 20% decrease in the emptying rate when the blood glucose level was increased from 4 to 8 mmol/L (72 to 144 mg/dl).

Non-strenuous exercise (like walking) leads to unchanged or more rapid emptying of the stomach, while strenuous exercise or physical exertion stops the stomach from emptying for 20–40 minutes after muscular activity finishes.

What is our food made of?

The food that we eat is mainly made up of a mixture of:

Carbohydrates	Fat	Protein
Sugar	Butter	Meat
Bread/flour	Margarine	Fish
Biscuits	Oil	Egg
Potatoes	Cream	Cheese
Pasta	Milk	Milk
Rice	Yoghurt	Yoghurt
Fruit	Cheese	
Cereals		
Sweetcorn, taro		
Milk, yoghurt		

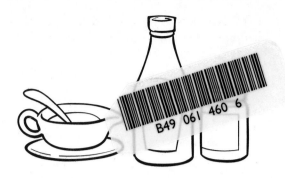

You can have a modest amount of sauce or ketchup with your food without any problems. However, be aware that many commercially produced sauces contain a lot of sugar. You need to keep a count of how much additional sugar you are eating.

A possible explanation for this delayed stomach emptying after physical exertion is an increased secretion of adrenaline and morphine-like hormones (endorphins).

Stomach emptying can also be delayed if you have gastroenteritis. This may explain why when some people develop diarrhoea and vomiting, their blood glucose levels remain low for the duration of the illness.

Gastroparesis is a serious complication of diabetes caused by damage to the nerves that control the automatic muscular activity of the stomach. This disrupts the normal emptying process, and the stomach ends up behaving like a floppy bag. Food is normally squeezed out of the stomach in a matter of hours, but if there is gastroparesis, stomach emptying is very variable and food may remain in the stomach for days. Gastroparesis may lead to heartburn, vomiting of undigested food and bloating of the abdomen (See also Chapter 31 on Microvascular complications).

Sugar content in our food

From a nutritional point of view, we do not actually need pure sugar at all. The liver is quite capable of producing the 250–300 g of glucose that a healthy adult normally needs per day.

Small amounts of glucose along with a meal (in the form of, for example, ketchup or another sauce) do not cause a rise in blood glucose. The recommendation to decrease the sugar content in food is based on more general factors:

1 Sugar gives 'empty calories', i.e. sugar gives only energy and contains no other nutrients. This energy will cause you to gain weight, while reducing your appetite for more healthy foods. Many patients with Type 2 diabetes have a particular problem with over-eating sugary foods, and it is important to reduce these where possible.

2 Sugar is bad for your teeth.

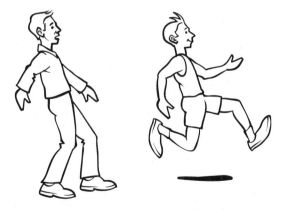

A moderate degree of exercise will not stop the stomach emptying, and may even speed it up. Strenuous exercise will stop the the stomach emptying while your muscles are working hard.

It used to be common practice to decrease the carbohydrate content in a diabetes meal plan at all costs. Unfortunately, this approach usually

Aims of nutritional management

➡ To provide appropriate energy and nutrients for optimal health.

➡ To maintain or achieve an ideal body weight.

➡ To achieve the best possible control of your blood glucose, by balancing food intake with oral medication or insulin, energy requirements and physical activity.

➡ To prevent and treat acute complications of insulin or sulphonylurea therapy, for example hypoglycaemia, crises with high blood glucose, illness and exercise-related problems.

➡ To reduce the risk of long-term complications through optimal glucose control.

➡ To reduce the risk of heart complications and blood vessel disease.

➡ To preserve your quality of life and your social and psychological wellbeing.

How can this be achieved?

➡ Healthy eating principles should be involve partners and other family members too.

➡ Your total calorie intake should allow you to maintain an ideal weight which, in turn, reduces insulin resistance.

➡ Cut down the amount of saturated fat.

➡ Eat more fruit and vegetables on a regular basis (the Department of Health recommends 5 portions a day of fruit or vegetables).

How is the emptying of the stomach affected?

More quickly	More slowly
Small bites	Large bites
Liquid food	Solid food
Drink with food	Drink after food
	Fatty food
	Food rich in fibre
	Extremely hot or cold food
Hypoglycaemia	High blood glucose
	High levels of insulin
	Smoking
	Gastroenteritis
Light exercise	Heavy exercise

causes an increase in fat intake, which in itself is less healthy than a normal diet. Nowadays the same dietary advice apples to people with and without diabetes, with the recommendation to eat less refined (high GI) carbohydrate and compensate with more low GI carbohydrate. Some people do lose weight by keeping to an ultra-low carbohydrate diet, Atkins-style diet but they must avoid eating extra fat in compensation. If you decide to give it a try, you will need to reduce your dose of insulin or sulphonylurea and should take medical advice. A recent study showed that the Atkins diet causes more weight loss than other commercial weight loss programmes at 2 months, but by 6 months the effects of different 'diets' are the same.

Taking fluids with food

You can affect your blood glucose level considerably, depending on what you have to drink with your meals. Sweet drinks like fruit juice can be used to raise your blood glucose if it is in the low range. If you are going to drink alcohol, don't forget that alcoholic drinks can contain a lot of calories too (see also Chapter 24). But if your blood glucose level is high, it is better to have water. It seems a bit repetitive, but people with Type 2 diabetes are often overweight, and any calorie reduction is beneficial.

It is a good idea to drink plenty of calorie-free drinks between meals if your blood glucose is high as this will help to bring it down (part of the excess glucose will be excreted into the urine). Water will be the best for this – you should be wary of too many drinks containing artificial sweeteners, and careful not to let your caffeine intake rise too high either.

Dietary fats

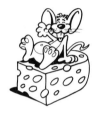

If you have diabetes, a key goal should be to decrease your total fat intake and thus reduce your risk of arteriosclerosis and heart disease (see Chapter 30 on Complications of the cardiovascular system). You need to be particularly careful with saturated fat and so-called 'trans fats'. Foods that contain large amounts of saturated fats include dairy products and red meats. They are also found in many snack foods such as chocolate, cakes and pastries and sometimes in crisps. Trans fats are often listed as 'partially hydrogenated vegetable oil' or 'vegetable shortening' on the food label. Try to use monounsaturated and polyunsaturated fats where possible instead of saturated fats. An increased intake of monounsaturated fats (MUFA) may even improve your HbA_{1c}. The softer the fat the better. Liquid margarine and oil contain no trans fats and also have a low content of saturated fatty acids. Be careful of palm, vegetable and coconut oil, which are high in saturated fat and used widely in different products (e.g. peanut butter, or many ready-made curry meals).

Today, dietitians promote MUFA which have a protective effect against heart disease. Ordinary margarine and butter are high in saturated and

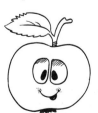

If you do have a snack, try a piece of fruit as a healthy option.

> ## Food rules of thumb
>
> ➡ Snacks taken between meals are often high-calorie, high-sugar foods which won't leave you satisfied and increase your weight.
>
> ➡ Eat fresh fruit as a snack rather than drinking fruit juice.
>
> ➡ Cut down on snacks and portion size at every meal if you have weight problems.
>
> ➡ Aim for a high fibre content in your food.

trans fats, so choose a margarine that contains MUFA if possible, for example one containing olive oil. Olive oil and rapeseed oil contain large amounts of monounsaturated fat and are useful for frying. However, if the frying pan is very hot, the unsaturated fat can be broken down and some types of light margarine cannot be used for frying. Sunflower oil, on the other hand, is good for frying as it is not broken down as readily as olive oil.

Many people mistakenly believe that fat directly increases the blood glucose level since people with diabetes are usually advised to cut down on fat in their diet. However, fatty food has no direct effect on the blood glucose level. As fat yields more energy than carbohydrate, the stomach is emptied more slowly when the fat content is high. A meal with a high fat content will therefore cause the blood glucose level to rise more slowly in the initial period. In the long term though, the higher calorie load in fatty food will lead to increased weight gain and worsen your blood glucose level.

It is the total amount of fat over time that is important in the long run. As long as you observe a healthy diet for the majority of the time, an occasional celebratory meal out won't cause you too much harm. It is worth remembering that fat substitutes may well contain carbohydrate. This will be just another source of energy and raise your blood glucose levels.

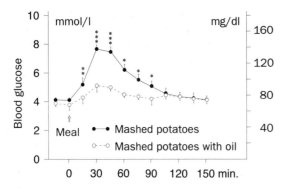

If your meal contains fat, this will delay the emptying of your stomach and cause your blood glucose level to rise more slowly. In this study (Welch, Bruce, Hill & Read), two helpings of mashed potatoes (50 g of carbohydrate) were given with or without corn oil (approximately 30 ml or two tablespoonfuls). The study was done in adults without diabetes, who can increase their amounts of insulin very fast. Notice that the blood glucose level increased very quickly despite this, with a significant change appearing in 30 minutes in the group of people whose mashed potatoes did not contain oil. If you have weight problems, you need to be careful about adding fat to your food.

Dietary fibre

The fibre content of food is healthy for many reasons. There are two kinds of fibre, soluble (gel-forming) and insoluble. Both help to prevent constipation, but only the soluble fibres (found in fruit, vegetables, legumes and oats) affect glucose control. You will feel full for longer after eating coarse rye or wholemeal bread with a high soluble fibre content than you would after eating the same amount of white bread without fibre. A high soluble fibre content will also decrease the cholesterol level in your blood. Adding fibre (such as oats and barley) to

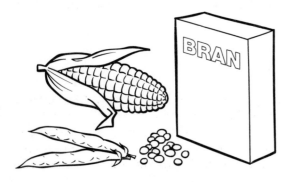

a meal will increase its bulk, causing the contents of the stomach and intestines to empty more slowly. The fibre forms a thin film on the intestinal surface, causing the glucose to be absorbed more slowly.

When a glucose solution is mixed with large amounts of water-soluble, gel-forming fibre (e.g. guar or ß-glucan) the expected rise in glucose concentration will be reduced. Soluble dietary fibre probably has the greatest impact on food intake with a high glucose content (such as many snacks) since it has been difficult to show in long-term studies that the addition of dietary fibre has resulted in a better HbA_{1c}. These studies have mainly been done on individuals with Type 2 diabetes. An Italian study of adults with Type 1 diabetes compared a low-fibre diet with a high-fibre diet rich in fruit, legumes and vegetables. Both diets contained exclusively natural foodstuffs. The high-fibre diet resulted in lower blood glucose levels, 0.5% lower HbA_{1c} and a decreased frequency of hypoglycaemia. In a European study on 2065 adults with Type 1 diabetes, the HbA_{1c} in people whose fibre intake was high was found to be approximately 0.3% lower than for the group with a low fibre intake.

Glycaemic index

The glycaemic index is an attempt to describe the blood glucose-raising effect of different foods. A certain amount of carbohydrate (usually 50 g) is given, and the area under the blood glucose curve is measured for 2 hours. Glucose is used to give a baseline GI index of 100. The GI can be misleading if you want to know how the blood glucose level is affected during a shorter period of time (e.g. 30–60 minutes) or if the food has a low, but easily accessible, sugar content. The list overleaf is based on work by Foster-Powell, Holt and Brand-Miller.

The GI of a mixed meal can be predicted from the GI of single foods. It may be difficult to estimate the GI for some combined meals from the GI of the single ingredients since the fat content also affects the speed with which carbohydrates are absorbed. A foodstuff with a low but easily

Glycaemic index

High glycaemic index	GI	50 g carb. in
Glucose	100	50 g
Instant mashed potatoes	85	375 g
Potato, baked	85	250 g
Corn flakes	81	60 g
Jelly sweets	78	65 g
White bread (gluten free)	76	100 g
Waffles	76	135 g
French fries	75	260 g
Weetabix	75	70 g
Oatmeal porridge	74	80 g (dry)
Rice, puffed	74	180 g
Potato, boiled	74	440 g
Water melon	72	1000 g
Popcorn	72	90 g
White bread	70	110 g
Sugar soda	68	370 g
Sucrose (sugar)	68	50 g
Rice, white	64	210 g
Average glycaemic index		
Rye bread (wholemeal)	58	110 g
Cola	58	480 g
Rice, long grain	56	180 g
Gluten-free pasta	56	64 g
Honey	55	70 g
Banana, all yellow	51	230 g
Pasta	46–52	200 g
Lactose (milk sugar)	46	50 g
Grapes	46	330 g
Rye bread (whole grain)	46	135 g
Low glycaemic index		
Milk chocolate	43	90 g
Banana, yellow and green	42	240 g
All Bran	42	65 g
Orange	42	550 g
Apple	38	400 g
Ice cream	37–61	190–280 g
Yoghurt	36	1100 g
Lentils, green	30	440 g
Kidney beans	28	300 g
Milk, 3% fat	21	1000 g
Fructose (fruit sugar)	19	50 g
Soya beans (dried)	18	1250 g
Peanuts	14	415 g

See also **www.mendosa.com/gilists.htm** for an extensive list of foods.

accessible sugar content (e.g. carrots) has a high glycaemic index but you must eat a great deal if your blood glucose is going to be increased. Although the use of low-GI food may reduce blood glucose levels after meals, more research is required before GI can be used as a general tool in diabetes care. The Diabetes and Nutrition Study Group of the European Association for the Study of Diabetes recommends the substitution of high-GI with low-GI foods to improve glycaemic control. A summary of many studies (called a meta-analysis) found that a low-GI diet reduced HbA_{1c} by 0.43% compared with conventional or high-GI diets. In Australia, the GI concept is much more accepted and widely used than, for example, in the US or the UK.

Potatoes (GI 74) give a faster blood glucose response than pasta (GI 46–52). Adding a small amount of oil or polyunsaturated or monounsaturated margarine to mashed potatoes (GI 85) will delay the glucose peak. If you replace one item in a meal with another (e.g. potatoes with pasta), the GI of the individual foods will help you determine the likely effect on the blood glucose. For example, it may be a good idea to have something with a low GI for supper as this could lower the risk of night-time hypoglycaemia if you are an insulin user.

GI is very useful when you are looking at eating between meals (single items of food often, such as yoghurt, an apple, a bun, ice cream, crisps, etc.). When you're considering something you shouldn't, the GI can often provide you with visual clues as to why a cream bun or a chocolate bar is worth avoiding.

Glucose tablets have a GI of 100 and can be used for treating hypoglycaemia when symptoms are pronounced or the blood glucose level is lower (3.5 mmol/L, 65 mg/dl).

Milk

If you can tolerate it, you should switch your milk from whole-fat to skimmed milk. The lower fat content in skimmed milk is associated with a reduced calorie burden. Skimmed milk contains a similar content of lactose (milk sugar) and is likely to have the same effect on blood sugar in the short term.

Vegetables

You can eat freely from this food group (except sweetcorn) as the carbohydrate content is very low (see the table opposite). Vegetables are also high in dietary fibre, which helps to smooth blood sugar peaks associated with food intake.

Potatoes

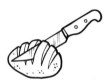

Potatoes, sweet potatoes, taro and yam belong to this type of foodstuff. The carbohydrate content of raw potatoes is absorbed slowly, but boiling causes the cell walls to burst. This allows the carbohydrates to be absorbed more quickly from the intestines. The carbohydrate content of mashed potatoes is absorbed as quickly as pure glucose (see graph on page 42). If you change the surface of a potato (e.g. by frying, deep frying or storing it in the refrigerator), the glucose will be absorbed more slowly than if you eat it freshly boiled. The manufacturing process and the high fat content of potato crisps cause the glucose contained in these to be absorbed very slowly; avoid them though because of the

Vegetables

	Quantity	Carb.	% fibre
Bamboo shoots, canned	100 ml	4 g	50%
Broccoli, frozen	100 ml	5 g	60%
Carrots, raw	100 ml	5 g	27%
Corn, canned	100 ml	20 g	30%
Corn on cob, cooked	1 medium	19 g	10%
Cucumber	250 ml	3 g	<1 g
Lettuce	250 ml	1 g	<1 g
Onions, cooked	100 ml	11 g	18%
Peas, green, cooked	100 ml	13 g	31%
Peppers, green, raw	100 ml	3 g	33%
Radishes	100 ml	2 g	50%
Tomatoes, raw	100 ml	4 g	25%

Data from work by Holzmeister, 2000.

increased energy and fat content, which will ultimately promote weight gain.

In one study of adults, chocolate cake was substituted for a baked potato without an increase in blood glucose levels. If the chocolate cake was added to the baked potato, the glucose level increased. However, remember that chocolate cake and baked potato are very different in nutritional and energy value!

Bread

At one time, people with diabetes were strongly advised to eat unsweetened bread. Today, we know that white bread raises the blood glucose level every bit as rapidly as ordinary sugar. However, margarine and something with a high fat content (e.g. cheese) on the bread will slow the rise in blood glucose by delaying the emptying of the stomach. Bread (such as whole grain) that is high in fibre will also slow down any rise in blood glucose levels.

If you bake your own bread, it is perfectly acceptable to use an ordinary recipe. It should

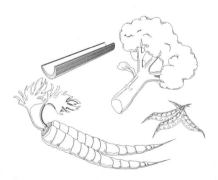

The starch in vegetables is broken down more slowly than other types of starch. Vegetables also contain soluble fibre, which is good for the digestion and prevents constipation.

How quickly is the blood glucose increased?

Puffed rice
Corn flakes
Mashed potatoes
Boiled potatoes
White bread
Whole-grain bread
Rice
Pasta
Potato crisps
Beans, lentils, peas

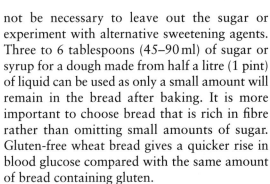

not be necessary to leave out the sugar or experiment with alternative sweetening agents. Three to 6 tablespoons (45–90 ml) of sugar or syrup for a dough made from half a litre (1 pint) of liquid can be used as only a small amount will remain in the bread after baking. It is more important to choose bread that is rich in fibre rather than omitting small amounts of sugar. Gluten-free wheat bread gives a quicker rise in blood glucose compared with the same amount of bread containing gluten.

Nutritious meals do not always need to be hot. A sandwich or roll with tuna, egg, lean meat, chicken or cheese and salad, along with yoghurt, fromage frais or fruit can be very enjoyable.

Unsweetened breakfast corn cereal (corn flakes) contains 90% starch, most of which rapidly becomes available as glucose. Sweetened (sugar-frosted) flaked corn cereal, on the other hand, contains around 50% starch and 50% sugar. Initially, both give the same blood glucose rise but sweetened corn flakes give slightly lower blood glucose levels after 3 hours. It comes as a surprise that corn starch raises the blood glucose faster than ordinary sugar. The best cereal to choose is one higher in fibre, such as bran flakes or All Bran. The amount of energy for a given weight of such a cereal is smaller, and the higher fibre content means that the GI is lower.

Pasta

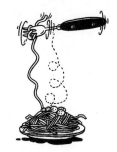

Pasta gives a slow rise in blood glucose since it is prepared from crushed or cracked wheat, and not wheat flour, which causes the starch to be enclosed within a structure of protein (gluten). This makes pasta a suitable food for people with diabetes. Wholewheat pasta is an even better choice.

Thinner pasta, such as macaroni, gives a quicker blood glucose response than spaghetti. Cooking time does not affect the rate with which the blood glucose is raised by spaghetti, except in extreme cases of overcooking. Tinned spaghetti increases the blood glucose as quickly as white bread. Because the gluten content of pasta contributes to the slow rise in blood glucose, gluten-free pasta allows blood glucose levels to rise more quickly.

Meat and fish

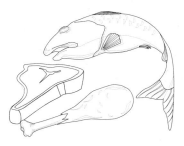

Meat and fish have a high protein content, and in some cases the fat content is also high. However, since they lack carbohydrates, they will not cause a direct increase in your blood glucose levels. Dietary protein does not slow the absorption of carbohydrate, and adding protein to a carbohydrate snack does not prevent late-onset or night-time hypoglycaemia.

Eating protein does not increase blood glucose levels in people who do not have diabetes. However, proteins stimulate the release of glucagon, which in turn helps to convert protein into glucose (a process called gluconeogenesis).

High-protein foods such as lean meat can make you feel full, which may be a real advantage if you have Type 2 diabetes and are watching your weight. If you have diabetic kidney disease, however, you may need to reduce the amount of protein in your diet. Your doctor and dietitian will be able to advise you about this.

Pizza

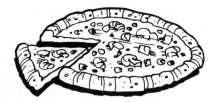

Pizza contains bread, cheese, meat or fish and possibly vegetables. However, a pizza usually contains more bread than most meals and often includes lavish helpings of fat – either cheese as a topping or fatty cuts of meat to add flavour. So an occasional pizza as a treat is fine, but if you eat it regularly you will put on weight.

Salt

Salt intake is generally far too high. In Western countries, it is difficult to decrease this as salt is added to many processed foods (only 20% of total intake is added at the table and in cooking). Extra salt in the form of sodium chloride (table-salt) will increase blood pressure and can be a risk factor, especially as diabetes itself increases the risk of heart and vascular diseases (see Chapter 32). Eating salty food can cause glucose to be absorbed more effectively from the intestine. Salt is also available as potassium chloride, but this is more expensive than common table-salt and tastes rather different. Sea-salt and herb-salt usually contain the same amount of sodium as table-salt. In many countries, including the UK, iodine is often added to table salt in order to prevent iodine deficiency. If this is available, it is a good choice since iodine is important for the function of your thyroid gland.

Herbs and spices

Herbs will not affect your blood glucose at all. However, it is important to be aware that some herbal 'seasoning' preparations also contain a lot of salt. If the flavouring is strong enough to make you drink more, your stomach may empty more rapidly, resulting in a quicker rise in your blood glucose level.

Fruit and berries

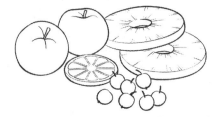

Fruits and berries have a high carbohydrate content (see table opposite). The higher the fibre content, the less effect they will have on the blood glucose level.

Mealtimes

Each family has its own routines for mealtimes, and these are likely to be the ones that particularly suit them. A dietitian should use the family's own eating habits and routines as a starting point when drawing up dietary advice for a person with diabetes. As discussed previously, too much snacking is to be avoided, and regular balanced meals are to be encouraged. If you live on your own and aren't interested in cooking, this may be difficult, but the effort of cooking a balanced meal will be rewarded in long-term glucose levels.

Special 'diabetic' food?

Diabetic food is to be avoided where possible. It quite often contains more calories than 'ordinary' substitutes, and fat may replace missing sugars. It also often contains sorbitol as a sweetener, which may produce side effects such as abdominal pain and diarrhoea. It is much better to learn how to handle ordinary food if you have diabetes.

'Fast food'

Many children, teenagers and adults like fast food, and it has become a fixture of modern life. Taking children or grandchildren out to a fast food eating place can be part of a family's social life. However, fast food often contains a lot of fat, so it should be eaten sparingly. Limit your eating of fast food to special occasions, such as a grandchild's birthday or a family reunion. The social and relationship benefits you will enjoy from eating fast food in this way once in a while should outweigh any potential problems.

Vegetarian and vegan diets

A pure vegetarian or vegan diet may result in a disturbed balance between the amount of

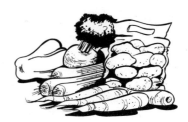

If you are a vegetarian, you will need to talk to your dietitian about your meal plan so that you will get enough of all kinds of essential nutrients.

protein and carbohydrate in the diet. This is because vegetarian nutrients contain much less protein than animal nutrients. A lactovegetarian diet includes milk products, which result in a higher protein intake but also an increased fat intake, unless you are careful. A vegan diet including a high proportion of fruits and berries may even have a higher content of sugar than a mixed diet. However, if reasonable attention is paid to achieving a balanced diet, most vegetarians keep very fit and avoid vitamin and mineral deficiencies.

In vegan or lactovegetarian diets, the animal products are mostly replaced by products from

Fruits

	Quantity	Carb.	Fibre	Fibre/ carb.		Quantity	Carb.	Fibre	Fibre/ carb.
Grapes	100 g	17 g	1.6 g	9%	Honeydew melon	100 g	8 g	0.9 g	11%
Blackcurrants	100 g	16 g	4.9 g	32%	Banana	1 fruit	21 g	1.5 g	7%
Blackberries	100 g	16 g	7.2 g	46%	Pear	1 fruit	16 g	3.0 g	19%
Pineapple, canned	100 g	16 g	1.0 g	6%	Apple	1 fruit	14 g	1.9 g	13%
Redcurrants	100 g	13 g	3.4 g	27%	Kiwi fruit	2 fruits	8 g	0.9 g	11%
Pineapple, fresh	100 g	12 g	1.2 g	9%	Orange	1 fruit	13 g	2.0 g	16%
Cherries, sweet	100 g	12 g	1.7 g	13%	Plums	2 fruits	9 g	1.2 g	13%
Strawberries	100 g	10 g	2.4 g	24%	Grapefruit	1 fruit	9 g	2.0 g	22%
Watermelon	100 g	9 g	0.6 g	7%	Raisins	1 tbs	8 g	1.0 g	12%
Rasberries	100 g	8 g	3.7 g	46%					

A higher percentage of fibre will cause the glucose to be absorbed more slowly. Bananas contain very little dietary fibre and will raise the blood glucose level more quickly than other fruits. They are therefore suitable fruits to take if your blood glucose is low, or during exercise. When counting grams of carbohydrate, the fibre content should be subtracted if it is 5 g or more.

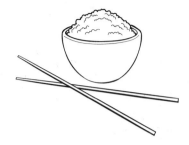

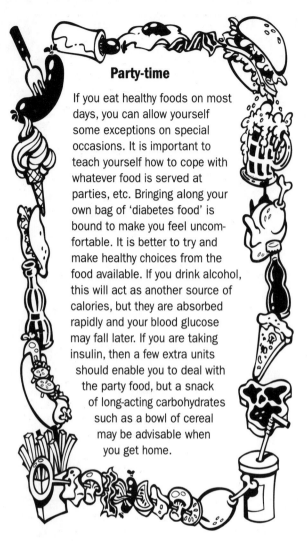

Party-time

If you eat healthy foods on most days, you can allow yourself some exceptions on special occasions. It is important to teach yourself how to cope with whatever food is served at parties, etc. Bringing along your own bag of 'diabetes food' is bound to make you feel uncomfortable. It is better to try and make healthy choices from the food available. If you drink alcohol, this will act as another source of calories, but they are absorbed rapidly and your blood glucose may fall later. If you are taking insulin, then a few extra units should enable you to deal with the party food, but a snack of long-acting carbohydrates such as a bowl of cereal may be advisable when you get home.

leguminous plants. The intake of vitamin B12 will be cut in half when the vitamins in animal products are not replaced. B12 deficiency leads to a number of different medical conditions, including anaemia, and most vegans accept the importance of taking supplements containing B12. You should talk to your dietitian or doctor if you are planning major changes in your diet.

Different cultures

Families from different cultures and different religions often have quite different eating habits. The number of meals can be fewer, and some-times certain foods are excluded due to religious reasons (Muslims and Jews do not eat pork and Hindus avoid beef). South Asian families often use ghee (clarified butter) for cooking, which is very high in saturated fat and must be reduced or omitted where possible.

In every case, it is of course important to take the family's customary food habits into consideration when discussing nutrition with a person who has diabetes.

Religious fasting days

Special religious fasting days, such as Yom Kippur for Jews, can easily be accommodated by careful monitoring and reducing doses of insulin or sulphonylureas for the period of the fast. Consult your diabetes healthcare team if you are at all unsure about how to handle the situation, and keep records in your logbook for the next time!

You can find more information about fasting for Yom Kippur on the Diabetes UK website (see page 220).

Ramadan: the fasting month

During Ramadan, the ninth month of the Islamic year, Muslims fast from dawn until sunset. Sick people, and women who are pregnant, breastfeeding or menstruating are exempt, as are young children. You can find more information about fasting for Ramadan on the Diabetes UK website (see page 220).

Fasting accelerates the breakdown of fat and ketone production, by increasing glucagon levels.

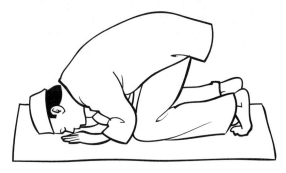

People with diabetes are generally exempt from fasting during Ramadan. If you still want to take part in the fast, it is very important that you seek advice from your doctor before doing so.

In addition to the problem of fasting, there is risk of overeating high-calorie sweets in the evenings during Ramadan. Although it's difficult to balance your meals during the evening following the fast, you should, where possible, make a healthy choice from the celebration food available.

Sweeteners

Sugar free?

When manufacturers state that a product has 'no sugar added', this does not always mean it is completely devoid of sugar. It usually implies that no sugar is added, whereas the natural sugar from berries or fruits is still present. No-added-sugar chocolate or ice cream can contain more calories than ordinary alternatives. Sweet foods like this often contain sorbitol, which will eventually be transformed into glucose in the liver. Check the food label carefully.

Non-nutritive sweeteners

Aspartame

Aspartame (E951) is 200 times sweeter than sugar and is used in such small amounts that the energy content is negligible. It can lose its sweetness through cooking and baking.

Free from sugar?

⮕	Unsweetened	No compound with a sweet taste has been added to the product. However, it can contain natural sugar (fruit sugar or milk sugar).
⮕	Without added sugar No added sugar No sugar added	No sugars have been added. However, it may contain sugar naturally, e.g. pure fruit juice.
⮕	Sugar free	No more than 0.2 g sugar per 100 g or 100 ml.
⮕	Reduced sugar	At least 25% reduction on the original product.

Aspartame is made up of two amino acids called aspartic acid and the methyl ester of phenylalanine. Amino acids and methyl esters are found naturally in foods like milk, meats, fruits and vegetables. When digested, the body handles the amino acids in aspartame in the same way as those in foods we eat daily. Although aspartame can be used by the whole family, individuals with a rare genetic disease called phenylketonuria (PKU) need to be aware that aspartame is a source of the protein component phenylalanine. Those who have PKU

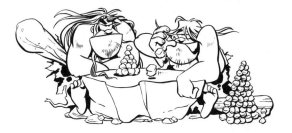

Since prehistoric times, humans have craved sugar. This is believed to be because sweet natural products are seldom poisonous, while many bitter ones can be so.

cannot properly metabolize phenylalanine and must monitor their intake of phenylalanine from all foods, including foods containing aspartame. In many countries, including the UK, every infant is screened for PKU at birth.

Unfortunately, many myths about aspartame are circulating, scaring people with diabetes and others who use 'diet' drinks. The fact is that aspartame has been studied extensively in humans. The safety of aspartame has been well established, and it has been shown that eating or drinking products sweetened with aspartame is not associated with adverse health effects. A 240 ml (8 ounce) glass of milk has six times more phenylalanine and 13 times more aspartic acid than an equivalent amount of soda sweetened with NutraSweet. An 8-ounce glass of fruit juice or tomato juice contains three to five times more methanol than an equivalent amount of soda sweetened with NutraSweet.

The UK's Committee on Toxicity of Chemicals in Food, Consumer Products and the Environment (COT, a committee of independent experts who advise the government on the safety of food chemicals) recently concluded that there is no evidence to suggest a need to revise their earlier statement confirming that aspartame is safe for use or revise the previously established acceptable daily intake (ADI) of 40 mg/kg body weight/day. An adult would have to consume 14 cans of a sugar-free drink every day before reaching the ADI, assuming the sweetener were used in the drink at the maximum permitted level. In practice, most drinks use aspartame in combination with other sweeteners so that the level is considerably lower. Aspartame intakes have been shown to be considerably below the recommended maximum level, even among children and people with diabetes who consume large quantities of sugar-free drinks.

Saccharin

Saccharin (E954) is a synthetic product. It is 300–500 times sweeter than sugar and contains no energy. It gives a slightly metallic taste when heated above 70°C (158°F) and should therefore be added only after cooking.

Acesulfame K

This sweetener (E950) is 130–200 times sweeter than sugar. It withstands heating well and can be used for baking. It is mixed with milk sugar (lactose) but in amounts too small to give any significant amount of energy.

Sucralose

Sucralose (E955) is 600 times sweeter than ordinary sugar. It is made from sugar but does not affect blood glucose. Sucralose tastes like sugar and is heat stable. It can be used both for baking and for cooking.

Cyclamate

Cyclamate (E952) is 30–50 times sweeter than sugar and contains no energy. It is stable at high temperatures and therefore suitable for cooking and baking. It is often used in soft drinks, dairy

---

Hot and cold drinks

	Quantity	Carb.	Fat	Kcal
Low-fat milk	200 ml	10 g	1 g	75
1.5%-fat milk	200 ml	10 g	3 g	96
3%-fat milk	200 ml	10 g	6 g	120
Chocolate milk*	200 ml	~20 g		
Orange juice	200 ml	~25 g	—	100
Squash	200 ml	~15 g	—	60
Soft drinks	200 ml	~20 g	—	100
Lemonade	330 ml	~30 g	—	120
Diet Fanta	330 ml	0 g	—	1
Diet cola	330 ml	0 g	—	1
Coffee	200 ml	~0.3 g	—	2
Tea	200 ml	0 g	—	2
Herb tea	Can have a high sugar content			

Carb. = carbohydrates; kcal = kilocalories

*The fat and energy content of chocolate milk depends on how much fat there is in the milk used.

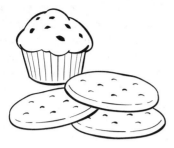

Some artificial sweeteners can be used for baking.

products and chocolate. The UK Food Standards Agency is advising parents to give young children no more than three beakers (about 180 ml each) a day of dilutable soft drinks, or squashes, containing the sweetener cyclamate. Drinking more than this amount could lead to children aged 1½ to 4½ years taking in more than the ADI for cyclamate. The Agency is also recommending that, when preparing dilutable soft drinks containing cyclamate for young children, parents should dilute them more than they would for an adult.

Nutritive sweeteners

These all contain energy, which should be considered if weight is a problem.

Fructose

Fructose is almost twice as sweet as sugar. Even if fructose does not affect your blood glucose level directly, it is transformed into glucose in the liver, and the calorie content can cause weight gain. Because of this, fructose is not considered as a suitable sweetener for people with diabetes in some countries. In other countries (such as Finland and Germany), many 'diabetes products' containing fructose are sold.

Sugar alcohols

Sugar alcohols (also called polyols) are used by food manufacturers to lower carbohydrate and/or fat content and are often used in chewing gum, 'sugar-free' sweets, ice cream and pastry. Sugar alcohols provide approximately half the energy (2.5 kcal/g) as other carbohydrates (4 kcal/g). Chemically, they are neither sugars nor alcohols, but eventually they will be converted into fructose and glucose by the liver. The names of sugar alcohols usually end in '-ol', for example sorbitol, xylitol, mannitol, maltitol and lactitol. Hydrogenated starch hydrolysates and isomalt are also sugar alcohols. The sweetness of sorbitol is about half that of sugar. When counting carbohydrates, it is currently suggested that only half the amount of sugar alcohols should be included.

Sorbitol (E420) is a natural component of plums, cherries and other fruits and berries. Sorbitol and other sugar alcohols absorb water from the intestines and provide nourishment for intestinal bacteria. Large amounts of sorbitol can cause abdominal pains and diarrhoea, which may put an automatic limit on the amounts eaten.

Sweeteners without energy		
Substance	**Trade name**	**Common in**
Acesulfame K	Sunett Hermesetas Gold (aspartame + acesulfame K)	Beverages, jams, sweets baked goods
Aspartame	NutraSweet Equal	Chewing gum Soft drinks Tabletop sweetener
Cyclamate	Sucaryl, Sugar Twin	Tabletop sweetener
Saccharin	Sweet'n Low	Tabletop sweetener
Hermesetas	Original	Tabletop sweetener
Sucralose	Splenda	Tabletop sweetener, drinks, baked goods, frozen and canned fruit

Diet drinks and 'light' foods

Diet drinks are usually sweetened with aspartame and do not contain any sugar. Most of these drinks are 'unrestricted' for people with diabetes in the sense that they do not raise the blood glucose. However, cola drinks often contain caffeine so it is not healthy to drink large amounts of them.

When a foodstuff is labelled 'light', the situation is more complex. Such products are not necessarily sugar free. In some countries, a foodstuff may be described as 'light' if the sugar content is decreased. Products containing fat can be labelled 'light' if the fat content has been decreased. Most countries have regulations to ensure that terms such as 'light' or 'low fat' are explained on food labelling. As the rules for labelling may vary from country to country, you should check with your dietitian about what is applicable where you live.

Light (low-fat) ice cream contains around one third of the fat content found in regular ice cream. 'Fat free' means the product contains no fat, while 'no sugar added' may mean sugar alcohols are added instead.

Weight control

Many people with Type 2 diabetes have spent their lives battling against being overweight. They have often spent years trying to lose weight by themselves, as well as being told by friends, family members and health professionals that they must lose weight. This chapter looks at the benefits of losing weight and the effects of a number of different diets as measured in randomized controlled studies. We hope that, by the time you have finished reading this chapter, you will be able to come to some practical conclusions about taking control of your weight. If you can find a strategy for losing weight that works for you, you will feel healthier and your diabetes will be easier to manage into the bargain.

What is 'overweight'?

The measure most commonly used to define healthy weight, overweight and obese is the body mass index, or BMI. This is based on a calculation involving your weight and your height. A BMI of between 20 and 25 is generally considered to be healthy, a BMI of 26–30 indicates overweight, whereas a BMI over 30 is a sign of obesity, which is a cause for real concern.

Your body shape is also important. People who are naturally 'pear-shaped', storing fat on their bottom and thighs, are at a lower risk of developing Type 2 diabetes than people who are 'apple-shaped' and store fat around their middle. This is called central obesity and is a risk for diabetes. This is also the reason why waist measurements can also be taken as a 'risk indicator' for developing Type 2 diabetes.

$$\text{Body mass index} = \frac{\text{weight (kg)}}{\text{height (m)} \times \text{height (m)}}$$

How to calculate your body mass index (BMI).

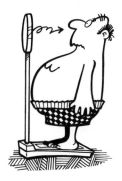

Younger women are more likely to be 'pear-shaped' than 'apple-shaped', although this is not always the case. Unfortunately, hormonal changes around the time of the menopause can change the way fat is distributed so some women may find they change from 'pears' to 'apples' as they get older, thus increasing their risk of developing diabetes.

Is weight always a problem?

It is important to point out that although the majority of people who develop Type 2 diabetes have a tendency towards overweight, there are exceptions. If you are of normal weight, or underweight, when you are diagnosed, this does not mean the diagnosis is wrong, though it may

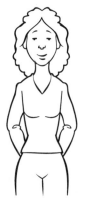
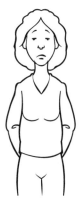

perhaps come as more of a surprise. In some cases, weight loss will be recent and one of the symptoms leading up to diagnosis. This is because glucose, the main fuel for your body, cannot be used or stored by the body in the normal way if you have uncontrolled diabetes. The unused glucose builds up in the bloodstream and overflows into the urine (where it will show up on a dipstick urine test). As much as 500g of glucose can be lost in the urine over in just 24 hours. This is equivalent to 2000 calories per day and, naturally, causes a drain on the body's resources.

Definition of central obesity

Population group	Waist measurement
Caucasian (white) male	102 cm (40 inches)
Caucasian female	88 cm (35 inches)
Asian male*	88 cm (35 inches)
Asian female*	80 cm (32 inches)

*Asian people have a higher risk than Caucasians of developing Type 2 diabetes, so the waist measurement is lower.

Body mass index (BMI) chart

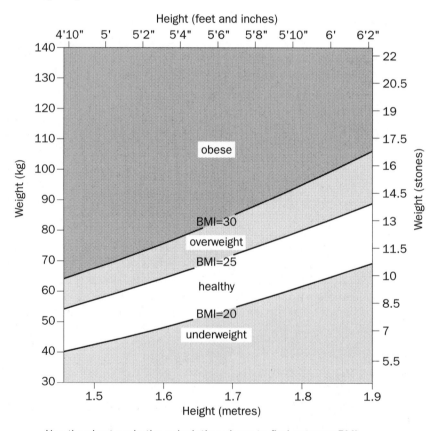

Use the chart or do the calculation above to find out your BMI.

Your BMI score:
below 20: underweight
20–25: ideal/healthy
25–30: overweight
30+: seriously overweight (obese)

People who are thin, especially if they have lost weight before diagnosis, are more likely to need tablets as soon as they are diagnosed. They are also more likely to need insulin treatment sooner rather than later.

Metabolic syndrome

Some people have a combination of insulin resistance, central obesity, raised blood pressure and high levels of cholesterol in their blood. This is referred to as the 'metabolic syndrome', and often leads on to full-blown Type 2 diabetes. If you have this syndrome, your doctor will be particularly keen to encourage you to do everything possible to bring your weight under control.

Weight loss: the benefits to your health

If you can manage it, a reduction of 5–10% in body weight will make your diabetes substantially easier to manage, reducing your HbA_{1c} by between 1 and 2% on average. While this won't halt progression of your diabetes, it will slow it down significantly. It will also reduce your total body fat content, particularly central fat, which is a major contributor to insulin resistance. The resulting improvement in insulin sensitivity leads to a reduction in blood pressure and increases the level of good cholesterol (HDL) in the bloodstream as well as being responsible for the improved blood sugars.

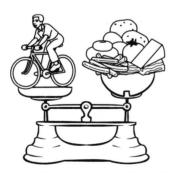

To regulate your weight, you need to balance the number of calories you eat against the calories you use through daily exercise.

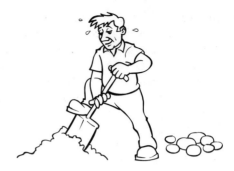

Exercise can take many forms. Gardening, for example, can be very energetic. Growing your own food can have the added benefit of encouraging healthy eating.

Exercise and weight loss

Unfortunately, there is no magic answer to losing weight or keeping it stable. Put quite simply, weight loss or weight gain depends on balancing the calories you eat against the calories you expend in your day-to-day activity. If you eat more than you expend, then you will put on weight. You might not be very keen on joining the gym or starting an exercise programme, but you would be surprised to find that many successful gym attendees started with just that frame of mind. Of course, the cost may be putting you off. Some GPs now offer prescribed exercise, and while this might not make your visit entirely free, it should reduce the cost substantially. If the gym just isn't for you, then you can try walking. Just getting off the bus one stop earlier, or walking to the paper shop may be enough to create a calorie deficit. Gardening is another efficient way to burn energy. If you have a garden big enough for a vegetable patch, try and rediscover a passion for healthy eating and exercise at the same time.

Are low carbohydrate diets useful?

This is an area in which there has been quite a lot of research over the last couple of decades, and the results do appear encouraging for a significant proportion of people. However, although they help people lose a large amount of weight, like most diets, the weight loss is not always maintained and there may be a yoyo effect. If you are on insulin, you will need to reduce the doses dramatically while you restrict your intake of carbohydrate (see Research findings box on this page).

If you are able to follow a low carbohydrate diet, the results in terms of reduction in insulin resistance, improvement in blood glucose levels, and other problems linked to excess weight such as high blood pressure can be spectacular. However, many people do find it difficult to cut out carbohydrates such as bread, pasta or rice. If this applies to you, it may be that this type of weight loss programme is not your best choice. A conventional low fat diet or meal replacement programme may be better for you. If you do feel this type of regime is appropriate for you though, there are a number of different websites or books available which can help you with carbohydrate reduction.

Are conventional low fat diets useful?

A more conventional low fat diet has been recommended for weight reduction in Type 2 diabetes for a number of years. Many people find it easier than a low fat, low carbohydrate diet as the food bears more relation to a 'normal' diet. Put simply, a reduced intake of saturated fat, with an increased intake of oily fish, complex carbohydrates such as wholemeal pasta or bran and fruit and vegetables is recommended. Meat should be a lean cut if possible. Studies of conventional low fat diets in Type 2 diabetes suggest that weight loss is around 3–7% at the one-year stage.

There are a number of varied recipes and meal plans that can be downloaded free from the Internet, or found in a suitable low fat diet book.

Partial meal replacement diets

Partial meal replacement implies replacing up to two meals in a structured way with lower calorie alternatives fortified with vitamins and minerals.

Research findings: low carbohydrate diets

➡ A number of research studies have shown that, in the short term at least, switching some of the carbohydrate component of a conventional low fat diet to protein appears to accelerate weight loss. It also seems to lead to preferential loss of body fat and a greater improvement in insulin sensitivity.

➡ A few longer-term studies are now beginning to appear which compare weight loss, body fat composition, glucose control and cardiovascular risk factors in people on low carbohydrate diets with a more traditional low fat diet containing a higher proportion of carbohydrate.

➡ One good long-term study comes from Adelaide, Australia. Researchers compared two diets, one high protein and low carbohydrate diet and the other a conventional low fat diet containing a higher proportion of carbohydrate. Participants were followed up for a period of 68 weeks in total. Although people on both the conventional low fat diet and the low fat, low carbohydrate diet lost weight, those on the the low-fat, low-carbohydrate diet lost more: on average 5.8% versus 3.6% over the course of the study. The low carbohydrate diet people had a greater fall in insulin resistance and their blood pressure was more likely to fall.

➡ In both groups, people found it increasingly difficult to stick to their diets after around 3 months of the study. This goes to show how difficult it can be to keep to a diet. If this is the case within a clinical trial, it is likely to be much more difficult without the support of the trial.

An example of this type of diet is the Slimfast programme. The weight loss achieved appears to be in the region of 7–8% within a year, which is generally slightly more than is seen in conventional reduced calorie diets.

Using the glycaemic index (GI) in dietary planning for weight reduction

Low glycaemic index (GI) diets are now a new dietary trend, following on from Atkins and reduced carbohydrate diets (see Chapter 8 on Nutrition). Low GI foods essentially contain more complex carbohydrate (starches) and more soluble fibre. This means that any glucose peaks after the food is digested occur over a longer period of time and the overall peak reached is also less. A group of researchers tested out the effects of a low GI diet in Type 2 diabetes. Although the study was very short, they did find that glucose control, lipid profiles and blood thickness were significantly better after only one month of following the diet.

Group therapy

A number of organizations, such as Weight Watchers and Slimming World, promote the idea of dieting and lifestyle change through group work. This approach can be very effective in encouraging people to stick to any diet or diet and exercise programme. If you have a friend or

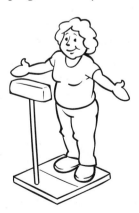

> ### Weight loss: summary points
>
> **1** The majority of people with Type 2 diabetes are significantly overweight.
>
> **2** Many will have tried for many years to modify diet, exercise and general lifestyle to try to encourage a slow loss of weight. A diagnosis of Type 2 diabetes can provide an opportunity to try again, with new impetus.
>
> **3** All diets in which the total number of calories taken by mouth is less than the number of calories expended will promote weight loss.
>
> **4** No diet is right for everyone. If you've tried one type of diet before and it hasn't worked, try another.
>
> **5** Group therapy helps many people, as the support of others can often help them achieve better results than working at weight loss on their own.
>
> **6** No matter how hard changing your life seems, it is worth it for the sake of your long-term health. Even modest weight loss can promote great improvements in your glucose control, blood pressure and other risk factors linked to complications of diabetes.

another member of the family who is overweight who can attend meetings with you, so much the better. There is no doubt that companionship in dieting makes long-term success much more likely.

This approach often involves inviting visiting speakers to talk to groups after the regular 'weigh-in' sessions. They may tell motivational stories, give recipe and meal-planning ideas, advise on exercise regimes or reinforce listeners' awareness of the long-term health benefits of weight loss.

Drugs for weight loss

Two drugs which suppress appetite have now been approved for use by people with diabetes. Both must be used in conjunction with a calorie-controlled diet in order to achieve the desired weight loss.

Rimonabant

Rimonabant (trade name Accomplia) is the more recent of these. It works by suppressing the urge to eat more. It appears to have few side effects. However, some recent work suggests it might be associated with an increased risk of depression. For this reason, rimonabant is not recommended for use by anyone who has a history of depression or other mental illness.

Sibutramine

Sibutramine (trade name Reductil) has been available for longer. It may be given to people with diabetes provided their BMI is under 27. Sibutramine is not suitable for everyone, and cannot be used by people with heart disease. It can cause blood pressure to rise, so if you are prescribed it your doctor or nurse should check your blood pressure more frequently than before. Your weight will also be monitored carefully, and the medicine discontinued if you have not lost 5% of your body weight in the first 3 months. Sibutramine is not suitable as a long-term treatment, and you should not take it for more than one year.

Orlistat

Orlistat (trade name Xenical) is another drug that can be used by people with Type 2 diabetes. Unlike the two drugs mentioned above, it is not an appetite suppressant; rather it works by acting on the stomach and small intestine in such a way that less than the usual amount of fat can be digested. This loss of fat is a loss of calories, and this is what leads to the weight loss. If you are prescribed orlistat, it is important that you follow a low-fat diet as far as you can, otherwise you can have some unpleasant side effects. You will also be given an information package to help you make changes in your lifestyle and access to a telephone helpline. It is very important you make full use of both of these while you are taking this medication.

Exercise

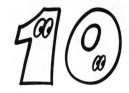

If you have Type 2 diabetes, it really is a good idea to take some form of regular exercise. It can help your diabetes by increasing your body's insulin sensitivity. It can also delay the onset of Type 2 diabetes if you have impaired glucose tolerance (see page 13) and are therefore at increased risk of developing it.

In addition, exercise encourages the burning of circulating energy fats (triglycerides) if the period of exercise is long enough. It encourages weight loss and leads to improvements in HbA_{1c}, blood pressure, and the profile of fats in the blood. Low blood sugars aren't normally a problem unless you take sulphonylureas or insulin, a dose reduction in either before a long period of exercise should usually avoid the need for a top up of carbohydrate and promote better weight loss.

What happens during exercise?

Regular exercise stimulates a series of events in the body that result in changes in body composition. It reduces the amount of fat and increases the amount of lean tissue: muscle, fibres and bone. This increases your metabolic rate and improves your fitness, which is the amount of exercise that you can do without getting tired or exhausted. This not only makes you feel better, it also reduces blood pressure and the 'bad' cho-

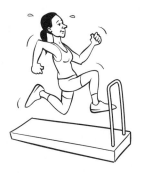

lesterol (low density, LDL) and increases the 'good' cholesterol (high density, HDL). Increasing fitness also increases the body's sensitivity to insulin and lowers blood glucose levels. It may increase the tendency to develop hypoglycaemia, and you might be able to reduce your insulin dose as your fitness improves.

Planning and maintaining exercise

Exercise should be fun. Find what you enjoy doing, and let you doctor know you are changing your lifestyle.

The first thing about making changes to your lifestyle to increase the amount of exercise in your daily routine is to find a fitness programme that you enjoy. Your aspirations can be very limited, such as going to football coaching with your children. Or you might set yourself a goal to look forward to such as a fun run or a walking holiday. This will require serious training.

Exercise does not have to involve sports, and you can usually find something suitable to suit your lifestyle. The staff at your local fitness centre are specially trained to help you with this, and these centres are a good place to start. They will work out an exercise programme with you and show you how to improve your fitness.

Before you undertake a new exercise programme, check first with your doctor or nurse. They will know about any underlying medical problems which might limit your capacity to exercise. Even if you don't have any associated conditions, if you're taking a mixed insulin or sulphonylurea tablets, you may need to reduce your dose before exercise. As a rough rule if you plan to do substantial exercise in the day, you should reduce your morning insulin by about 20–30%, or take half your sulphonylurea dose. This avoids the problem of hypoglycaemia in reaction to exercise, which necessitates snacking,

The effects of exercise on the blood glucose level

➡ Exercise increases absorption of insulin from the injection site that you move during exercise, for example the thigh when running or playing football.

➡ It increases the consumption of glucose without increasing the need for insulin.

➡ BUT – insulin must be available or the muscle cells will not be able to take up the glucose!

➡ Beware! Be careful with exercise when there is not enough insulin available in your body (blood glucose above 15–16 mmol/L, 270–290 mg/dl and elevated levels of ketones). You might need an extra insulin injection (0.05–0.1 units/kg, 0.25–0.5 units /10 1b) and abstain from exercise for 2–3 hours until the blood glucose level has gone down.

➡ You will be at risk of hypoglycaemia many hours afterwards (in the evening or during the night) because you have used the liver's store of glycogen after a lot of exercise.

➡ If you exercise regularly, you will know how much your blood glucose is affected. But if you exercise occasionally only, your blood glucose may drop much more than you expect during and after exercise.

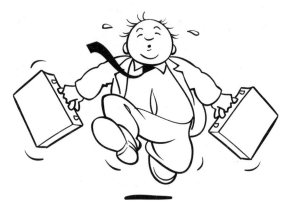

The heavier you are, the more energy you will use when you exercise.

with. The heavier you are, the more energy you use, like a horse running with weighted saddle bags! It is worth remembering that something which might not seem like a sport, such as digging the garden or walking the dog, may be an efficient way of burning calories.

Exercise and mood

Everyone remembers doing a period of hard exercise, usually something you didn't want to do at school, like a game of rugby or a long run. We all know the feeling of intense exhaustion that you feel during the game and the elation that you experience after the event. You may well not have experienced those feelings for many years, but even modest exercise can bring about a marked improvement in psychological wellbeing.

limiting any weight loss or glycaemic benefit from the hard work that you have done. Hypoglycaemia only occurs during exercise in people with good control. If your HbA$_{1c}$ is high, exercise may even lead to an increase in blood glucose.

In general, endurance exercise is most effective if you can manage it: 1 hour of walking will burn up 400 calories, jogging 600 and rowing on a machine nearer 700. Of course, the amount you burn up will depend on your weight to start

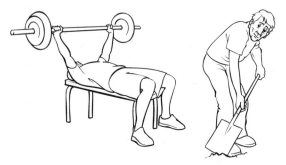

Not everyone likes the same sort of activity. It is important to find a form of exercise you enjoy so you will stick with it.

Ways of introducing exercise into your daily life

➡ Walk whenever you can, and avoid using the car.

➡ Climb stairs rather than take the lift.

➡ Walk to and from work.

➡ Take your dog for more or longer walks.

➡ Consider buying a bicycle or exercise bike.

➡ Make a point of taking at least three half-hour walks a week at a fast pace.

➡ Enrol for a dance class.

➡ Take up swimming.

Exercise advice for people who have complications arising from diabetes

A careful medical history and physical examination can minimize risks associated with competitive sports for people who have long-term complications of diabetes. In many cases, a formal graded exercise test will be helpful to determine the appropriate level of exercise.

Groups of people who need a gentle graded approach to exercise:

➡ Age > 50 years.

➡ People who know they have had Type 2 diabetes for more than 10 years.

➡ Presence of any additional risk factors for heart disease (overweight, hypertension, high lipid levels).

➡ Presence of eye damage (so-called proliferative retinopathy) or kidney damage (including microalbuminuria).

➡ Diabetes complications in the feet.

➡ Damage to the autonomic nervous system (see Chapter 31 on Microvascular complications).

One study compared the effect on mood of exercise training versus conventional anti-depresssants in a group of around 150 patients with major depression. After around 16 weeks of exercise training the response in terms of mood and depression scores was the same for the exercise group as it was for the group treated with drugs The amount of exercise undertaken was pretty modest, only three thirty minute sessions per week, but clearly exercise is a very good way to restore positive mood.

Positive mood is also important in the context of Type 2 diabetes. A number of studies have shown that depression and low mood both predispose to getting Type 2 diabetes and are associated with worse blood sugar levels in patients who already have diabetes. The reason for this is very clear, we have all reached for the comfort foods we enjoy and not wanted to exercise when it seems the world is getting the better of us. See also Chapter 29 on Psychological issues.

Exercise and the cardiovascular system

Although most studies focus on the effects of exercise on blood sugar control in diabetes, a number have also looked at the effects on the cardiovascular system.

We know that insulin resistance in Type 2 diabetes causes increased blood pressure and

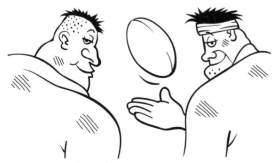

Exercise can have a really positive effect on your sense of wellbeing.

> ### Benefits of exercise in Type 2 diabetes: Research findings
>
> Exercise has been shown to have the following effects:
>
> ⇒ Improve blood glucose control.
>
> ⇒ Reduce central body fat.
>
> ⇒ Increase sensitivity to insulin.
>
> ⇒ Reduce blood triglycerides levels.
>
> ⇒ Help prevent the development of Type 2 diabetes in those at risk.

increased stiffness of arteries. It also impairs the ability of your arteries to relax, preventing greater blood flow to parts of the body that may need it, such as exercising muscles.

One of the best ways to reduce insulin resistance is to exercise. Regular endurance exercise, such as walking for a prolonged period, swimming, cycling or jogging for 20–30 minutes three times per week can have very positive effects.

Exercising in this way leads to a reduction in energy fats in the blood, an improved uptake of glucose into muscles and a reduction in blood pressure, particularly the lower (diastolic) figure. In addition it allows the walls of your arteries to relax, so allowing blood flow to get to where it's needed in times of exercise or physical work. At least some of the improvement seen is thought to be because levels of a chemical called nitric oxide are restored, and this is crucial in signalling to the muscular cells which line arteries to relax, making the lumen of the arteries bigger.

Exercise and its effects on blood sugar

One recent study from Germany confirmed a substantial benefit of exercise on reducing insulin resistance. A group of people with diabetes were asked to exercise for a period of 50 minutes 3 times per week as part of a fitness programme which lasted for 12 weeks. Although the VO2 max (a measure of fitness) didn't change substantially, insulin resistance was reduced by 92% and HbA_{1c} fell by 0.5% at the end of the programme. A highly significant reduction of 5 mmHg in systolic blood pressure and a fall in triglycerides were also seen.

Considering this happened in only 12 weeks, the reduction was very impressive. This demonstrates that, by taking up a modest exercise programme, you may be able to avoid the addition of an extra diabetes medication. Thus, small lifestyle changes can be seen to have a substantial impact on blood sugar levels.

Exercise and muscle strength

Fairly modest exercise in Type 2 diabetes can also have substantial effects on your physical strength. One study looked at 22 patients with Type 2 diabetes who were given a strength training exercise programme of repetition weight lifting on static machines in a gym, for 3 days each week. They had to lift weights for each major muscle group in three sets of 10. Over the course of 4 months the level of weights lifted was slowly increased.

In this short time their muscle strength improved by around 30% when taking into account all muscle groups. In addition, HbA_{1c} improved by 1.2%, with substantial changes in lipids and blood pressure.

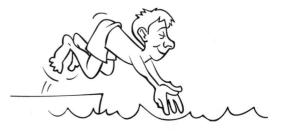

Regular endurance exercise, such as swimming, helps to reduce insulin resistance.

Monitoring

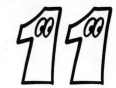

Venture into any chemist shop and you are bound to see a row of fancy glucometers that measure your blood glucose level at home, store the last 100 results and come with a CD-rom computer program that allows you to compare and contrast your results over the past 20 years. The debate centres around whether people who have monitored their blood glucose actually see an improvement in glycaemic control. This chapter takes a brief look at monitoring, the evidence for doing it, the methods you can use, and the key pitfalls or problems you may encounter.

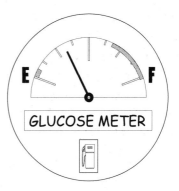

Measuring your blood glucose level is like checking the fuel gauge in your car. The difference is that you don't just need to be careful to avoid running out of petrol (sugar): you also need to make sure that the level doesn't go too high either.

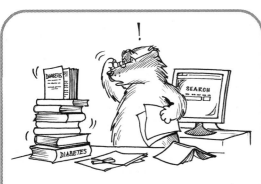

Key questions to ask yourself:

- Do I need to monitor at all?
- How many blood tests should I take, and when?
- What are the most common pitfalls and problems with the equipment?

The blood glucose testing dilemma

Diabetes is a condition in which the main problem is a raised blood glucose. We believe that it is of value for someone with diabetes to be able to measure their blood glucose and thus discover how they can best keep this under control. Used intelligently, blood glucose testing can help someone find out the effects of different activities such as eating various foods, drinking different types of alcohol and taking exercise. It is also an important way of identifying the problem if the blood glucose is either too high or too low.

On the other hand, most doctors know of individuals who check their blood regularly 3 or 4 times a day but never make any changes if the results are abnormal. It almost seems as if they are testing their blood for the benefit of their doctor or nurse but not to provide themselves with useful information.

Most properly conducted studies designed to investigate the value of blood testing in people whose diabetes is controlled by diet or tablets have not shown that testing leads to improved diabetic control.

Unfortunately, blood glucose test strips are expensive and, in an NHS which is trying to save money, it is not surprising that the people who hold the purse strings are keen to restrict the use of this process, for which there is no scientific proof of benefit.

BLOOD GLUCOSE SELF-MONITORING GUIDELINES

These guidelines were developed by Coventry PCT

Education and lifestyle	· Advice on diet, exercise and smoking habit key interventions at diagnosis and beyond. · If necessary, patients should receive education relevant to **appropriate** testing, **understanding when** to test and **what** to do with the result.	ALL PATIENTS WHO ARE SELF-MONITORING SHOULD BE ENCOURAGED TO USE THE MINIMUM NUMBER OF TESTS REQUIRED TO KEEP CONTROL.	
Newly diagnosed Type 2 patient + diet control only Recommended regime: **A**	· Self-monitoring may be required at diagnosis or as necessary depending on overall diabetes control and management plan. Self-monitoring may **not be necessary** if control is acceptable (e.g. HbA_{1c} to target). · Healthcare professional should advise patient when self-monitoring becomes necessary.	Urine testing may be appropriate for some patients in this group provided HbA_{1c} targets are achieved.	Typical weekly strip usage **0–6**
Type 2 patient, prescribed oral therapy Recommended regimes: **A, B, C**	· Re-assess patient need and educate prior to initiation of single oral therapy or combined treatment. · If self-monitoring is necessary, the healthcare professional should tailor monitoring regime to individual patient need, depending on diabetes control. · Special focus on testing to prevent hypoglycaemia, especially in sulphonylurea therapy.	If starting self-monitoring at this stage teach patient before initiating new therapy.	Typical weekly strip usage **0–6**
Type 2 patient, prescribed insulin Recommended regimes: **B, D, E**	· Self-monitoring is recommended in all cases with daily testing on initiation of insulin · Once a patient is stable, frequency of profiles can be reduced to 1–2 days a week or daily at varying times (week profile).	Stable patients are those whose blood glucose varies little from day to day and who are not having intensive changes of treatment.	Typical weekly strip usage **4–28**
Type 1 patients Recommended regimes: **E, F**	· Self-monitoring is strongly recommended in all cases. · Self-monitoring should be used to adjust insulin dose before meals where this is appropriate (e.g. basal bolus regime, pump therapy). · Self-monitoring in Type 1 diabetes may only be required on 1–2 days per week in stable patients and depending on patient's daily routine.		Typical weekly strip usage **8–28**

Examples of typical self-monitoring regimes

Regime **A**	One or two tests a week.
Regime **B**	Once daily at various times (week profile).
Regime **C**	Two tests daily.
Regime **D**	Four tests at different times on one day (day profile).
Regime **E**	Day profile twice a week.
Regime **F**	Test before meals and at bedtime each day.

- Urine testing is appropriate in those:
    where blood glucose monitoring is not possible
    or the patient has a preference not to blood test.
- HbA_{1c} target = below 7.5%.
- Increase testing frequency during:
    pregnancy
    times of illness
    changes in therapy
    changes in routine
    times of poor control
    when at risk of hypoglycaemia
    also to rule out hypoglycaemia, especially when driving.

Blood glucose monitoring targets

Fasting	4–6 mmol/L	Bedtime	5–10 mmol/L
Pre-prandial	4–6 mmol/L	Post-prandial	<10 mmol/L

- Self-monitoring does not replace regular HbA_{1c} testing, which remains the gold standard test, and should only be used in conjunction with appropriate therapy as part of integrated care.

Thus, there is disagreement between the scientists and NHS funding bodies on the one hand and people with Type 2 diabetes on the other. Some family doctors believe strongly that blood glucose testing is unnecessary in people with Type 2 diabetes on tablets. Most professionals agree that people with Type 2 diabetes treated with insulin should have the means to measure their own blood glucose levels

Do you need to monitor at all?

When glucometers were first launched for checking blood glucose at home, doctors believed they would be useful for educating people with Type 2 diabetes. Of course, you may well have a problem with eating too much, eating the wrong types of foods or exercising too little. But the theory went that, by checking your blood glucose after eating a Mars Bar or taking a cross-country run, you would learn how to maintain a pattern of good behaviour. Unfortunately, however, all of the studies reported so far appear to indicate that increased blood glucose monitoring in Type 2 diabetes isn't associated with improved glucose control.

This means one of two things: if you are on diet and exercise or tablets, you may well not need to monitor your blood glucose levels at home at all. If you do choose to monitor, then use it as an educational tool: see what happens when you over-eat and your sugars rise. Equally, watch the improvement in blood sugar levels at home if you lose weight or manage a sustained period of exercise.

Timetable of monitoring	
Test	Reflects the blood glucose levels over:
Blood glucose	Minutes
Urine glucose	Hours
Fructosamine	2–3 weeks
HbA$_{1c}$	2–3 months

How many tests should you take?

If you are on diet and exercise, metformin or glitazone treatment

It is probably not necessary to monitor your sugars at home. Your GP will be able to see what is happening from your HbA$_{1c}$, the long-term

---

Home monitoring tests can be divided into:

1 Immediate tests
Tests that you can perform at any given moment, in order to measure your blood glucose.

2 Routine tests
Tests that you perform regularly, and which help you to make long-term adjustments in your insulin doses, eating habits and other activities.

3 Long-range tests
Tests that reflect your diabetes control over a long period of time. These include such tests as fructosamine and HbA$_{1c}$.

---

mmol/L and mg/dl

mmol/L	mg/dl	mg/dl	mmol/L
1	18	20	1.1
2	36	40	2.2
3	54	60	3.3
4	72	80	4.4
5	90	100	5.6
6	108	120	6.7
7	126	140	7.8
8	144	160	8.9
9	162	180	10.0
10	180	200	11.1
12	216	220	12.2
14	252	250	13.9
16	288	300	16.7
18	324	350	19.4
20	360	400	22.2
22	396	450	25.0

(rows 4–9 marked ACCEPTABLE)

The numbers in this book refer to plasma glucose unless otherwise stated, as this is what most meters now display. Plasma glucose is approximately 11% higher than whole blood glucose.

If you are taking insulin, then home blood glucose monitoring will be useful in terms of titrating to the right insulin dose and confirming that any symptoms of hypoglycaemia are backed up by a low reading on the meter.

In the UK, blood glucose monitoring guidelines have been drawn up by Primary Care Trusts in association with GPs. These are shown in the box opposite.

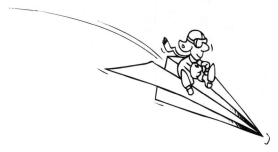

Send your blood glucose charts by mail or fax to your diabetes healthcare team and you can discuss them over the telephone. It may also be possible to send them by e-mail. Check this with your clinic.

measure of blood glucose levels. If you do have a monitor, you could use it two or three times a week, at different times and after different activities to get a feel for how particular activities make your blood sugar rise. You can then discover the effect on the blood sugar of foodstuffs that you have been warned against.

If you are on sulphonylureas

Sulphonylureas are more likely to cause hypoglycaemia, therefore you may need to test more often than two or three times per week if you are having symptoms of hypoglycaemia. Your doctor will advise on this and will want to see the results. You may need a lower dose of sulphonylurea.

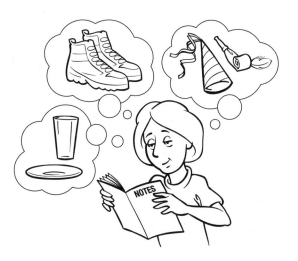

If you are on insulin

If you are on insulin, it is likely that you will need to watch your dose carefully, at least during the initial stages. Your diabetes specialist nurse will advise, but usually you should aim to check it 2–3 times per day when treatment first starts and up titrate your insulin until your sugars are in an acceptable range, (e.g. 5–7 mmol/L in the morning or around 10 mmol/L 2 hours after a meal).

Urine tests

Although urine glucose monitoring is no longer recommended as the primary method of glucose monitoring, it does have its advantages. Urine glucose monitoring can be useful in situations where blood glucose monitoring is difficult or impractical. In Type 2 diabetes, it may be used in some elderly patients although, generally speaking, it is not widely used.

'Good' or 'bad' tests?

It is common to refer to normal blood glucose readings as 'good' and high readings as 'bad'. A young person who hears these terms used frequently may begin to look upon him or herself as 'bad'. 'High blood glucose' sounds more neutral and is a more appropriate term. Test results are just pieces of information, and do not reflect on the quality of the person with diabetes.

All the research projects looking at the risk of complications use the average blood glucose, which is reflected in the HbA_{1c}. Everyone with diabetes has an occasional high blood glucose result, and it is important to realize that an isolated high peak does not do any harm.

Are some things forbidden?

We are often asked whether you are allowed to do this or that when you have diabetes. The best answer is that nothing is totally forbidden. It is important, however, to experiment in order to find out what you as an individual can and cannot do. It is a good idea to experiment with food, exercise and medication, provided this is done in conjunction with blood glucose monitoring. The only risk you are running is of having a temporarily high or low blood glucose.

Always write in your logbook the results of your tests, along with details of the activity you were participating in. Next time you go for a hike, out for a meal or to a party, you will find your notes really valuable.

Blood glucose

When you take a blood test, it will reflect your blood glucose level at that moment. However, the blood glucose can go up or down very quickly, and you may have quite a different reading 15 or 30 minutes later. Always check your blood glucose level when you are not feeling well so that you can avoid eating extra just to be on the safe side when you suspect hypoglycaemia. This is especially important in the early days of being diagnosed with diabetes, when you are not yet fully familiar with all the symptoms of hypoglycaemia. Later on, you will become more confident about these.

Recognizing symptoms of high blood glucose is usually more difficult. Always try to guess

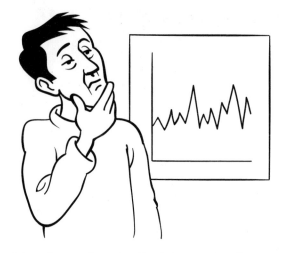

It is easier to estimate low blood glucose values than high ones.

your blood glucose level before checking it, and you will eventually become familiar with the way your body reacts when your blood glucose level is low or high.

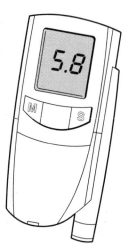

An example of a blood glucose monitoring device.

Lancets for blood glucose tests

Brand	Diameter of needle	Fits to device
BD Micro-Fine+	0.20 mm	Standard
BD Micro-Fine+	0.30 mm	Standard
Monolet Thin	0.36 mm	Standard
Surelite	0.66 mm	Standard
ComforTouch	0.45 mm	Standard
Unilet G Ultralite	0.36 mm	Standard
MediSense lancet	0.36 mm	Standard
Softclix II	0.36 mm	Softclix
Soft Touch	0.36mm	Standard
Cleanlet Fine	0.36 mm	Standard
Microlet	0.50 mm	Standard

Standard = Autoclix P, BD Lancer-5, Glucolet, Microlet, Monojector, Penlet II among others.
All lancets can be used for finger-pricking without using them in a device.
All the names mentioned above are ® or ™ of respective company. Other lancets may be available in your region.

How to take blood tests

Wash your hands with soap and water before taking a blood test. This is not just to ensure hygiene (though of course that is important), but to ensure there is no sugar on your fingers giving a false high reading, for example from glucose tablets or fruit. Use warm water if your fingers are cold. Do not use alcohol for cleaning your hands as this will make your skin dry. The risk of an infection from a finger prick is minimal.

There are a variety of different finger-pricking devices for taking blood glucose tests. With some you can adjust the pricking depth. Pricking devices and lancets can vary considerably in size and the way they puncture the skin. Try different types to find out which suits you best. From the point of view of hygiene, you can use the same lancet for a day's blood tests assuming that your fingers are clean. However, the lancet will be very slightly blunted every time you use it, so the pricks might become more painful with repeated usage.

If you prick the sides of your fingertips, your sensitivity will be less affected, which may be important if you play the piano or guitar, for example. Don't use your thumbs and right index finger (or left if you are left-handed) for finger pricking. You need the sensation of touch most in these places, and sometimes you will even feel pain the day after a finger prick.

Most blood glucose meters have memories for storing test results and can show the average of your readings over 2–4 weeks. This will give you a good picture of how your blood glucose levels have been during this time. The stored information can be transferred to a computer to view, analyse and print. Some newer meters have built-in blood glucose graphing programmes for summarizing patterns of blood glucose control.

Borrowing someone else's finger-pricking device

Borrowing another person's device for pricking your fingers is not a good idea. This is because one small drop of blood left on the device can cause contamination if it is infected. For

---

Why take blood tests?

Advantages

- You can take a test instead of eating 'just to be on the safe side'.
- Helps you learn about hypoglycaemia and its symptoms.
- Lets you know when you need to change insulin doses, e.g. with infections, stress, physical exercise, or going to a party.
- The only way to find out if you have night time hypoglycaemia.
- Blood glucose monitoring is necessary to get good glucose control and in the long run lessen the risk of complications as much as possible.

Disadvantages

- Pricking your finger can be painful.
- Monitoring takes time and extra effort.

Sources of error when measuring blood glucose

False high reading	False low reading
Glucose on fingers	Drop applied too late
	Finger removed too quickly
	Not enough blood on the strip
	Water or saliva on finger

Regular use of the control strip or control solution provided with your meter for calibration is very important to get and maintain reliable values.

example, an outbreak of hepatitis B in a hospital ward was caused by using the same pricking device (Autolet) despite switching lancets between each test.

Does the meter show the correct value?

The margin of error in a correctly used blood glucose meter is approximately 10%. This means that with a blood glucose level of 20 mmol/L (360 mg/dl), the meter can show 2 mmol/L (36 mg/dl) above or below the correct value. However, at a blood glucose of 3 mmol/L (54 mg/dl) the error should not exceed 0.3 mmol/L (5 mg/dl). It is very important to apply enough blood to the strip. Too small a drop will give a false low reading. Don't rub the blood onto the strip. If you have sugar on your fingers when you take the test, this will cause a false high reading.

Ask your diabetes nurse for advice about the available meters and their prices. You can often get a discount on the cost of a new meter if you hand in your old one at the time of purchase.

Comparing different meters can be confusing as they often show different readings. For example, one may show a blood glucose level of 12 mmol/L (215 mg/dl), while another (used at the same time on the same patient) shows a level of 14 mmol/L (250 mg/dl). However, this difference is well within the error margins stated by the manufacturers of the meters. It is advisable to stick to one meter that works well, as the difference of 1–2 mmol/L is not particularly significant at high readings. Bring the meter with you when you come to clinic, and ask your diabetes nurse to check your meter with glucose control solution at regular intervals. Make sure you calibrate your meter regularly according to the manufacturer's advice. Use the reference test strip and make sure the code numbers correspond.

In hospital, blood for glucose monitoring is often taken through an intravenous needle to lessen the pain. In people without diabetes, venous blood tested after a meal has about 10% less glucose than capillary blood. This is logical

Alternative site testing

- Some new meters are used for testing blood glucose at alternative sites. This may be helpful if you play the piano, for example, and do not want to keep pricking your fingers.

- In the fasting state, the glucose readings from the forearm are similar to the fingertip.

- After an intake of 75 g of glucose, the rise in blood glucose in adults was 2.6–7.6 mmol/L (47–137 mg/dl) lower on samples taken from the forearm compared with the fingertip.

- When blood glucose fell quickly after an insulin injection, the values from the fingertip were 3.4–6.6 mmol/L (61–119 mg/dl) lower than the values from the forearm.

- Blood glucose changes appeared on average 35 minutes later in forearm tests compared with the fingertip. By rubbing the skin vigorously for 5–10 seconds before pricking, the accuracy from a forearm test was considerably improved, but with large individual differences.

- In another study in which tests were taken after a meal, lower glucose readings were produced from the forearm and thigh compared with the fingertip, in spite of vigorous skin rubbing.

- The differences are caused by a greatly increased blood flow in the fingertip. To be on the safe side, it seems best to rely on fingertip tests when checking for hypoglycaemia, (e.g. when driving a car or after exercise).

if you remember that venous blood has already delivered some of the glucose it contains to the body tissues. This can probably be explained by the lack of fine-tuned insulin release in response to the blood glucose level.

Self-monitoring around mealtimes

Because of problems with the design of studies, a great deal of debate exists in the medical press about the value of blood glucose monitoring in Type 2 diabetes. This relates particularly to pre-prandial (before meal) and post-prandial (after meal) testing. What is known is that both pre-prandial and post-prandial levels of blood sugar contribute significantly to your overall blood glucose load, and hence any risk of long-term diabetes complications. In particular, it seems that the post-prandial blood sugar level correlates strongly with the risk of cardiovascular disease in Type 2 diabetes. Post-prandial blood sugars are normally taken around 2 hours after a meal.

We will examine the value of self-monitoring in patients who are and are not taking insulin and the studies which are available to help us make a decision on this.

Self-monitoring around mealtimes if you are not taking insulin

One recently published study examined the effect of self-monitoring on HbA_{1c} in patients with relatively good control of their diabetes (average HbA_{1c} at the start of the study was around 7.3%). What researchers found was that the group who monitored their blood sugars had a reduction of nearly 0.2% in their HbA_{1c} over a year, versus no change in a control group. This difference seems small, but the groups were relatively well controlled at the beginning of the study and were given instruction to monitor and alter their lifestyle only. In addition to the percentage drop in HbA_{1c}, the patients in the intervention group showed a reduction in cholesterol, reinforcing the fact that they may have made other positive interventions in their lifestyle.

It would have been interesting to test out the effects of blood glucose monitoring in a group of individuals with less good control, or where the study included an intervention that individuals could make themselves, such as increasing the dose of their metformin tablet. Other studies looking at the impact of self-monitoring which did include an educational component showed a reduction in blood glucose of between 0.3 and 0.4%, but again readings were from a relatively well-controlled population of patients. In short, if you choose to monitor your blood sugar and you are controlled on tablets only, then this shouldn't be like rearranging the deck chairs on the *Titanic*.

Significant icebergs lie ahead in the shape of complications due to a chronically raised blood sugar. Work with your doctor or nurse to draw up a structured plan for making changes to your lifestyle and medication regime and you might be able to navigate a path between them.

For instance, if your pre-meal sugars are too high in the first few weeks, work out how you can increase the amount of exercise you take. Can you build in time for a walk in the morning, or in the afternoon? If your blood sugars are raised after you have eaten, try reducing your portion size, increase the fibre content of your meals and avoid sauces containing a lot of carbohydrate.

If you have already made changes to your diet and lifestyle, and are taking metformin, a sulphonylurea or both these drugs together, talk to your nurse or doctor as soon as possible. Together, you will need to work out a plan to increase the medication you are taking, according to the pattern of your blood sugars. Of course if you lose a lot of weight and your blood glucose levels are well controlled, you should be able to reduce your medication. Proactive working like this can help you and your doctor or diabetes nurse get the most out of your glucose meter.

Self-monitoring around mealtimes if you are taking insulin

If you take insulin for Type 2 diabetes, the rationale for self-monitoring is much clearer. As

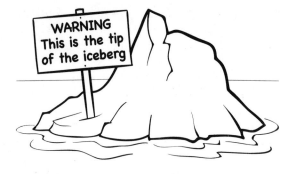

with patients not taking insulin, before and after meal blood sugar levels both contribute significantly to your average HbA_{1c}.

For patients on twice-a-day insulin injections, pre-meal blood sugar levels help you decide if you are on the correct dose of long-acting insulin. Post-meal blood sugar levels tell you if you're eating the right amount of food, and whether your dose of short-acting insulin is appropriate. When you're taking morning and evening mixed insulins, it's usual to take a pre-meal blood sugar in the morning or before the evening meal, and a post-meal sugar after breakfast or the evening meal. If both your pre- and post-meal sugars are too high, you should increase the total insulin dose. If one is relatively higher than the other, different mixes of twice a day insulins exist, and your doctor or diabetes nurse may vary the ratio of short- to long-acting insulin.

For individuals taking mealtime insulin doses with one long-acting injection per day, (basal bolus), pre- and post-meal glucose monitoring can be very instructive. According to exercise and activity in the day, as well as meal size, you can use monitoring to adjust the amount of insulin you take. You may also learn how your insulin requirements alter at certain times of the week, for example if you are at work or having time off at home.

Self-monitoring around mealtimes: what it means for you

Too many people have been asked to monitor blood sugars at home without having proper guidance on how to act on the results. We know that, with proper education and a management plan, monitoring your blood glucose levels can help improve your overall blood sugar control. It can also help with insulin adjustments related to exercise and healthy eating. If you are able to work out a titration plan for medication, it will allow you to take ownership of your diabetes and make decisions without having to check out everything with your doctor or nurse. If you are offered blood testing equipment and feel that you are not likely to make good use of it, it is better to put it off till later. It is not good to let unused blood glucose strips gather dust in a cupboard.

Continuous glucose monitoring

The Medtronic MiniMed CGMS (Continuous Glucose Monitoring System ®) is a device that monitors glucose levels (2.2–22 mmol/L, 40–400 mg/dl) every 10 seconds and records an average value every 5 minutes. It measures through a thin plastic tube placed in the subcutaneous tissue, and can be worn for up to 3 days. The latest models allow you to read glucose values in real-time. When the monitor is connected to a computer, the data can be downloaded and viewed on screen. Using this method has made it easier to see patterns of glucose fluctuation, which has in turn led to changes in treatment and improved glucose control in people of all ages.

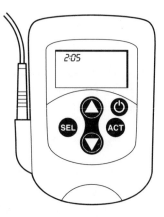

The CGMS monitor measures glucose continuously for up to 3 days through a small cannula that is inserted into your subcutaneous tissue.

Does continuous finger-pricking cause loss of feeling?

A lot of people are afraid that constantly pricking their fingers to test their blood will cause them to lose all feeling in them. Fortunately, all the evidence suggests that this won't happen. When fingers that had been pricked an average of 1000 times were compared with control fingers not used for pricking, it was only pressure sensitivity that was affected (due to an increased skin thickness). There were no signs of decreased sensitivity to heat or touch.

Ketones

Ketones are produced by the body when the cells do not have enough glucose energy. The body then breaks down fat to produce energy and the breakdown products are called ketones. Ketones can be used as fuel by the muscles, heart, kidneys and brain.

If a person has diabetes, ketones are produced in excess when there is a lack of insulin and the blood glucose levels are usually high. Diabetes ketones therefore indicate high blood glucose levels and the need for extra doses of insulin. Due to insulin resistance, the pancreas has over compensated for many years by increasing insulin production. As even a tiny amount of insulin avoids you developing ketones, and people with Type 2 diabetes usually have some reserve of insulin production, problems with ketones are very rare in Type 2 diabetes. However, pregnant women should check for ketones each morning, using urine strips or blood strips, and more often if they feel sick, vomit or have an infection with a raised temperature (see Chapter 21 on Coping with sickness).

Acting on the information

It is important to reflect on the reasons for your blood glucose values and, if necessary, to take action and change your insulin doses after having evaluated the tests. The blood glucose level will not improve by merely measuring it. Remember that the tests are for your own sake, not just to show your diabetes nurse or doctor. Studies on home blood glucose monitoring in Type 2 diabetes tend to suggest that it does not make an impact in terms of improving average blood glucose levels. Many healthcare organizations are now refusing to pay for test strips if patients are not taking insulin. If you have a series of high home blood glucose test results, make sure you talk to you doctor or diabetes nurse.

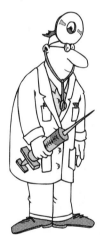

Do you take the tests for your own sake or do you take them to have something to show your doctor or diabetes nurse when you come to the clinic?

Glycosylated haemoglobin (HbA$_{1c}$)

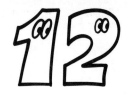

Glycosylated haemoglobin or HbA$_{1c}$ is the name for the test used to measure average glucose control over a longer period of time. It is named after a subgroup of adult haemoglobin, the red pigment in blood cells, which binds and transports oxygen in the red blood cells. Glucose molecules become attached to the haemoglobin molecules in the red blood cells, which have a lifespan of 120 days. During the life of the red blood cell, the amount of glucose bound to haemoglobin in the red cell depends on the level of glucose in the blood at any one time. The percentage of haemoglobin that is bound to glucose provides an estimate of the average blood glucose level over the life of the red cell. Since red cells last for 120 days, the average age is 60 days or 2 months.

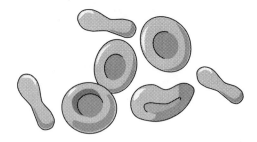

Haemoglobin in the red blood cells takes up oxygen in the lungs and transports it to the cells. The red blood cells also take carbon dioxide from the cells back to the lungs. During their lifetime in the blood circulation, glucose also sticks to haemoglobin, which can be measured by HbA$_{1c}$.

HbA$_{1c}$

⟶ Glucose is bound to haemoglobin in the red blood cells.

⟶ The level of HbA$_{1c}$ depends on the blood glucose levels during the lifespan of the red blood cells.

⟶ A red blood cell lives for about 120 days.

⟶ HbA$_{1c}$ reflects the average blood glucose during the previous 2–3 months.

HbA$_{1c}$ is a measure of the percentage of the haemoglobin in the red blood cells that has glucose bound to it. This reflects an average measurement of the blood glucose levels during the last 2–3 months. The blood glucose levels from the week prior to testing will not be included in the reading as this fraction of HbA$_{1c}$ is not stable. If HbA$_{1c}$ is monitored at regular intervals (at least every 3 months) at the diabetes clinic, the results will provide a good summary of how your glucose control has been throughout the year.

It is important to remember that HbA$_{1c}$ reflects an average of your blood glucose levels. You can get an acceptable HbA$_{1c}$ reading with a combination of high and low blood glucose values. More often than not, you will feel better when your blood glucose level is relatively even. However, there is no scientific evidence that you will have more complications as a result of your diabetes if your blood glucose level is unstable than if your blood glucose readings are all the same, assuming that HbA$_{1c}$ is unchanged too. There is some evidence that HbA$_{1c}$ goes up with age, due to an increase in glucose bound to proteins such as haemoglobin. This may account for the fact that the HbA$_{1c}$ in some elderly patients seems too high when compared with their blood glucose test results.

HbA$_{1c}$ and blood glucose

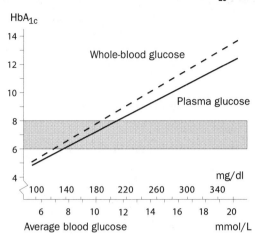

Association's Clinical Practice Recommendations 2003. The solid line shows the relationship between HbA$_{1c}$ and plasma glucose (11% higher than blood glucose in this study). Aim to have an HbA$_{1c}$ value of 7% or below if possible. If it is above 8%, you and your diabetes team have some work to do together, assessing and revising your diabetes care.

Your HbA$_{1c}$ value depends on the average blood glucose levels during the last 2–3 months. A 1% increase in HbA$_{1c}$ (measured with the DCCT-equivalent method) means that you have had an average increase of approximately 2 mmol/L (35 mg/dl) in blood glucose levels compared with when your last test was taken. The graph shows readings from the American DCCT study and is redrawn from American Diabetes

HbA$_{1c}$	Plasma glucose		Whole-blood glucose	
%	mmol/L	mg/dl	mmol/L	mg/dl
5	5.6	103	5.1	92
6	7.6	138	6.9	124
7	9.6	138	8.6	156
8	11.5	208	10.4	188
9	13.5	243	12.2	219
10	15.5	278	13.9	251
11	17.5	314	15.7	283
12	19.5	349	17.4	314

This table (from the Rohlfing et al. reference) shows the mean glucose values that a certain HbA$_{1c}$ value represents.
Most meters used nowadays display plasma glucose.

What level should HbA$_{1c}$ be?

Unfortunately, different laboratories have different reference values for HbA$_{1c}$ but they are slowly becoming more standardized. The American Diabetes Association recommends that the goal of therapy in adults and adolescents should be an HbA$_{1c}$ below 7% and that the treatment regimen should be re-evaluated in patients with repeated HbA$_{1c}$ above goals. The Canadian Diabetes Association recommends that adults and adolescents should aim for an HbA$_{1c}$ below 7%. The International Diabetes Federation (IDF) now recommends an even lower HbA$_{1c}$ target of 6.5%.

Many studies have shown that with an HbA$_{1c}$ value of less than 8% the risk of long-term blood vessel complications will be considerably lower. If your HbA$_{1c}$ is above 9% we feel that this is unfair to your body since we know that in the long run it will sustain damage from this.

Studies of adults have shown that those with a lower HbA$_{1c}$ experience better levels of psychological wellbeing. This includes less anxiety and depression, improved self-confidence and a better quality of life.

The risk of severe hypoglycaemia makes it difficult to achieve very low HbA$_{1c}$ levels. If someone with Type 2 diabetes has an HbA$_{1c}$ within the range for individuals without diabetes, this usually means they are at high risk of severe hypoglycaemia and/or hypoglycaemia unawareness. In the DCCT study, patients with low HbA$_{1c}$ had a significantly higher risk of severe hypoglycaemia. However, the risk decreased during the years of the study.

Why check your HbA$_{1c}$?

Is checking your HbA$_{1c}$ worthwhile? For whose benefit is the HbA$_{1c}$ test being done? Many individuals feel as if they are visiting a 'control station' and being examined by health professionals to see how well they have 'behaved themselves'. From the professional point of view, however, the HbA$_{1c}$ test is most valuable to you yourself. When you see the reading, you will know if your way of life over the last three months has allowed you to achieve the average blood glucose level you want for the future.

When the HbA$_{1c}$ method was introduced, 240 adults with diabetes measured it every third month without otherwise changing their diabetes treatment. After a year, the average HbA$_{1c}$ value was unchanged but it turned out that those with very low values had increased them and those with high values now had lower values, showing the benefit of knowing your HbA$_{1c}$ level.

HbA$_{1c}$ goals

	DCCT method and equivalent
Normal value person without diabetes	4.1–6.1%
Adolescents and young adults	< 7.5%
Adults	< 7.0%
Needs improving and re-evaluation of treatment	8–9%
Not acceptable: High risk of complications	>9%
May have high risk of severe hypoglycaemia	< 6%

There may be individual differences in the HbA$_{1c}$ value it is realistic to achieve. Discuss with your diabetes team what value may be realistic for you.

For how long do blood glucose levels affect HbA$_{1c}$?

Your recent blood glucose level affects HbA$_{1c}$ much more than that from 2–3 months ago. However, your values during the last week will not show on most methods since this fraction of HbA$_{1c}$ is very unstable. For a given HbA$_{1c}$ value, the contribution of the blood glucose is (counting backwards):

Day 1–6	very low
Day 7–30	50%
Day 31–60	25%
Day 61–90	15%
Day 91–120	10%

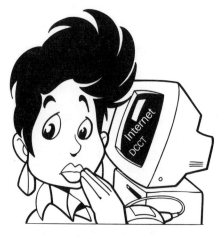

Many countries (US, Australia, UK, Denmark, France, The Netherlands among others) have standardized their HbA$_{1c}$ monitoring methods to show DCCT-equivalent numbers. This means that if you read about studies on the Internet, you can compare like with like between one study and another.

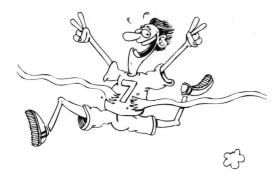

Set up your own personal goal for your HbA$_{1c}$ in collaboration with your diabetes team. This goal will be different for different people and perhaps also different during different times of your life. It may be more difficult to achieve the same HbA1c level for example at times when you are having problems at home or at work. By competing with yourself and setting a reasonable goal you will have a fair chance of winning your race.

How often should you check your HbA$_{1c}$?

Everyone with Type 2 diabetes should check their HbA$_{1c}$ regularly, every 3–6 months. A high level (8–9% with DCCT numbers or an equivalent method) is not acceptable, considering the risk of future complications. In older people, it may be up to 0.5% higher simply due to increasing patient age.

After a visit to your diabetes healthcare team, you may feel more motivated to 'get your act together' and keep your blood glucose readings low. Use this motivation to address any problems with diet, lifestyle, your medication or insulin regimes.

Some clinics send their HbA$_{1c}$ tests to the laboratory, so it may be some days before you get the result while others ask you to send in a blood sample a week before the clinic. Others use a desktop method that gives a result after a few minutes.

Even if your blood glucose control is improving and your tests are showing lower readings, it will still take some time for this to show in your HbA$_{1c}$. Half the change will show after about a month, and three quarters of the change after 2 months. If you start with a very high HbA$_{1c}$ (12–13%) and normalize your blood glucose levels completely (as often happens at diagnosis) it will go down by approximately 1% every 10th day.

Can your HbA$_{1c}$ be 'too good'?

If you have a very low HbA$_{1c}$ your average blood glucose is low and you may have a high risk of developing serious hypoglycaemia without any warning symptoms. If you have a low HbA$_{1c}$ (6–7%) and problems with severe hypoglycaemia or hypoglycaemia unawareness, it may be a good idea to aim for a slightly higher blood glucose level.

Can the HbA$_{1c}$ measurement give false information?

The HbA$_{1c}$ result relies on the fact that red blood cells last about 120 days. Any medical problem which shortens the life of the red cell will tend to artificially reduce the HbA$_{1c}$ percentage. Such conditions include haemolytic anaemia, kidney failure and pregnancy.

Fructosamine

Monitoring fructosamine is a method of measuring the amount of glucose that is bound to proteins in the blood. The value reflects the blood glucose level during the last 2–3 weeks. Fructosamine can be good indicator during times of rapid changes in glucose control, for example when you start with a new method of treatment. However, if you take a fructosamine test every third month only, you will not get a representative measurement of your glucose control over a longer period of time. This method, therefore, is not recommended for routine monitoring of long-term glucose control.

Tablets for lowering blood sugar

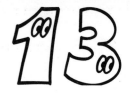

Although healthy eating is a cornerstone of management of Type 2 diabetes, and regular exercise plays an equally important role, it is still very likely that your blood sugar levels will begin to rise over time. Despite the importance of your doctor or nurse exploring every option for lifestyle improvement with you, many health professionals now believe it is a good idea for patients to start taking tablets much sooner after

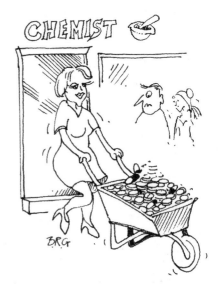

being diagnosed with Type 2 diabetes. Indeed, the most up-to-date advice is to take a tablet called metformin at the time that Type 2 diabetes is diagnosed.

You may feel perfectly well though, and this may make it difficult for you to understand why you may need tablets. So it is very important that your doctor or nurse talks you through the nine Key Points of your diabetes treatment. If your professionals are not honest with you, and do not communicate clearly, then why should you follow their advice? If you can't understand their explanations, do please tell them.

The following sections mention a number of characteristics and side effects of drug therapies used for lowering your blood sugar. This list can't be exhaustive and is almost out of date as soon as it is written. You can find the latest information on any drug treatment over the Internet from sites such as the electronic medicines compendium (see page 247 for website address).

Nine Key Points that you need to know when starting an oral treatment for Type 2 diabetes

- The name of the therapy, or tablet, that the doctor has prescribed for you.

- The dose you need to take.

- When is the best time of day to take the tablets.

- How the tablets work.

- Why the doctor has started you on this particular medication, and what evidence supports this choice.

- Whether the tablets can cause low blood glucose levels.

- Any other side effects you may experience.

- Possible interactions with other tablets or medications you may be taking (e.g. blood pressure drugs).

- What to do if you have problems (e.g. contact the surgery).

Tablet treatments for diabetes

At the present time, five groups of drug are used in for treating blood sugar levels in Type 2 diabetes, and a sixth group is in development.

1 Biguanides (metformin).

2 Glitazones (also called insulin sensitizers or thiazolidinediones).

3 Sulphonylureas.

4 Postprandial glucose regulators (PPGRs).

5 Alpha-glucosidase inhibitors.

6 Gliptins (DPP-4 inhibitors).

Biguanides (metformin)

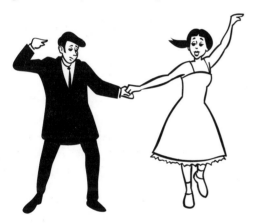

Metformin was first developed in the late 1950s.

Metformin is a member of the biguanide family of diabetes drugs, and it works by reducing the amount of sugar that is produced by your liver. It is recommended as initial drug treatment for anyone with Type 2 diabetes, unless other medical problems or side effects make its use unwise.

The insulin resistance associated with Type 2 diabetes tricks the liver into thinking that more sugar is required to satisfy the needs of the body. This causes the release of sugars from glycogen stores, and production of sugar from other energy sources such as lipids (fats). Metformin appears to be most effective in patients who are overweight.

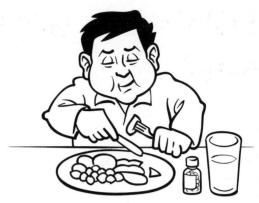

Metformin can cause tummy upsets but taking your tablets with food will help you avoid this.

One major advantage of taking metformin is that it is the only diabetes tablet which lowers blood glucose without causing weight gain; indeed, many patients manage a small loss of weight when they take metformin. You should take your metformin with food, as this may reduce the risk of gastrointestinal upset. If you find metformin causes a tummy upset, ask your GP to try the slow-release form.

Who should not take metformin

➤ Anyone with kidney problems, particularly if they have a raised creatinine level or a reduced eGFR (estimated glomerular filtration rate) either of which would indicate some degree of kidney damage.

➤ Anyone undergoing an X-ray involving contrast media or dyes.

➤ Anyone preparing for a surgical operation – tell the doctors you are on metformin.

➤ Women who are breastfeeding.

When should you not use metformin?

If you have significant problems with your kidneys, metformin will not be appropriate for you. Your family doctor will probably measure your serum creatinine (a measure of the amount of waste products from the body which are circulating in the blood). When patients have a creatinine level which is more than around 130–150 µmol/L, another drug should be used instead. This is because a very rare side effect of metformin, called lactic acidosis (to do with the acidity of the blood), may be more likely to occur if the kidneys aren't working properly.

Many patients with diabetes also need investigations of their blood vessels. Even if this does not apply to you now, it may do at some stage. These investigations are often done with injection of special liquid so that the blood vessels show up on X-ray pictures. When these contrast injections contain iodine, metformin should be stopped at least 24 hours before you have the investigation and not started again until you have recovered from the procedure. If your doctor has booked one of these investigations for you, it is very important to make sure that the X-ray department of the hospital knows you are taking metformin.

Similarly, if you need to have an operation under general anaesthetic, you should stop your metformin at least 48 hours before the surgery. You should not start it again until your doctors are happy that your kidneys are working properly again.

Metformin is now used for pregnant mothers, but should probably not be taken if you are breastfeeding. Women with Type 2 diabetes who are also insulin resistant can often take a while to get pregnant in the first place. Metformin may improve your chance of ovulation and pregnancy, so if you start metformin and don't want to get pregnant, remember you will almost certainly need to be careful about contraception.

Side effects

Gastrointestinal problems (tummy upsets) are the most common problem associated with taking metformin. These may include a combination of nausea, abdominal bloating and diarrhoea. There is every possibility that gastrointestinal problems can be minimised if you and your doctor work to increase the metformin dose gradually over the course of a few weeks. There is some evidence that if you do have problems with nausea or tummy upsets while you are taking metformin, switching to a 'once a day' preparation may reduce these side effects.

You may also find you lose your appetite, and this may well contribute to some of the weight loss which occurs in metformin users. More unusual problems may include a metallic taste in the mouth, and a lowering of your body's levels of the vitamin B12.

Lactic acidosis can occur very rarely in people taking metformin. Symptoms include lethargy, muscle pains and hyperventilation. Lactic acidosis is associated with increased acidity in the blood and is more likely to occur when metformin is used by people with kidney problems or with heart failure. It is almost unheard of in patients who have healthy kidneys and a well-functioning heart.

Side effects may develop soon after you start taking metformin, or may develop after several years. However, many people have taken metformin for decades without experiencing problems.

Evidence for using metformin to manage your diabetes

The main outcome evidence for using metformin comes from the UKPDS study. In this study,

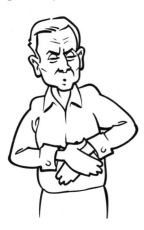

If you have significant problems with your liver, or tend to drink more alcohol than the Department of Health recommended limits (see Chapter 24), metformin may not be suitable for you.

Available metformin preparations		
Drug	Brand name	Normal dose
Metformin	Glucophage Glucophage SR (once a day formulation) *Also found in Avandamet, Janumet and Actoplusmet (combination tablets with rosiglitazone)*	500 mg–3 g for the multiple dose form of metformin, 2 g for the once-per-day drug. Evidence suggests that doses above 2 g, in combination with other blood glucose-lowering tablets, may cause more side effects, without extra glucose lowering. Should be taken with food.

metformin reduced the risk of cardiovascular disease and microvascular complications (kidney, eye and nerve damage). For this reason, it carries the strongest recommendation as initial drug treatment for diabetes. A few other studies have shown that, as well as lowering blood glucose, metformin also has positive effects on blood clotting (reducing the chance of thrombosis) and inflammation.

Other uses for metformin

Metformin is often used in women without diabetes who have polycystic ovarian syndrome (PCOS). In this condition, metformin helps with weight reduction and excessive hairiness and is used to induce fertility.

Side effects of metformin

- Gastrointestinal problems: tummy upsets, nausea, abdominal bloating, diarrhoea.
- Loss of appetite.
- A metallic or burning taste in the mouth.
- Reduction of the body's ability to store vitamin B12.
- Lactic acidosis in people whose kidneys are not functioning properly, or who have heart problems.

Glitazones (insulin sensitizers)

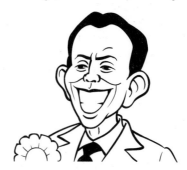

Glitazones were first developed in the 1990s.

Two glitazones, rosiglitazone and pioglitazone are currently available in the UK, Europe and the US. They act by helping sugar to get in to muscle and fat, where it can be stored or used for energy. Effectively, this is re-establishing the body's sensitivity to its own insulin. For this reason, glitazones combine well with metformin as they act at complementary sites in the body.

People who are overweight tend to have lower insulin sensitivity, so glitazones may be a good choice for them. Your doctor can use glitazones as initial treatment if you are unable to take metformin, or in combination with metformin, or with metformin and a sulphonylurea. If you are unable or unwilling to take insulin, triple-tablet therapy with metformin, a sulphonylurea and a glitazone may be the best option for you.

Both pioglitazone and rosiglitazone are usually taken once per day unless your doctor prescribes a combination treatment, Avandamet or Competact.

Glitazones

Drug	Brand name	Normal dose
Rosiglitazone	Avandia *Also available in combination with metformin* *as Avandamet* *and in combination with glimeparide as Avaglim*	4 mg daily if used alone or in combination with metformin may increase to 8 mg daily (in one or two divided doses)
Pioglitazone	Actos *Also available in combination with glimeparide* *as ACTOplus met*	15–45 mg once daily

When should you not use a glitazone?

If you have significant problems with your liver, your doctor will not be able to prescribe a glitazone for you. There is evidence, however, that if you have problems with fat accumulating in the liver, leading to less severe changes in your liver function tests, you might actually benefit from taking one of the modern glitazones. Some of the caution comes from liver problems which were associated with an earlier drug called troglitazone, but there is no evidence that either rosiglitazone or pioglitazone cause abnormal liver tests.

Because glitazones can increase fluid retention, they should be avoided if you have heart failure. Your doctor will be aware of this and if you have significant problems with heart failure or fluid retention, it is best that you avoid this class of drugs. There has also been some indirect evidence that rosiglitazone may carry a small increased risk of heart attack. This suggestion is open to question and is not a reason for people who are benefiting from the drug to stop taking it. This risk was seen most in patients who were taking nitrates, tablets normally used for treating angina.

Who should not take glitazones?

➡ Some people with liver problems. (Anyone who has problems with their liver should have their liver function tested before they start on a glitazone.)

➡ Anyone who has heart failure or a history of angina or chest pain from the hear.

➡ Anyone who has problems with fluid retention.

➡ Most people on insulin treatment, although it may be possible to take a glitazone with insulin in certain circumstances and if your doctor monitors you very carefully.

➡ Any woman who is pregnant or trying to get pregnant.

➡ Women who are breastfeeding.

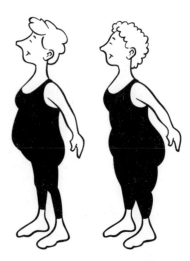

You may find that taking a glitazone tablet moves fat from around your middle (where it is more likely to cause you health problems) to your hips and thighs.

When glitazones were first developed, the clinical trials in patients with Type 2 diabetes who were taking insulin showed that some of these patients had an increased risk of fluid retention. Although not recommended by the National Institute for Health and Clinical Excellence (NICE), glitazone in combination with insulin is widely used in the UK and is licensed for use in the US.

Not enough information is available for these drugs to ensure that they are safe to be used in women with Type 2 diabetes who are pregnant or breastfeeding. For this reason they should be avoided in pregnant women or breastfeeding mothers. If you are a young woman with Type 2 diabetes, it is worth bearing in mind that taking glitazones may improve your chances of ovulation, and increase your chances of getting pregnant. So you will need to be careful about contraception.

Side effects

One of the main side effects associated with glitazones is increase in body weight. This is because the glitazones improve the way that the body stores fats and increases fat stores, particularly around the hips. Most of the weight increase happens in the first 6–12 months of treatment and is around 2–6 kg in total.

Fluid retention may also be a problem for some individuals, and tends to be worse if there are already problems with heart failure. This is why doctors will be unwilling to prescribe glitazones to anyone with a history of significant fluid retention. Exact numbers of people with Type 2 diabetes who develop fluid retention are difficult to determine, but it tends to be about 5–10% of those in clinical studies. You can be reassured that fluid retention problems are mild in most patients who take glitazones. Early symptoms of retention of fluid may include a rapid increase in your weight, shortness of breath and swollen ankles.

Another relatively common problem which may occur is anaemia. This is usually mild and occurs mainly because of fluid retention.

Evidence for using glitazones to manage your diabetes

Because these drugs are still new, there is only one outcome study that has reported so far. The PROactive Study showed that in addition to lowering blood sugars, pioglitazone had some protective ability against cardiovascular disease. This effect was very modest though, and patients did suffer increased fluid retention. One reassuring finding from PROactive was that pioglitazone appears to protect against worsening of blood glucose in some patients. Around half as many patients in the pioglitazone group needed to start insulin to control their blood sugar levels, compared with the group taking the placebo (dummy pill). Some clinical trials have looked at the effect of glitazones on cardiovascular risk factors and have shown effects that lead to blood pressure lowering, improvements in blood clotting and an ability to raise levels of good cholesterol. The DREAM study, which reported in 2006, investigated the effect of ramipril and rosiglitazone in preventing progression to diabetes in a cohort of 5269 people with two different forms of pre-diabetes. It showed that while ramipril had no protective effect, rosiglitazone 'prevented' diabetes in 66% participants. However, it has been pointed out that since rosiglitazone is an effective drug in the treatment of diabetes, the findings hardly come as a surprise. Perhaps it would have been more accurate to describe the effect as delaying rather than preventing the onset of diabetes in this at risk group. More recently, the ADOPT study has shown that rosiglitazone used as a single treatment can reduce blood glucose levels for almost 5 years. See Chapter 36 for more information about these and other studies.

Sulphonylureas

Sulphonylureas act by making the beta cells of the pancreas release insulin. They do this by binding to a receptor on the surface of the insulin-producing beta cells. This leads to a change in the balance of salts inside the beta cells,

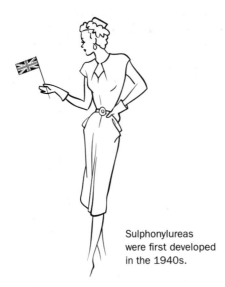

Sulphonylureas were first developed in the 1940s.

normal or below average and you have diabetes symptoms. But if you are overweight, a glitazone (insulin sensitizer) may be a better choice.

The main side effects of sulphonylureas are hypoglycaemia and weight gain. About 20% of patients taking a sulphonylurea have one or more hypoglycaemic attack in a year. These are usually mild. However, in the course of a year, up to 1% of patients on a sulphonylurea have a hypoglycaemic attack that is sufficiently severe for them to need to be given glucose by another person. The risk of hypoglycaemia is much greater in the first year and decreases with time.

Some of the sulphonylureas may be particularly suitable if the kidneys are damaged due to diabetes. For example, gliclazide is broken down by the liver and not the kidneys. When taking a sulphonylurea, you should have the lowest dose possible to control your blood sugar.

which causes insulin to be released. Release of insulin happens even when blood sugar levels are low, which explains why hypoglycaemia (low blood sugar) may occur with sulphonylureas.

The most commonly prescribed sulphonylurea in the UK is gliclazide. Alternatives include glibenclamide, glimipiride, glipizide, gliquidone and tolbutamide. Chlorpropamide and glibenclamide are less less widely used now as their longer duration of action increases the risk of hypoglycaemia.

Generally, sulphonylureas are no longer recommended as the first choice therapy for Type 2 diabetes. When your doctor is thinking about adding in another tablet to metformin, a sulphonyurea would be preferred if your weight is

When should you take a sulphonylurea, and how much?

Your doctor should generally advise you to take short-acting agents such as glipizide before main meals. Once a day preparations such as gliclazide MR or glimepiride should be taken once daily before breakfast. Small doses of glicazide can be taken once a day, but larger doses need to be taken twice a day. Evidence suggests that most effect is seen with increases in sulphonylurea dose at the lower end of the range, and the benefit diminishes a little as the

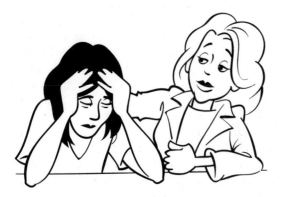

During any year, around 1% of patients taking a sulphonylurea will suffer a hypoglycaemic attack that is severe enough for them to need help from someone else.

Who should not take sulphonylureas?

➡ Anyone who has problems with their liver.

➡ Anyone who has problems with the function of their kidneys.

➡ Most women who are pregnant or breastfeeding, although it may sometimes be possible for them to take a sulphonylurea drug instead of insulin provided their doctor monitors them closely.

Commonly used sulphonylureas in the UK

Drug	Marketing names (examples from the UK)	Dose range
Gliclazide (Once or twice a day)	Diamicron Diamicron MR – lower dosing regimen	40–160 mg daily With breakfast Divide higher doses
Glimepiride (Once a day)	Amaryl	1–4 mg daily With first main meal
Glipizide	Glibenese Minodiab	2.5–20 mg daily Before breakfast or lunch up to 15 mg as single dose; higher doses divided

doses are increased. Hence rather than push your sulphonylurea to the highest possible dose, your doctor might consider adding in another medication instead. Generally over time there is a slow drift upwards in HbA_{1c} in patients taking sulphonylureas. For this reason, your doctor will almost certainly need to increase the dose of your medication over time.

When should you not use a sulphonylurea?

Sulphonylureas shouldn't be used if you have severe problems with your liver or kidney function, but your GP will be aware of these contraindications. In addition, it isn't generally advisable to take a sulphonylurea for control of diabetes during pregnancy or breastfeeding. One small study has shown that glibenclamide may be an acceptable alternative to insulin for some pregnant women with Type 2 diabetes.

Side effects

Hypoglycaemia associated with sulphonylurea use tends to be more frequent with the longer-acting sulphonylureas such as glibenclamide, where your eating patterns are erratic (such as if you work shifts) and where your blood glucose levels are close to target. In the elderly, sulphonylureas may lead to severe prolonged hypoglycaemic attacks. These may lead to symptoms of confusion or stroke and the diagnosis may be missed if the doctor fails to realize that they are taking a sulphonylurea and omits to check the blood glucose level. As stated above, the annual risk of hypoglycaemia varies from 20% (mild) to 1% (severe).

You are likely to put on weight after you start taking a sulphonylurea. This is usually between 1 and 4 kg, but the increase in weight is at its greatest during the first 6 months of treatment.

Hypersensitivity reactions can occur with sulphonylureas, as they can with all drugs, but these are rare. They may be manifest as jaundice, skin rashes or problems with the manufacture of blood cells.

Evidence for using a sulphonylurea to manage your diabetes

Evidence from the most robust long-term outcome study for Type 2 diabetes, the UKPDS study, suggests that reducing blood sugar using a sulphonylurea impacts on microvascular problems to do with your diabetes. These are complications such as retinopathy (diabetic eye disease), neuropathy (nerve damage due to diabetes) and nephropathy (kidney damage due to diabetes). The same study suggests that taking a sulphonylurea does not reduce your risks of cardiovascular disease due to diabetes. It is therefore important that health professionals take a holistic approach to treating your diabetes, looking at all risk factors including blood pressure and cholesterol.

Postprandial glucose regulators (PPGRs)

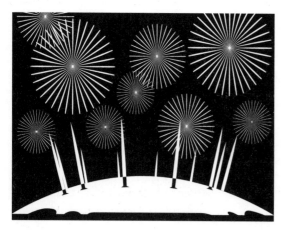

PPGRs were first developed in the late 1990s.

These drugs work in a similar way to sulphonylureas but have a very short duration of action and are usually taken before each meal. They may be useful if you work shifts or eat your meals at odd times of the day. Limitations are similar to those of the sulphonylureas, in that they stimulate release of insulin but do not improve glucose uptake into muscle or fat (improve insulin sensitivity). Two post-prandial

glucose regulators, nateglinide and repaglinide, are currently available.

When should you avoid PPGRs?

PPGRs shouldn't be used if you have severe problems with your liver, are pregnant or are breastfeeding. They may be more useful than sulphonylureas where you have a history of kidney problems, because they have a much shorter duration of action and as such are less likely to cause hypoglycaemia.

Side effects of PPGRs

Hypoglycaemia does still occur in patients taking PPGRs, but is less likely than with sulphonylureas because of the shorter duration of action of these drugs. This is more likely when the drugs are used in combination, for instance with metformin.

Weight gain with PPGRs is thought to be less than with sulphonylureas. This may be due to the fact that insulin release is stimulated to a lesser extent because of the shorter duration of action.

Who should not take PPGRs?

⟹ Anyone who has severe problems with their liver.

⟹ Women who are pregnant or breastfeeding.

Postprandial glucose regulators (PPGRs)

Drug	Brand name	Normal dose
Repaglinide *Can be used on its own or in combination with metformin*	Prandin	500 g–16 mg Within 30 minutes before main meals Up to 4 mg as a single dose
Nateglinide *Can only be used as combination therapy*	Starlix	60–180 mg three times daily Within 30 minutes before main meals

Evidence for using a PPGR to manage your diabetes

Evidence for using a PPGR to manage your blood sugar is limited. A number of studies show positive effects of these drugs on blood sugar, particularly during the early stages of diabetes, but there are not a lot of longer-term data on sustained blood sugar control. There are no outcome studies showing a benefit on cardio-vascular disease.

Alpha-glucosidase inhibitors

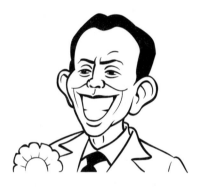

Alpha-glucosidase inhibitors were first developed in the 1990s.

When you eat starches or complex sugars, such as those you find in a pasta meal, these are broken down by enzymes in the gut called glucosidases. These produce shorter chain sugars which can be more easily absorbed by the body and used for energy. One of these agents, acarbose, is currently used in the UK.

Who should avoid taking acarbose?

Using acarbose isn't recommended in patients with significant bowel troubles. If you have a hernia, or have had abdominal surgery or inflammatory bowel disease such as Crohn's or ulcerative colitis, then acarbose may not be a good idea for you. Also, if there are problems with the function of your kidneys or liver, you are unlikely to be prescribed this drug. Acarbose shouldn't be used by women who are pregnant or breastfeeding.

Side effects of acarbose

The main problems associated with acarbose tend to be with gastrointestinal side effects. Some of the sugars which are prevented from being digested by acarbose pass into the large bowel. When they are there, they provide a very readily available food source for the naturally occuring bacteria that live in your large bowel.

Who should not take acarbose?

➡ Anyone who has bowel problems such as inflammatory bowel disease.

➡ Anyone who has a hernia or has had abdominal surgery.

➡ Anyone who has severe problems with the function of their liver or kidneys.

➡ Women who are pregnant or breastfeeding.

Alpha-glucosidase inhibitors		
Drug	*Brand name*	*Normal dose*
Acarbose *May be used alone or in combination with other drugs*	Glucobay	50–600 mg The dose should be increased slowly to improve tolerability and reduce problems due to gastric upsets

The bacteria that use them as a food source then produce large amounts of gas. This gas leads to abdominal wind and bloating, pain because of distension of the colon, flatulence and 'blowy' diarrhoea.

If acarbose is used in combination with other drugs, then there is the possibility of hypoglycaemia occurring. Many of the products to treat hypoglycaemia contain sucrose, the absorption of which is blocked or slowed by acarbose. If you are taking acarbose in combination with other drugs then you may need to carry glucose as a treatment for hypoglycaemia.

What is the evidence for using acarbose to treat Type 2 diabetes?

There is evidence that acarbose is effective in reducing blood glucose, particularly in early Type 2 diabetes. But it has not been a popular choice, due to the potential side effects described above. Studies in pre-diabetes show that acarbose can both prevent progression to Type 2 diabetes and reduce cardiovascular events in this important group of patients.

Gliptins

DPP-4 inhibitors (gliptins) act by blocking an enzyme which breaks down glucagon-like peptide-1 (or GLP-1). This is quite a new development but more data are becoming available. An alternative to blocking the breakdown of GLP-1 is by injection: one GLP-preparation that is available as an injection is exanetide.

DPP-4 inhibitors appear to lower the blood glucose by between 0.8 and 1.2% in the short term, depending on the blood glucose level you start with. Studies have been published showing that this effect persists for around a year, but some longer-term data should be available soon.

Additionally, some limited information is beginning to come out showing that the class has mild positive effects on blood pressure and blood fats.

The DPP-4s will, at the very least, not cause you to put on weight. Exanetide has been shown

in people who respond to it actually to lead to weight loss over a number of months.

Another advantage is that they don't cause fluid retention (like glitazones). And they don't cause hypoglycaemia as often as sulphonylureas do.

Experience is still limited with the two drugs in the class, sitagliptin (Januvia) and vildagliptin (Galvus), and some reports of skin rashes have occurred in conjunction with their use. More data on their long-term safety will become available over the next few years.

A combination tablet containing sitagliptin and metformin (Janumet) is available, and a combination containing vildagliptin and metformin is also proposed.

Oral treatment pathways for blood glucose: what is the best form of treatment?

The International Diabetes Federation (IDF) has published guidelines recommending the gold standard way to manage blood glucose with tablets in Type 2 diabetes. Evolving evidence has confirmed the need to lower the blood glucose

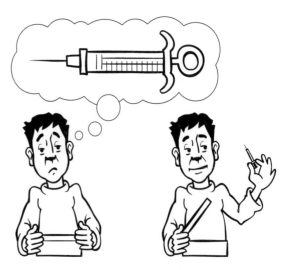

It is natural to feel afraid of starting insulin therapy, but the reality will be much more positive than you may expect.

target for Type 2 diabetes, and therefore a target level of HbA$_{1c}$ 6.5% is recommended. This is much lower than the target level your family doctor may have been used to in the past.

These IDF guidelines support the use of metformin as initial drug therapy and then recommend that either a sulphonylurea or a glitazone be added next. They also underline the importance of managing your diet and lifestyle to the best degree that you possibly can, as good work in this area can really improve control of your blood glucose.

Once your control has escaped recommended levels when you are taking two blood glucose-lowering drugs, the guidelines suggest that you start insulin or consider triple oral therapy. They stress the importance of considering insulin therapy earlier though, if your symptoms are increasing or your blood glucose levels are becoming harder to control.

Other diabetes experts recommend tailoring treatment according to the weight of the patient concerned. There is evidence that, if you are overweight and taking metformin, you may benefit more from addition of a glitazone rather than a sulphonylurea to metformin.

Unfortunately, no tablet treatment for blood glucose in Type 2 diabetes has yet been shown to stave off insulin therapy for ever. Your doctor will need to broach the subject of starting insulin treatment with you at some stage. Insulin may be used on its own, or in combination with tablets. When you are first using insulin, it may only be one injection a day to supplement the tablets. It this does not appear to be working sufficiently, then two or more injections of insulin per day may be used. Do please remember that there is nothing to fear from going onto insulin therapy, and any problems that appear insurmountable in the early stages can usually be overcome.

Insulin treatment

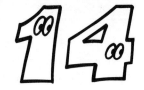

The pancreas of a person without diabetes always secretes a small amount of insulin into the bloodstream, constantly throughout the day and night (called basal secretion). After a meal, a larger amount of insulin is secreted to deal with the glucose coming from the food (called the bolus secretion; see graphs on page 92). As time progresses, if you have Type 2 diabetes, your pancreas will cease to be able to produce enough insulin to overcome the resistance to its action, or to respond to the rise in blood glucose after a meal. As Type 2 diabetes is a progressive disease, this happens eventually to everyone. The goal of all insulin replacement treatment is to mimic this function and provide insulin to the bloodstream in the most appropriate way.

Animal and human insulin

In the past, bovine (beef) and porcine (pork) insulin were the only forms of insulin available. Nowadays, human insulin is the most commonly used, with a few people deciding to remain on animal insulin. This has a chemical structure identical to the insulin produced by the human pancreas, and manufacturers are now withdrawing production of animal insulins. Human insulin is produced using gene technology, which involves the insertion of human

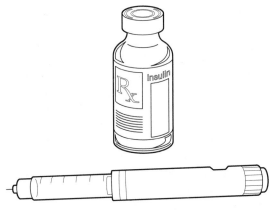

insulin-producing genes into a yeast cell or bacterium. In this way the yeast cells or bacteria are tricked into producing insulin instead of their own proteins.

Short- and rapid-acting insulins are pure insulin without any additives. They are in the form of a clear liquid and do not require stirring or mixing before use. Different additives are used to make the insulin longer acting, and these make it cloudy. The cloudy component collects as sediment at the bottom of the bottle or cartridge. This sediment should be mixed again

---

Production of human insulin: biosynthetic DNA-technology method

Production from baker's yeast	Novo Nordisk insulins.
Production from coli-bacteria	Eli Lilly insulins. Sanofi-Aventis insulins.

Methods of slowing the action of insulin

NPH insulin	Binds to a protein from salmon (protamine).
Lente insulin	Excess of free zinc.
Lantus	Clear solution but precipitates (becomes cloudy) after injection due to a higher pH in the subcutaneous tissue.
Levemir	Binds to a protein in the bloodstream (albumin).

with the rest of the contents by turning over or rolling (but not shaking) the cartridge 20 times before use. The newer basal insulins are clear because they are both solutions. These types of insulins have a prolonged effect because of changes to the molecular structure which slow down their absorption, rather than added molecules such as zinc or protamine.

In intravenous insulin therapy, short-acting insulin is given directly into the bloodstream. This is the most effective way to treat diabetic ketoacidosis. It can only be given in hospitals as an intravenous drip or in a motorized syringe. There is no advantage in giving rapid-acting insulin intravenously, since the blood glucose-lowering effect is no quicker than for regular short-acting insulin. Since the half-life of insulin is very short, only about 4 minutes, the blood glucose will increase sharply if intravenous insulin is stopped. If it is being used, the blood glucose must be checked every hour (even during the night) to monitor the correct dosage.

Intravenous insulin is often used during surgery or if a person is suffering for any length of time from diarrhoea and vomiting. It also gives us a practical way of working out how much insulin the person needs over a 24-hour period, for example when starting treatment with an insulin pump.

Rapid-acting insulin

Normally, insulin molecules stick together in groups of six (so called hexamer formation; see illustration on page 93). These groups must be broken up before the insulin can be absorbed into the blood. If the insulin molecules could be injected in a solution of single molecules (monomeric insulin), the action would be much quicker. Due to the shorter action span, it would also be possible to achieve more normal insulin levels between meals, lessening the need for snacks. Regular short-acting insulin is actually a bit too slow in action. The insulin level in your blood is not high enough during the meal. Rather, it is higher than necessary a couple of hours later, which is what causes you to need a snack.

By changing the protein building blocks in the insulin molecule, the problems of hexamer formation are considerably reduced. The rapid-acting insulin analogue (lispro or Humalog) introduced in the 1990s, takes effect very soon after injection and enters the bloodstream at about the same rate as food is absorbed. Other similar rapid-acting insulins are NovoRapid (aspart) and Apidra (glulisine). These are used by many people with diabetes.

NPL is a new intermediate-acting insulin originating from Humalog. The longer effect is achieved by adding protamine, in the same way as for ordinary NPH insulin. NPL has the advantage of being stable for at least a year if mixed with Humalog. It has the same action profile as ordinary NPH insulin.

Basal insulin

People without diabetes always have a low level of insulin in their body between meals and even during the night (see graphs overleaf). This steady release of insulin from the pancreas takes care of the glucose that is released between meals from the store in the liver. This constant low level of insulin is known as basal insulin or background insulin. People with diabetes do not have this steady production of insulin and need to take intermediate or long-acting insulin to replace it. This basal insulin controls release of glucose from the liver in the time between meals.

New basal insulins

Once a day injections of existing intermediate- or long-acting insulin preparations do not provide an appropriate 24-hour basal insulin level (between meals and during the night) in most people with diabetes. The long-acting analogue Lantus (glargine) was introduced in 2000. By altering the insulin molecule, the blood glucose-lowering effect has been spread more evenly over up to 24 hours, resembling the background insulin secretion in a person without diabetes. The subcutaneous uptake of

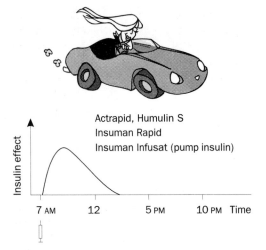

Actrapid, Humulin S
Insuman Rapid
Insuman Infusat (pump insulin)

Regular short-acting insulin

Regular short-acting insulin (also called soluble insulin) is given as a bolus injection before meals. The listed brand names are examples of insulins.

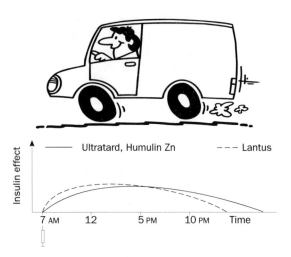

Ultratard, Humulin Zn   - - - Lantus

Basal insulin analogues

Basal insulin analogues have effect for up to 24 hours. Older forms have been superseded by new long-acting insulins Levemir and Lantus which give a more stable insulin effect and are injected once or twice daily.

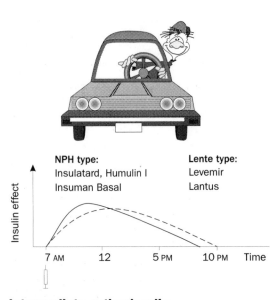

NPH type: Lente type:
Insulatard, Humulin I   Levemir
Insuman Basal   Lantus

Intermediate-acting insulin

Intermediate-acting insulin is used as basal (background) insulin when injecting twice daily and once or more daily in a multiple daily injection regimen. There are different types. NPH insulin (- - -) and lente (zinc-depot) insulin (—). The new basal insulins Levemir and Lantus are classified as both intermediate and long-acting.

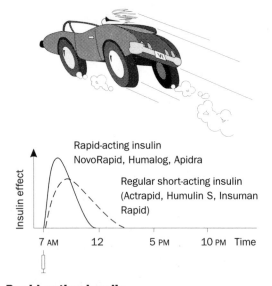

Rapid-acting insulin
NovoRapid, Humalog, Apidra

Regular short-acting insulin
(Actrapid, Humulin S, Insuman
Rapid)

Rapid-acting insulin

The new rapid-acting insulin analogues (NovoRapid, Humalog, Apidra) have a much more rapid action than regular short-acting insulin. You can inject them just before a meal and still get a good insulin effect at the time when the glucose from the food reaches the bloodstream. However, the insulin will have less effect after 2–3 hours, and the blood glucose may therefore rise before the next meal. Because of this, a basal insulin that takes effect during the day is usually given.

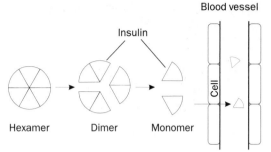

Insulin is always in a so-called hexamer form when it is injected. It must then divide into dimers and monomers before it can pass between the cells of the blood vessel to enter the bloodstream. The new rapid-acting insulin analogues (NovoRapid or Humalog) dissolve much faster than regular short-acting insulin, thus making the time of action much faster. Massage of the injection site can also enhance the dissociation, into monomers causing a faster absorption of the injected insulin. The addition of zinc (as in lente insulins) stabilizes the hexamer, delaying the absorption.

insulin is more stable from day to day with Lantus compared with NPH insulin.

Levemir (detemir), another basal insulin, was introduced in 2004. A 6-month study of adults using NovoRapid as pre-meal insulin showed that, with Levemir, the same HbA_{1c} levels (7.6%) as with NPH insulin were obtained, but with a lower risk of hypoglycaemia, especially during the night. Overnight glucose profiles

were more even with Levemir, and body weight was significantly lower after 6 months in the Levemir group. In another study the variability of insulin effect from day to day was smaller with Levemir compared with NPH and Lantus. More recent studies have shown that Levemir appears to be associated with strikingly less weight gain than other long-acting insulins. One possible explanation is that Levemir may have a greater effect on the liver and less effect on places where fat is laid down.

A review of several studies comparing Levemir and Lantus in adults found the duration of action to be very much the same (21.5–23 hours for Levemir and 22–24 hours for Lantus) but Levemir gave a more stable insulin effect from day to day in the individual person. A paediatric study also found less variation in effect for Levemir when comparing the two insulins. A 6-month study in adults comparing Levemir (given twice daily) and Lantus (given once daily) as basal insulin found no difference in HbA_{1c} or weight

Research findings: Levemir

- A study of adults using Levemir (detemir) found the time of action to be between 6 and 23 hours when doses between 0.1 U/kg and 0.8 U/kg were given.

- The use of Levemir is associated with less weight gain than NPH insulin.

- One possible explanation for this is that Levemir's chemical structure causes it to have a greater effect in the liver than conventional insulins. This may increase the glycogen store and affect hunger signals.

Research findings: Lantus

- Lantus has been shown to give similar levels of basal insulin over 24 hours to an insulin pump.

- In one study, adults with Type 1 diabetes compared Lantus (given once at bedtime) with NPH (given once or twice daily). Fasting glucose was 2.2 mmol/L (40 mg/dl) lower when using Lantus.

- In the group using NPH once a day, the doses of Lantus were similar. But Lantus doses for the group using NPH twice daily were 6–7 units lower than the sum of the NPH doses.

- A recently published study of treating to target with Lantus in Type 2 diabetes has shown neutral or only slight weight gain, with acceptable levels of nocturnal hypoglycaemia.

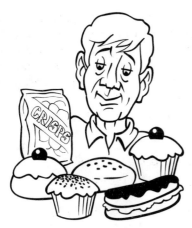

Snacking to deal with hypoglycaemia will lead to weight gain.

gain, but the Levemir group had a lower fasting glucose level and less severe and night time hypoglycaemia.

Pre-mixed insulin

The cartridges of pre-mixed insulin that are available for insulin pens contain different proportions of rapid-acting and intermediate-acting insulin of NPH type. You can also find cartridges containing mixtures of short-acting and intermediate-acting insulins. With pre-mixed insulins, the proportions of the two insulins cannot be adjusted. If you change the dose you will get more or less of both types of insulin. It is important to assess the use of different mixtures depending on your meal schedule. For example, the prolonged effect of the intermediate-acting part in a 30–50% mix with rapid-acting insulins may be useful if you have a long wait between lunch and dinner/tea.

Units and insulin concentrations

Insulin is measured in units, abbreviated to U (international units, previously abbreviated IU). One unit of insulin was originally defined as the amount of insulin that will lower the blood glucose of a healthy 2 kg (4.4 lb) rabbit that has

fasted for 24 hours to 2.5 mmol/L (45 mg/dl) within 2.5 hours. Quite a complicated definition, don't you think? With better analytical methods, one unit has been defined as 6 mmol or 29 mg of insulin.

Today, the most common insulin concentration around the world is 100 units/ml (U-100). In some countries other concentrations are used, mostly 40 units/ml (U-40).

Insulin units are counted in the same way, regardless of the concentration. A weaker insulin will be absorbed more quickly. Insulin of 40 units/ml gives approximately 20% higher insulin levels 30–40 minutes after injection compared with the same number of units of 100 units/ml. People taking insulin need to be aware that it will take effect more quickly if they switch from 100 units/ml to 40 units/ml.

Twice-daily treatment

Twice daily injections are still widely used in Type 2 diabetes. It is often difficult to adjust mentally to taking insulin during the early stages of insulin therapy, and injections twice daily help a high percentage of people with Type 2 diabetes to reach their targets. However, a twice daily injection regimen usually means that there is less flexibility for planning mealtimes. When targets aren't achieved, increasing twice daily insulin to deal with mealtime glucose loads causes a risk of hypoglycaemia during the late afternoon or night. Snacking to deal with late hypoglycaemia will cause weight gain.

Multiple injection treatment

Multiple injection treatment implies taking rapid-acting (NovoRapid, Humalog, Apidra) or short-acting (Actrapid, Humulin S, Insuman Rapid) insulin before each main meal, and one or two doses of intermediate-acting (Insulatard, Humulin I, Insuman Basal) or long-acting (Lantus, Levemir) insulin to cover the need for insulin between meals and during the night.

Multiple injection treatment has been used

since 1984, and the first insulin pen was introduced in 1985. Studies in adults with Type 1 and Type 2 diabetes have shown that it is possible to improve glucose control with this regimen. If using multiple injections doesn't give you an improved HbA$_{1c}$, it may at least give you more flexibility with your day-to-day living, rather than planning your day around your insulin. This arrangement is particularly easy to use in people who do shift work. Programmes such as DAFNE for people with Type 1 diabetes have encouraged patients to tailor their treatment to their lifestyle rather than their lifestyle to their treatment. This has proved to be very motivating for many.

Injections before meals (bolus insulin)

Bolus insulin is the rapid- or short-acting insulin taken before a meal. Rapid-acting insulin begins to act after 10 minutes and is at its most effective after just one hour. If you are using rapid-acting insulin, you will not need to be as strict about mealtimes if you also have a dose of basal insulin in the morning (see page 97). Short-acting regular insulin (Actrapid, Humulin S, Insuman Rapid) begins to act 20–30 minutes after a subcutaneous injection and has its maximal effect after 1.5–2 hours. The blood glucose-lowering effect lasts for about 5 or more hours.

One difference between rapid- and short-acting insulins for multiple injections is that with rapid-acting insulin you may notice a rise in your evening blood sugars if you eat a large afternoon snack, unless you are playing sport, digging the garden or doing some other activity. With short-acting insulin, the opposite is the case and activity may mean that you need a sandwich in the middle of the afternoon to avoid hypoglycaemia. Check your blood glucose level to help you decide what dose you need.

Results from the Lantus 'treating to target' algorithm study suggest that intensive treatment with a long-acting insulin analogue regime results in improved control and only a small rise in the incidence of hypoglycaemia, accompanied

by little significant weight gain. Previously clinicians accepted a degree of compromise with respect to insulin use in Type 2 diabetes. With the use of modern analogue insulins and the possibility of combination with insulin sensitizing agents such as metformin or the glitazones, most people can reach their targets.

When should you take your pre-meal dose?

All three brands brands of regular short-acting insulin have the same time action and start to have an effect 15–30 minutes after injection. Rapid-acting insulins (Apidra, NovoRapid, Humalog) start working within a few minutes of injection. The abdomen is the most common

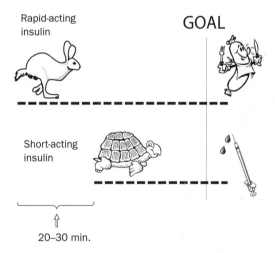

Rapid-acting insulin

GOAL

Short-acting insulin

20–30 min.

The rapid-acting insulins (NovoRapid, Humalog) are very quick to take effect and can be given immediately before the meal. However, since it takes 20–30 minutes for regular short-acting insulin (Actrapid, Humulin S, Insuman Rapid) to begin its action, you must give the insulin a head start or the race will be very uneven. The carbohydrates from your meal will enter the bloodstream first and raise your blood glucose level. The insulin will enter your bloodstream later, but will remain in the system after the food has been absorbed. This will lead to a high blood glucose initially but put you at risk of a low blood glucose before your next meal. Taking your injection 30 minutes before the meal is particularly important at breakfast time, but if you recognize these problems, you should take your injection 20–30 minutes before all meals.

Research findings: multiple injections

- Studies indicate that more than 90% of participants have found multiple injections acceptable.
- Results from the DCCT study in Type 1 diabetes show that starting an intensive treatment regimen can have positive effects, particularly on microvascular complications.

---

injection site for pre-meal injections. If you take regular pre-meal insulin in the thigh (or buttocks) you may need to add another 15 minutes to these time limits since insulin is absorbed more rapidly from the abdomen than the thigh. The time limits given in this chapter refer to abdominal injections of regular short-acting insulin if not otherwise stated. If you use rapid-acting insulin you must adjust the time intervals as indicated above.

Ideally, regular short-acting insulin should be administered 20–30 minutes before all meals since the blood glucose is not affected immediately. However, at lunchtime some of the short-acting breakfast insulin still remains in your body and the same holds true for the other meals. Because of this, the 30 minute insulin 'head start' is not as essential with other meals as it is with breakfast.

Can regular short-acting insulin injections be taken just before a meal?

To find out, take the injection just before your meal and measure your blood glucose before and 2 hours after the meal. The blood glucose should have risen 4.0 mmol/L (70 mg/dl) at the most. If it has risen more, the effect of your regular insulin is too slow.

Try the same thing when you take your insulin 15 and 30 minutes before eating, to find out which suits you the best. If the blood glucose

is too high, even when you have taken the insulin 30 minutes before the meal, you will probably need a higher dose.

If you inject regular short-acting insulin just before your meal, it is important that the food is not absorbed from the intestine immediately. If it is, your blood glucose will rise before the insulin reaches your bloodstream. Any fat content of the meal will slow down the gastric emptying rate. For example, ice cream made with milk products has a higher fat content and will therefore give a slower rise in blood glucose than water ice. See also Chapter 8 on Nutrition.

The blood glucose reading before a meal will indicate when it is appropriate to take the injection. If your blood glucose is high, you can wait 45–60 minutes before eating, if this is convenient. If you have a low blood glucose, you should leave the injection until it is time to eat or wait 15 minutes at the most (see table below).

If you use rapid-acting insulin (NovoRapid or Humalog) it should normally be injected just before the meal.

If you have background insulin lasting 24 hours (which should be the case), the timing of the bedtime dose won't matter.

When should I take my pre-meal insulin? (abdominal injections)

Meal	Rapid-acting insulins*	Regular short-acting insulin
Breakfast	Just before the meal	At least 30 min. before
Other meals	Just before the meal	0–30 min. before (see text)
Hypoglycaemia at mealtime	After the meal	Just before you eat
High blood glucose at mealtime	Wait 15–30 min. before eating	Wait 30–60 min. before eating

*NovoRapid, Humalog, Apidra.

Can I change my mealtimes?

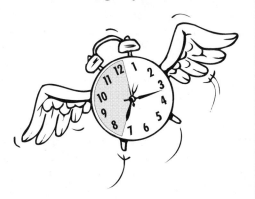

You can usually adjust your timetable for meals and injections by one hour in either direction. If you are using rapid-acting insulin (NovoRapid or Humalog) you won't need to be as strict about mealtimes if you take basal NPH insulin in the morning too, or if you use long-acting insulin (Lantus, Ultratard, Humulin Zn) as your basal insulin You should not go for more than 5 hours between meals and injections of regular short-acting insulin if you don't use a basal insulin during the day. Waiting more than 5 hours between injections of regular insulin puts you at risk of insulin deficiency.

Can I skip a meal?

Your body needs to have some insulin in the blood, even between meals, to take care of the glucose produced by the liver. If you use NovoRapid or Humalog and take basal insulin as well in the morning (or one daily dose of Lantus), you may try to skip both the meal and the corresponding NovoRapid or Humalog dose. If your blood glucose is high, you may need a small corrective dose of rapid-acting insulin. Increase the dose of NovoRapid or Humalog, if necessary, the next time you eat. A useful rule of thumb is that 1 unit of insulin lowers your blood glucose by about 3 mmol/L.

Bedtime insulin

The bedtime insulin injection is the most difficult dose to adjust. Although we do not eat during the night, our bodies need a continuous low level of insulin to prevent the liver releasing glucose freely into the bloodstream. The most common bedtime insulin with multiple injection treatment used to be intermediate-acting insulin of NPH type. Insulin with longer effect (Lantus or Levemir) is now used widely instead. Modern long-acting insulin analogues such as Lantus or Levemir are designed to have a true 24-hour profile, but in practice this is not always the case. Working out the correct dose of background insulin can have a great impact on HbA_{1c} and on your quality of life.

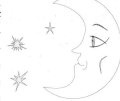

When should the long-acting injection be taken?

The long-acting insulin analogue Lantus can be taken at the evening snack, at bedtime or even in the morning. Because it has a long half-life, your levels of Lantus are likely to reach a steady state after the first few injections. Most people find one evening dose of Lantus is sufficient, but some may need to split the dose and give part of it in the morning. Levemir (detemir) has a similar long duration of action, requiring one or two injections per day. Both these newer analogue insulins are associated with much less hypoglycaemia at night than traditional intermediate-acting insulins.

Since long-acting insulins act for up to 24 hours, sometimes even longer, it is important not to change the dose more often than 2 (or 3) times a week.

Mixing insulins

Insulin of NPH type (Insulatard, Humulin I, Insuman Basal) can be mixed with both rapid-acting NovoRapid and Humalog and regular short-acting insulin. You should not mix the new long-acting insulin analogues Lantus and Levemir in the syringe.

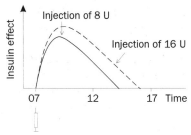

A larger insulin dose (dashed line) gives both a stronger and a longer-lasting insulin effect.

Depot effect

If only intermediate or long-acting insulin is used, a depot (store) of insulin is formed in the subcutaneous fat tissue, corresponding to about 24 hours of insulin requirements. If the dose of bedtime insulin is changed, the size of the insulin depot makes it necessary to allow 2–3 days for your body to adjust until you see the full effect of the change.

The disadvantage of a large insulin depot in Type 2 diabetes is that, if your levels of long-acting insulin have built up to too high a level over a long period, there may be problems with hypoglycaemia lasting for more than 24 hours. Differences in the rate of absorption can vary when you change injection position, for example from the top of the legs to the abdomen, where people with Type 2 diabetes may have rather more subcutaneous fat.

How accurate is your insulin dose?

If used correctly, an insulin pen will give a very accurate insulin dose with an error of only a few per cent. However, the effect of a given insulin dose also depends on a number of other factors. The effect of an identical dose of insulin, given to an individual at the same site, can vary by as much as 25%. It can vary by nearly 50% when the same dose is given to two different individuals. This explains the frustrating fact that you can eat the same food, do exactly the same things and give identical doses of insulin for two days in a row, but get quite different blood glucose results.

There is less variation in the action profile of the newer insulin analogues.

Insulin absorption

The absorption of insulin from the injection site can be influenced by a number of factors. Heat will increase the absorption. If the room temperature increases from 20° to 35°C (68–95°F), the speed of absorption of short-acting insulin will increase by 50–60%. Taking a bath or a sauna at a temperature of 85°C (185°F) may increase the absorption by as much as 110%! In other words, you could be at risk of hypogly-

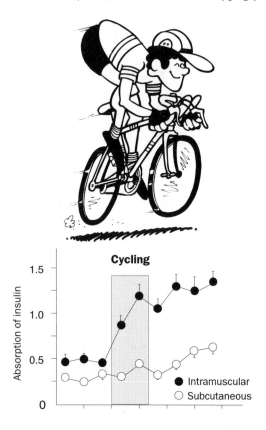

After an injection in your thigh muscle, the absorption rate will increase considerably when you exercise the muscles in your legs. Short-acting insulin (10 units) was given at 0 minutes. After an injection in the subcutaneous fat, you will only see a slight increase in the absorption rate, probably due to the subcutaneous insulin depot being 'massaged' by the moving muscles.

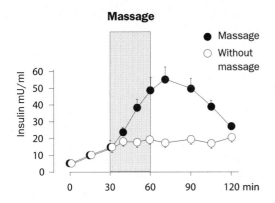

Massage

- ● Massage
- ○ Without massage

Massaging the injection site will considerably increase the absorption of insulin. Short-acting insulin (10 untis) was given at 0 minutes. You can utilize this if you want your short-acting insulin to take particularly rapid effect, for example if you have a high blood glucose.

caemia if you inject short-acting insulin shortly before taking a hot bath. A temperature of just 42°C (108°F) in a shower, spa bath or jacuzzi may double the insulin level in your blood, while a cold bath (22°C, 72°F) will decrease the absorption of insulin. Massage of the injection site for 30 minutes has been found to give higher insulin levels and lower blood glucose, with both short-acting and long-acting insulins.

The skin temperature is also important. In one study, the same insulin injection gave twice the concentration in blood after 45 minutes when a skin temperature of 37°C was compared with that of 30°C (same room temperature). In the same study, individuals with a thicker subcutaneous fat layer (10 mm) had lower insulin levels than those with a thin subcutaneous fat layer (2 mm). The above mentioned factors have less of an effect on the absorption of new insulin analogues.

What if you forget to take your insulin?

You can try the following suggestions if you have had diabetes for some time and are confident about how the insulin you inject works.

- If you are even slightly unsure, you should seek expert advice.

Forgotten pre-meal injection (multiple injection treatment)

It is unlikely in Type 2 diabetes that missing one mealtime injection of insulin will cause you much of a problem, but of course if this happens over a number of occasions, your average control will be poorer and your HbA_{1c} will begin to rise. The best thing to do may be to add 1 or 2 units to the insulin taken at your next mealtime. If your sugar is high before the next meal, you should correct it using the rule of thumb: take one extra unit of short-acting insulin for every 3 mmol/L above 10.

Forgotten bedtime injection (multiple injection treatment)

If you wake up before 2 am, you can still take your bedtime insulin (of isophane-type), but you should decrease the dose by 25% or 2 units for every hour that has passed since the normal time of injection. Unlike in Type 1 diabetes, it isn't likely that missing one night-time injection will cause you too much harm. Naturally, your blood sugar level may be significantly higher the following day.

If you have forgotten your evening or bedtime Lantus or Levemir dose, you can take it when you remember it, if only a few hours have passed. If you remember in the morning, take approximately half of the dose you should have taken in the evening. However, if you take Levemir or Lantus twice daily, just take your usual morning dose. In addition, if your blood glucose level is high, you should take extra mealtime insulin to correct this.

What if you take the wrong type of insulin?

At bedtime

Taking your pre-meal insulin instead of the bedtime insulin by mistake when going to bed is not uncommon. This may happen if your day and night pen injectors are very similar. Long-acting

Factors influencing the insulin effect

1 Insulin resistance

Insulin resistance probably has the most effect on insulin efficacy and the dose required for control in Type 2 diabetes. Resitance to the effects of insulin underpins the development of the disease in overweight patients.

2 Subcutaneous blood flow

(increased blood flow will give a faster insulin absorption).

Increased by	Heat, e.g. sauna, jacuzzi, hot shower, hot bath or fever.
Decreased by	Cold, e.g. a cold bath. Smoking (constriction of the blood vessels). Dehydration.

3 Injection depth

Faster absorption after an intramuscular injection.

4 Injection site

An abdominal injection of short-acting insulin will be absorbed faster than a thigh injection. The absorption from the buttocks is slower than from the abdomen but slightly faster than from the thigh.

5 Insulin antibodies

Can bind the insulin, resulting in a slower and less predictable effect. These are of much more clinical relevance in Type 1 diabetes.

6 Exercise

Increases the absorption of short-acting insulin even after you have finished exercising, particularly if the injection is given intramuscularly.

7 Massage of the injection site

Increased absorption of short-acting insulin, probably due to a faster breakdown of the insulin.

8 Subcutaneous fat thickness

A thicker layer of subcutaneous fat gives a slower absorption of insulin.

9 Injection in fatty lumps (lipohypertrophy)

Slower and more erratic absorption of insulin.

10 Concentration of the insulin

40 units/ml is absorbed faster than 100 units/ml.

Levemir and Lantus insulins are clear solutions so it can be easy to mistake short-acting or rapid-acting insulin for the long-acting variety if both are drawn from vials and given with syringes.

This can be very frightening, but it is not a catastrophe! You will need to check your blood glucose regularly during the night and it would be sensible to eat some long-acting carbohydrate (bowl of cereal and milk). If possible make a partner or other family member aware of the problem.

It would be a good idea to have food available to eat extra meals during the night, preferably food that is rich in carbohydrates but contains as little fat as possible. If you need to take glucose to counter hypoglycaemia, the effect will be much slower if you have a fat-rich meal in your stomach.

Taking the wrong type of insulin will only be dangerous if you take short- or rapid-acting insulin at bedtime without noticing it. If you are used to low blood glucose levels, your body might not give any warning symptoms until the blood glucose is dangerously low (see 'Hypoglycaemia unawareness' on page 131).

Remember that the effect of rapid-acting insulin usually diminishes after 4–5 hours (a little later if you have taken a dose larger than 10 units). Short-acting insulin will last a little longer. Because the shorter-acting insulin wouldn't last through the night, your morning blood sugar level is likely to be high. This isn't anything too much to worry about and will settle when you take your usual long-acting insulin the following evening.

During the day

If you happen to take a dose of intermediate-acting instead of rapid- or short-acting insulin during the day, it will not give you much of a blood glucose-lowering effect for that meal. The effect will come some hours later. It would be best, therefore, to factor in a mid-morning or afternoon snack to avoid hypoglycaemia.

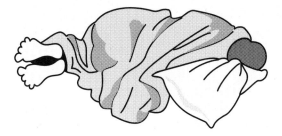

Having a lie-in at weekends

You may want to sleep in a little longer at weekends. This is rarely a problem but you will notice that your morning blood glucose is a little higher. This is unlikely to cause problems in practical terms in Type 2 diabetes.

Staying awake all night

Being up all night is not common practice, but it is sometimes unavoidable for shift workers or people who are travelling. During intercontinental flights, people often have to stay awake for long periods (see 'Passing through time zones when on insulin' on page 183).

If you stay awake all night, you should take your normal dose of Lantus or Levemir. However, you should probably not take your bedtime insulin if it is isophane. Instead, you inject pre-meal inulin when you eat every 4 or 5 hours. Adjust the dose according to how much you eat (compare the carbohydrate content of your meal with your usual lunch, dinner/tea or evening snack). You should not use the amount of insulin taken at breakfast for comparison because more insulin is commonly needed for breakfast (See 'Moving towards treatment by insulin alone'). If you use rapid-acting insulin (NovoRapid or Humalog), and twice daily intermediate acting basal insulin (Insulatard, Humulin I, Insuman Basal), you may need to take half the night time dose to cover your basal

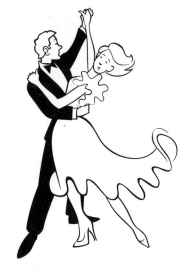

If you are out at a party, remember that dancing is exercise too. Don't forget to eat something during the evening. You may well need to reduce your bedtime injection of insulin or eat a bedtime snack, such as a bowl of cereal.

need of insulin during a long-distance flight. If you use long-acting insulin (Lantus or Levemir), this will probably give sufficient basal effect throughout the flight.

Shift work

It may be difficult to combine diabetes with shift work. After returning home from a night shift, you need insulin to cover both the meal you are about to eat as well as background insulin for the time you sleep during the day. Rapid-acting insulin (NovoRapid or Humalog) is a better mealtime insulin in this situation as its effect will be wearing off as the basal insulin takes effect. With regular short-acting insulin, there will be a risk of overlapping effects, which could cause hypoglycaemia after 3–4 hours. If you switch to a work pattern with lots of shifts, consider asking your diabetes nurse for advice first.

Administering insulin

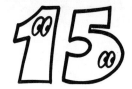

The only way insulin can work in the cells is by binding to the receptors on the cell surface. Because of this, insulin will take effect only when it has been carried to the cells in the bloodstream. Today, the only practical method of administration is by injection or infusion into a vein. However, a great deal of research is currently being carried out to explore alternative ways of administering insulin. Inhaled insulin has been developed but there is no commercial preparation available at the present time.

Injection technique

Having an injection is never going to be pleasurable. At best it is a nuisance, and at worst it can be painful, especially at the beginning. Most people can adapt to difficulties if they can take them at their own pace.

Taking the pain out of injections

Pain is generated by the pain receptors just under the skin and the sensation is carried along fine nerves to the spinal cord and up to the brain. The nerves spread like the branches of a

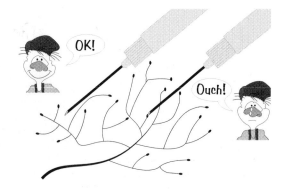

Nerve fibres look like thin branches of a tree. If you hit a nerve, you will feel more pain than if you inject between the nerve fibres.

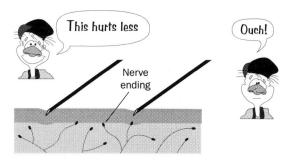

Try to find an injection site that hurts less when you press the needle against your skin.

tree. If you hit a pain receptor directly, this will be painful. You can test out the position of receptors by pressing the needle carefully against your skin, and feeling where it hurts more and where it hurts less. Certain areas on your abdomen and thighs will probably hurt less than others. However, the disadvantage of always using the same places for injections is that you will soon start to develop fatty lumps (lipohypertrophy; see page 124). Insulin will be absorbed more slowly from such lumps. If you insert the needle quickly with thrust, you will feel less pricking. However, some people prefer to push the needle slowly and carefully through the skin.

For many years people with diabetes have been using the same needle time and again but current advice is that for each injection, you should use a new needle. Needles are finer, shorter and lubricated to make injections as painless as possible.

Is it best to inject into fat or into muscle?

The recommendations for how to inject insulin have changed considerably over the years. With old (25 mm, 1 inch) needles it was natural to use a raised skin fold when injecting. When the

Research findings: injection technique

- Even with an 8 mm needle, there is a considerable risk of injecting into the muscle when using a perpendicular injection technique (despite lifting a skin pinch-up with a correct two-finger technique).

- The safest way to inject with the 5–6 mm needles is to lift a skin fold with two fingers and inject at a 90° angle.

Recommended injections sites

Rapid-acting insulin	Abdomen (tummy)
Short-acting insulin	Abdomen (tummy)
Intermediate-acting insulin	Thighs or buttocks
Long-acting Lantus or Levemir	Abdomen, thighs or buttocks

12–13 mm needles were introduced, it was thought that a perpendicular injection would deposit the insulin within the subcutaneous (fatty) tissue. However, as mentioned below, you risk injecting into muscle when using this technique, and people are now being advised again to inject at an angle into a raised skin fold, except when using the very short 5 or 6 mm needles.

Insulin should be given by subcutaneous injection, i.e. into the fat beneath the skin, not into the muscle. To avoid injecting into the muscle, it is important to lift a skin fold with the thumb and index finger ('two-finger pinch-up') and insert the needle at a 90° angle (see illustration on page 107). Lifting a skin fold is important, even if you are using an 8 mm needle. With 5–6 mm needles, injections can be given without lifting a skin fold if there is enough subcutaneous fat (at least 8 mm as skin layers may be compressed when injecting perpendicularly).

Some research has found that injecting into the muscle is not necessarily more painful, but the insulin is absorbed more quickly. An injection into the muscle is usually experienced as uncomfortable, even if it is not particularly painful. The uptake of short-acting and intermediate-acting insulin is increased by at least 50% from an intramuscular injection compared with a subcutaneous injection.

The thicker the layer of subcutaneous fat, the smaller the blood flow. This results in a slower absorption of insulin. In one study, short-acting insulin (8 units injected into the abdomen) was absorbed twice as fast from a subcutaneous fat layer of 10 mm compared with 20 mm. The same result was found in patients using insulin pumps. You can take advantage of this phenomenon by injecting where the subcutaneous fat is thinner, if you wish the insulin to take effect more quickly. Also, insulin that is injected above the navel will be absorbed slightly more quickly than insulin injected below or beside the navel.

Some people find it more convenient to inject themselves through clothing. Although this can cause unpleasant skin reactions, these seem to be unusual. However, it is more difficult to get hold of a proper skin fold through clothing, and this increases the risk of accidentally injecting into muscle. There is also a risk of blood staining your clothes.

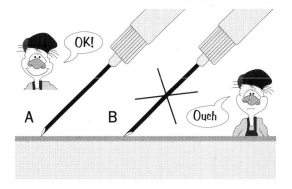

Look closely at the needle tip before pushing it through the skin. The tip of the needle is cut very sharp so that it will pierce the skin easily. If you prick the skin with the eye of the needle facing towards the skin (B), you will feel more pain than if you prick the skin with the sharp tip pointing towards the skin (A).

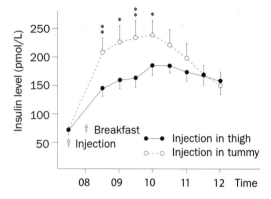

In an American study, adults took the same dose of short-acting insulin before breakfast in the tummy one day and in the thigh one day. The injection in the tummy gave both a faster onset of insulin action and a higher peak level of insulin in the blood.

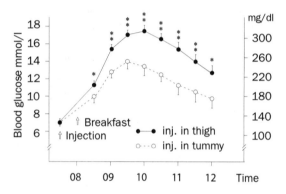

Blood glucose levels from the same study as above. Because insulin enters the blood more quickly after an injection in the tummy, this will cause the glucose content of the breakfast to enter the cells more effectively, resulting in a lower blood glucose level.

In the tummy or the thigh?

In adults, insulin is absorbed more rapidly after a subcutaneous injection into the abdomen or tummy, than after an intramuscular injection into the thigh, and the blood glucose-lowering effect is also increased (see illustrations opposite). This is caused by an increased blood flow in the subcutaneous fat in the tummy compared with that in the thigh. The insulin uptake from the buttocks is quicker than from the thigh but not as quick as from the tummy.

The absorption of intermediate-acting insulin (NPH insulin) is better balanced after an injection in the thigh and will give a lower insulin effect early in the night and a higher insulin effect later in the night, compared with an abdominal injection.

As insulin is absorbed faster from the tummy than from the thigh, we recommend giving the

Subcutaneous injection technique 8–13 mm needle

1 Eject a tiny amount of insulin (½–1 unit with a pen) in the air to ensure that the tip of the needle is filled with insulin.

2 Lift the skin with your thumb and index finger ('two-finger pinch-up').

3 Penetrate the skin at an angle of 90° to the skin surface.

4 Hold the skin fold and inject the insulin.

5 Count to 10 slowly.

6 Withdraw the needle.

7 Let go of the skin fold.

8 If you have problems with leakage, you can press a finger over the hole in the skin after the needle is withdrawn or consider using a longer needle.

When injecting into the buttocks, the subcutaneous fat layer is usually thick enough to inject even with 8 and 13 mm needles without lifting a skin fold.

Disinfection of the skin before injection is not necessary as the infection risk is negligible.

pre-meal doses of rapid-acting (or short-acting) insulin into the tummy and the bedtime injection of intermediate- or long-acting insulin into the thigh (or in the buttocks). We do not recommend changing the site of injection between the thigh and the tummy from day to day as this will vary the effect of the insulin.

Rapid-acting and short-acting insulin

The difference in uptake between injection sites is not as pronounced when using rapid-acting insulin. If you are using NovoRapid or Humalog, the uptake is only slightly faster from the abdomen than from the thigh. There was no difference in absorption between subcutaneous and intramuscular injections when using Humalog for thigh injections in a German study.

Long-acting insulin

The long-acting analogues Lantus (glargine) and Levemir (detemir) give the same effect when injected into the tummy, thigh or arm. Absorp-

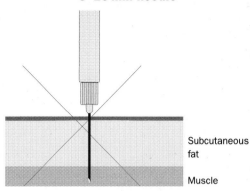

Subcutaneous injection technique 8–13 mm needle

Subcutaneous fat

Muscle

If you inject at a 90° angle with a 12–13 mm needle without pinching the skin, there is a considerable risk of accidental intramuscular injection. This risk is substantial even with the shorter 8 mm needle if you inject in areas with a thin subcutaneous layer, such as the outside of the thigh, the upper arms or the sides of your body. Insulin from an intramuscular injection is absorbed more quickly into the bloodstream, and this will give you a stronger but shorter insulin dose. However, you can take advantage of this type of injection in the thigh if you want your insulin to start working more quickly, or if you have problems with lipohypertrophy (see page 124).

tion of insulin is affected by many other factors as well (see Chapter 14 on Insulin treatment).

Is it necessary to disinfect the skin?

There is no need to disinfect your skin with alcohol before injecting with an insulin pen or syringe. The risk of skin infection is negligible, and alcohol disinfection often causes a stinging pain when the needle is inserted. Good hygiene and careful hand-washing are more important.

If you use an insulin pump or indwelling (Insuflon®) catheter, you should wash the skin

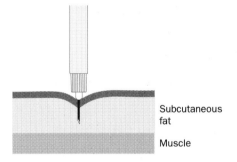

Subcutaneous injection technique 5–6 mm needle

Subcutaneous fat

Muscle

1 Eject a tiny amount of insulin (½–1 unit with a pen) in the air to ensure that the tip of the needle is filled with insulin.

2 The 5–6 mm needle can be used for perpendicular injections if the subcutaneous tissue is at least 8 mm thick, otherwise you need to pinch a skin fold.

3 Penetrate the skin at an angle of 90°.

4 Inject the insulin.

5 Count to 10 slowly.

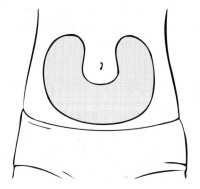

The abdomen is usually used for injections of short-acting and rapid-acting insulin (Apidra, NovoRapid or Humalog). It will be absorbed slightly faster above the tummy button compared with other areas of the abdomen. Always use the same area for a given type of insulin, e.g. the tummy for short-acting insulin, and the thigh for bedtime insulin. It is important to rotate the injection sites within each area to avoid the development of fatty lumps (lipohypertrophy, see page 124).

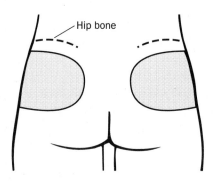

You can also use your buttocks for injections. Inject a few centimetres below the edge of the hip bone. The absorption of insulin is slightly slower from the buttocks than from the tummy. The illustrations are from the reference by Henriksen and colleagues.

with an antiseptic solution or use chlorhexidine in alcohol or a similar disinfectant if you have problems with skin infections. Some skin disinfectants contain skin moisturisers which may cause the adhesive to loosen more easily.

Storage of insulin

Insulin withstands room temperature well. Most manufacturers recommend that insulin in use

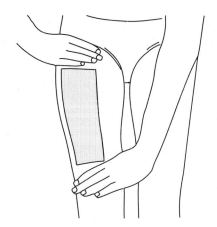

Put one hand above the knee and the other below your groin. The area between your hands is suitable for injections into the thigh. Remember that insulin will be absorbed more slowly from the thigh than from the tummy.

should be discarded after 4 weeks at room temperature (not above 25–30° C, 77–86° F).

Check the package leaflet for the type of insulin you are using and the expiry date on the bottle or cartridge. At room temperature, insulin will lose less than 1% of its potency every month. According to one study, regular, Lente and NPH insulin used for up to 110 days kept their insulin concentration at 100 units/ml. Even after a year or more of being stored at room temperature, as long as it is kept in darkness, the insulin will lose only 10% of its effect. Check the expiry date on the bottle or cartridge.

A practical routine is to have your spare insulin supplies stored in the refrigerator (4–8° C, 39–46° F), and the bottle or cartridge that is currently in use, stored at room temperature. Storing it at room temperature makes the preservatives more effective in killing any bacteria that may have contaminated the vial during repeated use for injections. Humalog that is diluted (with sterile NPH medium) to 50 units/ml (U-50) and 10 units/ml (U-10) is stable for one month when stored at 5° C and 30° C.

Don't put your insulin too close to the freezer compartment in the fridge as it cannot withstand temperatures below 2° C (36° F). Don't expose insulin to strong light or heat, such as the sunlight in a car or the heat of a sauna. Insulin loses its effect when it is stored at temperatures above 25–30° C (77–86° F). Above 35° C (95° F) it will be inactivated four times as fast as it is at room temperature. A practical way to keep your insulin cool on holiday is to store it in a cooled thermos flask or wrapped in moist flannel to keep it cool.

In very hot climates where there is no refrigerator available, insulin vials and cartridges can be stored in a box that is floating in an earthenware pitcher (matka) filled halfway with water without losing its activity. The pot should be kept in the shade. An Indian study showed that insulin stored in this way did not lose any of its effectiveness after 60 days with temperatures up to 40° C (104° F).

You need not store human insulin in the dark as it keeps just as well in daylight (but not sunlight). Human insulin carried in a shirt pocket for 6 months did not deteriorate significantly more quickly than when it was stored at room temperature. Never use insulin that has become cloudy if it usually is clear (applies to rapid- and short-acting, Lantus and Levemir). Intermediate-

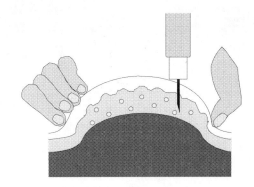

If you lift the skin with a whole-hand grip there is less risk of a superficial injection with a 5–6 mm needle. This technique, however, should not be used with the longer 8 and 13 mm needles since the muscle will be lifted as well resulting in a risk of intramuscular injection.

or long-acting insulin that contains clumps or that has a frosty coating on the inside of the vial should not be used either.

Syringes

Disposable syringes have been used since the 1960s and are still the standard injection device in many countries. They are graded in units for U-100 insulin, containing 30, 50 or 100 units.

Syringes are used when mixing two types of insulin into the same injection or for types of insulin that are not available in pen cartridges.

You will need to be careful when travelling, especially if you are visiting countries that use a different concentration of insulin. It is particularly important **not** to use U-40 insulin in a U-100 syringe or vice versa. In countries where pen injectors are less common, syringes are used for multiple injection therapy. In many countries

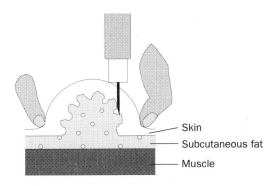

— Skin
— Subcutaneous fat
— Muscle

The safest way to inject with the 5–6 mm needles is to lift a skin fold with two fingers and to inject at a 45° angle. However, if you inject slightly to one side with a 5–6 mm needle, there is a risk of an injection into the superficial skin (intracutaneous injection; see figure) from which the insulin may be absorbed more slowly. With 5–6 mm needles, the injections can be given perpendicularly without lifting a skin fold to avoid intracutaneous injections if there is enough subcutaneous fat (at least 8 mm as the skin layers often are compressed when injecting perpendicularly). When injecting into the buttocks, the subcutaneous fat layer is usually thick enough to inject without lifting a skin fold.

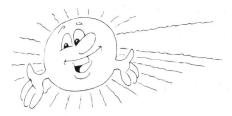

Insulin is sensitive to heat and sunlight, so don't leave it in the sun or a hot car.

Different ways of administering insulin

- Syringes   1–3 injections/day.
- Insulin pen   4–6 injections/day.
- Insuflon®   Indwelling Teflon catheter. Can be used if injection pain is a problem.
- Insulin pump   Delivers a basal rate over 24 hours and bolus doses at mealtimes.
- Jet injector   Injection without a needle. A thin jet stream of insulin is shot through the skin.
- inhaled insulin   Not available at present.

with lower economic standards, non-disposable glass syringes with needles that require manual sharpening are still used.

Injections with syringes

Cloudy insulin (intermediate- and long-acting) needs to be mixed before use. This is done by gently turning or rolling the bottle between the hands 10–20 times. Do not shake the bottle as this will lead to problems with air bubbles in the syringe. Start the injection by drawing air into the syringe corresponding to the dose of insulin you will inject. Then inject the air into the insulin bottle, turn it upside down and then draw up the correct dose of insulin. Hold the syringe with the needle upwards, and then tap on it a couple of times to get rid of the air bubbles.

Pen injectors

A pen injector (insulin pen) is a practical tool that is loaded with a cartridge of insulin for repeated injections. The standard cartridges contain 300 units (3 ml). Pen injectors will give a more accurate dosage compared with syringes, especially in the low doses. Some pens can be adjusted to half units.

Disposable pens are also available for most insulins. They are a practical alternative for carrying spare insulin, for example when you are travelling. Make sure that you have an extra disposable insulin pen at work, or anywhere else you go regularly.

Why aren't all insulins available for pens?

Traditional intermediate- and long-acting insulins are cloudy and the bottle must be turned or rolled (not shaken!) at least 20 times before the insulin is injected to mix it up well. The pen cartridge contains a small glass or steel marble that will help stir the insulin when the pen is turned.

Replacing pen needles

Sterile, disposable pen needles and syringes are designed for single use only. However, many patients reuse them for several injections. The risk of infected injection sites when reusing disposable needles seems to be negligible. However, the injections may hurt more since the needle becomes blunted due to tip damage after

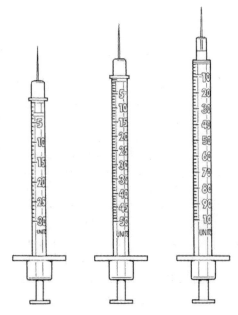

Insulin syringes: 0.3 ml, 0.5 ml and 1 ml

Mixing insulins in a syringe

Very few people actually mix their own insulin these days, but if you do, this illustrates how to do it.

➠ Gently roll the bottle containing cloudy insulin until it is mixed and there is no powder on the bottom of the bottle. Do not shake the insulin bottle because this can cause air bubbles.

➠ Clean the bottles of clear and cloudy insulin with an alcohol pad.

➠ Take the syringe out of its package and remove the needle cap.

➠ Pull the plunger of the syringe down to the number of units of cloudy insulin you need. The syringe will fill with air.

➠ Push the needle through the stopper of the cloudy insulin bottle.

➠ Push the air into the bottle by pushing the plunger all the way down. Putting air in the bottle makes it easier to get the insulin out.

➠ Take the needle out of the cloudy insulin bottle. The syringe will be empty. Set the cloudy insulin bottle aside.

➠ Pull the plunger of the syringe down to the number of units of clear insulin needed to fill with air.

➠ Put the needle into the stopper of the clear insulin bottle and push the air into the bottle.

➠ Turn the clear insulin bottle upside down with the syringe still in place. Support the needle so it does not bend.

➠ Pull the plunger down to the number of units of clear insulin you need.

➠ Check for air bubbles in the syringe.

➠ Pull down on the plunger and fill the syringe with the correct amount of insulin.

➠ Take the needle out of the clear insulin bottle.

➠ Put the needle into the rubber stopper of the cloudy insulin bottle.

➠ Be careful not to push any clear insulin into the cloudy insulin bottle.

➠ Slowly pull the plunger back to the total number of units needed. This lets the cloudy insulin fill the syringe.

➠ Take the needle out of the cloudy insulin bottle.

repeated use, and the silicon lubricant wears off. There is also some evidence that reusing needles with damaged tips causes repeated small injuries to the tissue when injecting. This can cause a release of certain growth factors that may lead to the development of fatty lumps (lipohypertrophy) which may affect the amount of insulin required and its absorption.

Isophane insulin may solidify in the needle, so either change the needle every time or at least eject 2 or 3 units into the air before each injection to make sure the needle is clear.

Different pens for daytime and night time insulin

It is easy to take the wrong pen injector by mistake if the pens for daytime and night time insulin are similar. To avoid taking the wrong type of insulin, we recommend that you always use two completely different pens for daytime and bedtime insulin, so that you can feel the difference even if it is completely dark. If you have experienced taking the wrong type of insulin even once, having two completely different pens can start to look like a cheap form of life insurance.

Air in the cartridge or syringe

When the cartridge warms up with the needle attached (e.g. when you carry it in an inner pocket), the liquid in the cartridge will expand

An insulin pen.

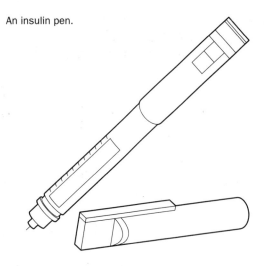

and a few drops will leak out through the needle. When the temperature falls again, air will be sucked in. In one study, the surrounding temperature was lowered from 27° to 15°C (81° to 59°F). This caused air corresponding to 4 units of insulin to be sucked into the cartridge.

A particular problem will occur with intermediate-acting insulin when the temperature is

Needles for insulin pens

Brand	Diameter of needle	Size of needle	Length
B-D Micro-Fine+	0.25 mm	31G	5 mm
NovoFine	0.25 mm	31G	6 mm
Penfine	0.25 mm	31G	6 mm
Unifine	0.30 mm	30G	6 mm
B-D Micro-Fine+	0.25 mm	31G	8 mm
Penfine	0.25 mm	31G	8 mm
Unifine	0.30 mm	30G	8 mm
NovoFine	0.30 mm	30G	8 mm
Omnican mini	0.30 mm	30G	8 mm
Penfine	0.33 mm	29G	10 mm
Penfine	0.33 mm	29G	12 mm
Omnican fine	0.33 mm	29G	12 mm
Unifine	0.33 mm	29G	12 mm
B-D Micro-Fine+	0.33 mm	29G	13 mm
NovoFine	0.36 mm	28G	12 mm
Optipen	0.36 mm	28G	12 mm

lowered. As the insulin is in the cloudy substance that sinks to the bottom of the cartridge, only the inactive solution will leak out through the needle. The result will be that the remaining insulin will become more potent, up to a concentration of 120 or 140 units/ml. If the pen is stored upside down, the problem will be reversed. The insulin crystals will then be closest to the needle and leak out when the temperature increases and the liquid expands. The remaining insulin will then be diluted. In one study, the insulin concentration in used vials and cartridges of NPH insulin that had not been mixed thoroughly varied between 5 and 200 units/ml.

The problem of altered concentration will not occur with clear insulins as the insulin is completely dissolved in the liquid. However, the air as such can cause problems of accuracy. You will be less likely to have problems if you remove the needle after each injection and store the pen with the top pointing upwards, for example in the pocket of your jacket. It is possible, on occasion, to accidentally inject a bubble of air from the syringe or cartridge along with the insulin. Subcutaneously placed air is quite harmless to the body and will soon be absorbed by the tissue. The real problem is that you will have missed out on a certain amount of insulin (as much as was misplaced by the air). You may need to take a unit or two extra to compensate for this. The same also applies if you are using an insulin pump (see below). Air injected through the tubing is completely harmless, but you will have missed a certain amount of insulin at the same time which may cause problems.

Insulin on the pen needle

Sometimes a drop of insulin will leak from the tip of the needle after it has been withdrawn from the skin. The drop contains up to 1 unit of insulin and is caused by air in the cartridge which is compressed when you press the pen mechanism. You can avoid this problem by waiting about 15 seconds for the air to expand before withdrawing the pen needle. You can also remove the needle after each injection, which will prevent air from being sucked into the cartridge. This problem will not occur when you are using a syringe because you inject all the insulin it contains. Remove the air in the pen cartridge according to the illustration on this page. Even if all air is removed, it is a good idea to hold the needle in for 10 seconds to prevent insulin dripping from the tip of the needle.

Used needles and syringes

Discard used syringes, pen needles and finger-pricking lancets in a special sharps box so that no one will be pricked by mistake. Sharps boxes and their disposal should be the responsibility of the local council. If you have trouble with this service, ask your diabetes specialist nurse for advice. You can get a special cutter (B-D Safe-Clip, see overleaf) to remove needle points.

Automatic injectors

An automatic injector will thrust the needle very quickly through the skin, and this keeps pain to a minimum. With one type (Injectomatic, Inject-Ease) the syringe needle is pushed through the skin automatically, but you have to push the insulin in yourself. A similar device (Pen-Mate)

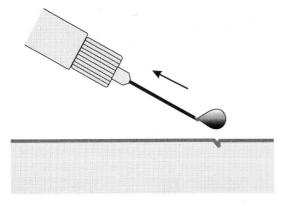

If there is air inside the pen cartridge, you may see a drop of liquid coming out from the needle-tip after your have withdrawn the needle from your skin.

How to get rid of the air in the insulin cartridge

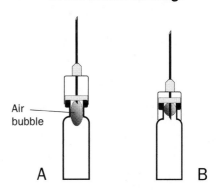

Air bubble

A   B

When you replace the needle you can get rid of the air by following these steps:

1 When the needle is removed, depress the pen mechanism a few times so that the pressure inside the cartridge will be increased. Tap on the cartridge to make the air rise.

2 Slowly push the needle through the membrane on the cartridge.

3 Air will leak out as soon as the needle penetrates the membrane. If you push the needle through the membrane too quickly an air pocket will remain in neck of the cartridge (see illustration).

Push the needle slowly through the membrane when you replace it to allow air to leak out (A). When the needle is pushed quickly all the way in, a small pocket of air is formed in the neck of the cartridge (B).

is available for the pen injectors from Novo Nordisk. With another type (Autoject) the syringe needle is pushed in and the insulin is injected automatically. The Diapen both inserts the needle and injects the insulin automatically. The Autopen is a pen injector that injects the insulin automatically after you have pricked the skin yourself with the needle.

Jet injectors

A jet injector uses very high pressure to form a thin jet stream (thinner than a needle) of insulin that penetrates the skin. The insulin is absorbed quickly, and the glucose control can be as good as it is with an insulin pump. Some people find the device less painful while others experience the pain of the jet injector as comparable with that of an ordinary injection needle. A jet injector might be a good alternative for people with pronounced needle-phobia if they are not helped by using an Insuflon.

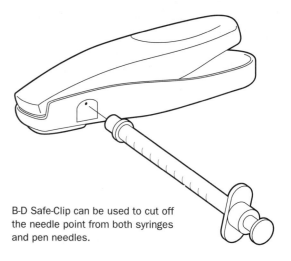

B-D Safe-Clip can be used to cut off the needle point from both syringes and pen needles.

Insuflon

An Insuflon is an indwelling catheter which makes multiple injection treatment much easier. It is used particularly for young children with Type 1 diabetes, but also has a role for older patients with Type 2 diabetes who are new to using insulin. It can be particularly helpful for those patients who find the idea of injections unduly distressing.

Insulin pumps

The rationale for using insulin pumps has been extensively studied for patients with Type 1 diabetes. There is good evidence that patients using them have better blood glucose control, and less weight gain, and a number of studies have shown an associated improvement in quality of life. Not surprisingly, as by far the greatest proportion of patients have Type 2 diabetes, clinicians have begun looking at the value of using insulin pumps in this group. Here we'll look at the rationale and evidence for using pumps, particularly in an older patient group with Type 2 diabetes.

What is an insulin pump, and why bother with one in Type 2 diabetes?

An insulin pump is a small battery-operated infusion pump which delivers insulin continu-

ously via a small catheter device under the skin. The pump is set up to deliver a background lower rate of insulin delivery to cope with requirements outside mealtimes, and there is a facility on the pump to deliver an extra burst of insulin to cope with a meal. The amount of insulin needed at mealtimes is estimated by the pump user according to the carbohydrate content of the meal. To deliver insulin in this kind of profile with separate injections would require you to inject several times a day.

We know from a number of different studies that whether you live in Germany, England or America, your blood glucose control isn't as good as it should be, no matter if you have Type 2 diabetes and are managed with diet, metformin or insulin. Many patients with Type 2 diabetes take their insulin as twice a day mixed insulin injections, this is a bit un-physiological (not like real life), and may be associated with worse blood glucose control and more weight gain compared with multiple injections or a pump. So if you need to take insulin for your

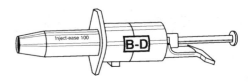

The Inject-Ease will insert the syringe needle automatically when you press the spring.

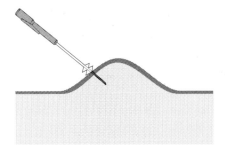

The catheter can peel backwards on the metal needle (called 'peel-back') if you penetrate the skin too slowly. This is a typical beginner's problem.

Type 2 diabetes, multiple daily injections or a pump infusion device may be a better way to deliver it.

What do the studies say about using pumps in Type 2 diabetes?

The best study to look at is one where older patients with Type 2 diabetes (above 60 years of age, with poor glucose control or on one or more insulin injections a day), were randomized to go onto either the Minimed insulin pump or onto multiple injections of insulin when they were failing on at least one injection of insulin per day to get their glucose to a target HbA_{1c} of 7%. Very overweight people with a body mass index (BMI) of more than 45 were excluded from entering this study. What the study showed was that both an intensive regime of lots of insulin injections and pump therapy achieved a significant improvement in HbA_{1c} of around 1.5% over a year. There wasn't a great deal of

Tips for using indwelling catheters

- Use topical anaesthetic cream (e.g. EMLA, lidocaine) when inserting the cannula, especially if you are new to the technique. Apply it 1–2 hours before insertion.

- Lift a skin fold and insert the Insuflon at a 45° angle. Lift the skin with three or four fingers if the subcutaneous tissue is thin.

- Insert with a slight thrust and there will be less risk of 'peel-back'.

- Apply the end of the adhesive that covers the insertion site first. Never try to remove an adhesive that is already stuck to the skin.

- Insert the injection needle with the opening turned towards the skin and it will not get stuck on the plastic wall. Rotate the needle gently.

- Use an adhesive of stoma-type (such as Compeed) if you experience itching or eczema from the enclosed adhesive.

- Use a 8–10 mm needle for both pens and syringes and there will be no risk of piercing the Teflon catheter by pushing the needle too far in. With the new Insuflon design, different needle lengths may be used – check the inserted instructions.

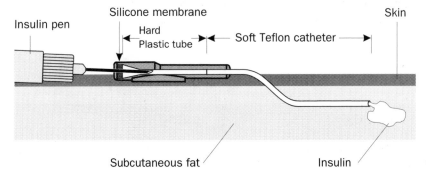

When using an Insuflon, you pierce a silicone membrane (instead of the skin) with the needle. The soft Teflon catheter is placed under the skin, and you inject the insulin through it. The catheter is replaced on average every 4–5 days. This can easily be done at home. If it is painful, you can use a topical anaesthetic cream before replacement.

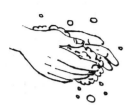

Hygiene is particularly important if you use an indwelling catheter or an insulin pump. Always wash your hands before replacing the catheter. We recommend using chlorhexidine in alcohol for disinfecting the insertion site.

difference between patient groups in how they scored quality of life, the amount of weight they put on or the number of times they suffered from low blood sugars. Several other case studies have been presented and suggest that pump therapy may be a good option for more obese people as there is less tendency to over-use insulin and end up having to eat to avoid a hypo, which causes more weight gain. Unfortunately, a good study like this one but in the very overweight doesn't actually exist.

What's the conclusion?

Insulin pumps are very expensive but they may suit some people with Type 2 diabetes. It's likely though that they will have been through lots of other options – tablets, single-dose insulin, dual insulin, multi-dose insulin, and so on. The evidence published so far suggests that in people who can cope with multiple injections, the data for blood glucose control are just as good. What we don't have is long-term data on blood glucose, or any data on the complications of diabetes. There is also no evidence for early introduction of the insulin pump in Type 2 diabetes as the majority of studies have been conducted with people already on at least one insulin injection per day.

Also, pump users have to be motivated, interested and have the skill to manipulate the machinery. It's necessary to have both the brains to take on the kit and the interest! Until the price of the technology reduces and the evidence base grows, pump therapy is likely to remain out of reach, certainly for most patients. In the longer term, as the technology for continuous glucose sensing improves, there may come a time when an integrated sensor for glucose can be built into

the insulin pump, with an algorithm for the computer to automatically regulate the insulin delivered. This would finally bring about the prospect of greater improvements in quality of life for a significant number of patients.

Unfortunately, pumps are not recommended by the National Institute for Health and Clinical Excellence (NICE) for people with Type 2 diabetes so you will probably have to fund the pump yourself. The approximate cost (2008 prices) is £2000 for a pump and a spare, plus £60–80 running costs per month.

New methods of insulin delivery

Inhaled insulin

Exubera inhaled insulin became available in 2006 and could be used in the UK by patients with severe fear of needles. However the take up was generally poor and the manufacturers (Pfizer) withdrew production and sales of Exubera in October 2007. Other insulin manufacturers are developing their own forms of giving inhaled insulin.

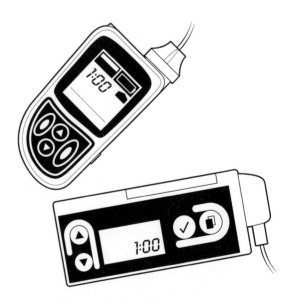

Modern insulin pumps are small and easy to manage.

As we learn more about this method of insulin delivery, it will become an important treatment option for patients unable or unwilling to take short-acting insulin injections. Currently, while further studies and information are awaited, NICE has placed quite severe restrictions on the use of the product.

In development

Other methods of insulin delivery under investigation include modified-release capsules, and delivery via an aerosol device which administers insulin via the skin lining the inside of the mouth.

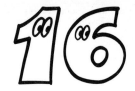

Changing insulin requirements

When insulin treatment is first suggested to people with Type 2 diabetes, they may be dismayed. But once they have started insulin, they are often pleased to discover how much better they can feel.

Tablets with insulin: what can you expect?

There may be an overlap of quite some time during which people with Type 2 diabetes continue to take their tablets even though they have started on insulin. So, what can you expect if you are receiving this type of treatment?

Insulin and metformin

Metformin is used in combination with insulin to reduce your total insulin requirements and minimize any weight gain associated with insulin treatment. One study of Type 2 diabetes (by Douek) involved starting people on insulin alone, or starting insulin and continuing metformin treatment. Those people who continued metformin gained less weight and required a smaller total daily dose of insulin. Additionally, the greater the dose of metformin, the more effective it was at reducing the insulin dose.

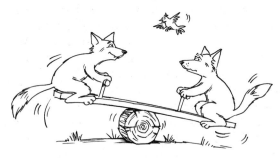

It's all a question of balance . . .

Unfortunately not everyone can take metformin, particularly if they have problems with their kidneys. Your doctor will advise if you have to stop metformin treatment when you begin insulin.

Triple regime

A triple regime with metformin, a glitazone and insulin treatment is becoming more popular. Insulin should be added to the glitazone rather than vice versa: adding the glitazone as a last resort is more likely to cause water retention. One study involved adding insulin to Avandamet – a combined tablet of rosiglitazone and metformin. This showed better control and a lower insulin dose than stopping all tablets and using insulin on its own.

Unfortunately, there are also restrictions on the use of glitazones, particularly in patients with heart failure. You should be carefully assessed before starting a glitazone. If you develop ankle swelling or shortness of breath, you should see your doctor as soon as possible for a review of your medication.

It is also possible to continue metformin and a sulphonylurea at the same time as starting insulin. This is usually done when a long-acting insulin is started at night. The sulphonylurea still provides some cover for the peaks of sugar which follow meals.

Moving towards treatment by insulin alone

In time, you may progress to being treated by insulin alone. The amount of insulin you need may also go up as time goes by. When you first

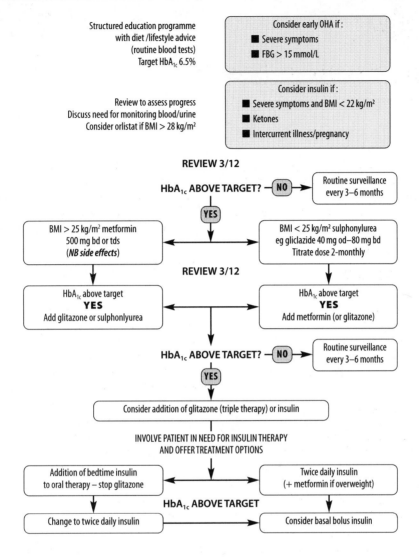

Structured education programme
with diet /lifestyle advice
(routine blood tests)
Target HbA₁c 6.5%

Consider early OHA if :
■ Severe symptoms
■ FBG > 15 mmol/L

Review to assess progress
Discuss need for monitoring blood/urine
Consider orlistat if BMI > 28 kg/m²

Consider insulin if :
■ Severe symptoms and BMI < 22 kg/m²
■ Ketones
■ Intercurrent illness/pregnancy

REVIEW 3/12

HbA₁c ABOVE TARGET? — NO → Routine surveillance every 3–6 months

YES

BMI > 25 kg/m² metformin
500 mg bd or tds
(NB side effects)

BMI < 25 kg/m² sulphonylurea
eg gliclazide 40 mg od–80 mg bd
Titrate dose 2-monthly

REVIEW 3/12

HbA₁c above target
YES
Add glitazone or sulphonlyurea

HbA₁c above target
YES
Add metformin (or glitazone)

HbA₁c ABOVE TARGET? — NO → Routine surveillance every 3–6 months

YES

Consider addition of glitazone (triple therapy) or insulin

INVOLVE PATIENT IN NEED FOR INSULIN THERAPY
AND OFFER TREATMENT OPTIONS

Addition of bedtime insulin
to oral therapy – stop glitazone

Twice daily insulin
(+ metformin if overweight)

HbA₁c ABOVE TARGET

Change to twice daily insulin

Consider basal bolus insulin

This chart is typical of the guidelines your doctor will be following in planning your care.
(BMI = body mass index).

start taking insulin (with or without tablets) and each time the doses change, you will be encouraged to be particularly careful about monitoring and reporting your own blood glucose levels. You should be kept under close medical supervision to see how the new regime suits you.

Your regime may be made up of different types of insulin, all acting at different speeds, so that your body's needs are supplied in an even manner throughout the day and night.

The first insulin to be made was clear soluble insulin, which was short acting. When short-acting insulin is injected under the skin, it works within about 30 minutes and lasts for 4–8 hours. Over time, various modifications have been made to this original insulin so that it will continue to work for longer after injection. When protamine or zinc is incorporated into soluble insulin, a single injection can last from 12–24 hours.

For many years, doctors advised people with

Five common insulin regimes

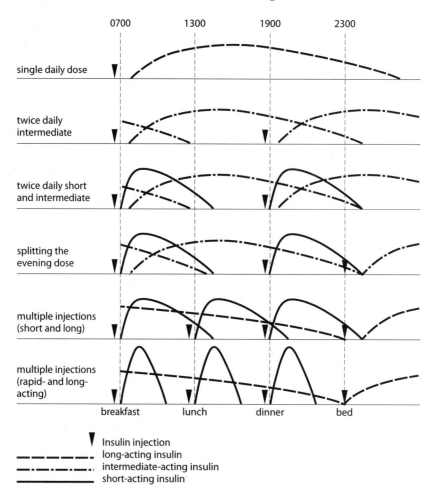

diabetes to take a single daily injection, but it became clear that this was not a good way of controlling the variations in blood glucose that occur during the day. Today, many people who need insulin take a mixture of short-, intermediate- and long-acting insulins during the day. Your doctor or nurse will work with you to find out what sort of pattern of insulin-taking, and what combination of different types of insulin, suits you and your lifestyle the best.

You may find there is a need for trial and error in your insulin regime early on but it should stabilize over the first few weeks or months. But all people on insulin go through periods when the amount of medication they need comes under review, for very good reasons.

Why might an insulin regime need changing?

A number of factors affect how much insulin you will need. These include:

- The length of time you have had Type 2 diabetes, as the body's ability to produce natural insulin gradually declines.

- Your weight, diet and general level of

fitness – keeping these at the best possible levels will mean that you need less insulin.

- Life changes such as retirement may have an effect on the amount and type of activity you carry out.

- Your general health: for example, if you are feverish, or have a surgical operation, you are likely to need additional insulin.

Some people also find that weather and how hot or cold they are affects their insulin requirements. This may be an indirect effect as being too hot makes people unwilling to exercise and being cold might encourage them to eat more. It may simply be a question of skin temperature. It is worth thinking about how these factors affect you and your blood glucose.

It is important that you monitor your blood glucose levels carefully (see Chapter 11) at any time when you are changing your treatment regimen. Ideally, the process of careful monitoring should be started a couple of weeks before any changes are made, and continue for several weeks after.

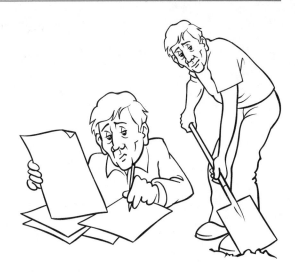

Your lifestyle can change dramatically when you retire; so can the nature and amount of activity you do.

and, possibly, the type of insulin you inject.

If you don't understand why your blood glucose reading turned out the way it did, try keeping to the same doses for another day or two. You will often see the pattern improve.

Blood glucose goals

The American Diabetes Association recommends that blood glucose goals should be individualized and that lower goals may be reasonable on benefit–risk assessment.

If you find a low blood glucose (less than 4 mmol/L) at a time when you have no symptoms of a hypo, you may have lost warning signs of hypoglycaemia, which is a potentially serious situation and affects your ability to drive. You need to discuss this with your doctor as there are strategies available to help you regain your warning signs. If you find you are low at 2 am, this has particular significance and may mean that this is happening regularly without you being aware of this. This low blood glucose at night is well recognized as a cause of high morning blood sugars caused by a rebound effect. If you discover that this is happening to you, it is important to correct this by changing your dose

Managing your insulin doses

When you're on insulin and there is need for a change in treatment due to suboptimal glucose control or increased hypoglycaemia, you need to monitor more often. Before altering doses though, you should check a range of values – some in the morning, some two hours after a meal, some directly before a meal and some before going to bed.

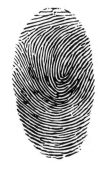

Just as all fingerprints are different, insulin doses vary, and unfortunately they often seem to work differently every day. This is perfectly logical if you think about it – we are all very different as individuals, and insulin must be adjusted to fit the individual lifestyle.

Keeping good records

Register all blood glucose readings in your notebook, otherwise you can never make an adequate judgement. If you have difficulties remembering to write them down, an electronic notebook can be a good alternative. Most blood glucose meters have memories and can be connected to a computer to be read. In an American study, patients who recorded their blood glucose readings properly had lower HbA_{1c} values (7.1% compared with 7.9%) than those who did not record their tests.

What to do if your blood glucose level is high

You should not worry if you have a single high blood glucose reading. It is important to look for patterns of blood glucose in the course of a day. Having done so, you should make a decision about changing insulin to correct the results that are outside target. If you constantly chase high and low blood glucose results with changes in your insulin dose, you may find you never know which insulin is causing the problem. You can end up chasing your tail. You also have to accept the irritating fact that sometimes, when you are trying very hard and doing everything according to the book, you will have an unexplained high or low glucose level.

Whatever the problem with your glucose control on insulin is, you can usually work with your doctor or diabetes nurse to rectify it.

A large number of individuals with Type 2 diabetes are on twice a day mixed insulin (short- and longer-acting insulins pre-mixed together). If the total insulin dose is insufficient to get the HbA_{1c} to target, increasing it may cause hypoglycaemia.

One solution to this difficulty is to move to mealtime injections of short-acting insulin accompanied by one injection of long-acting insulin. This allows your insulin to be tailored much more towards peaks of food intake.

Similarly, if you've been started on one insulin injection per day in conjunction with tablets, there may come a time when the amount that the insulin can be increased is limited by low blood sugars between meals, reducing the chance of getting your HbA_{1c} to target. This often coincides with reduced effectiveness of any tablets to lower your glucose at mealtimes. If this is the case, the best solution is to switch to two or four insulin injections per day.

Side effects and problems with insulin treatment

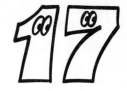

This chapter discusses some of the potential side effects and problems with insulin. The main problems for people with Type 2 diabetes are weight gain, particularly during the first few months, and hypoglycaemia. The chapter also discusses why people with Type 2 diabetes may need more insulin than those with Type 1 diabetes, along with problems which may affect your injection sites.

Many people are concerned about the idea of having to inject themselves, but this often proves to be much worse in anticipation than in reality. You can find more information about administering insulin, including injection techniques and other methods and equipment that are available, elsewhere.

Insulin and weight gain

By now, you will be well aware that Type 2 diabetes is closely associated with being overweight, particularly around the abdomen (central obesity). As described in earlier chapters, this results in insulin resistance, which in turn leads to failure of the beta cells in the pancreas. As a result, your glucose begins to rise and you find yourself with symptoms of diabetes.

Eventually, after a variable number of years, blood glucose-lowering tablets become less effective and your blood sugar can start to rise. Instead of being processed into energy stores, this sugar remains in the bloodstream and can accumulate, causing damage. It also passes out into the urine, which can of course be detected when the urine is tested. By reducing the amount of sugar lost in the urine, insulin prevents calorie loss by this route and converts glucose into energy stores, thus causing weight gain.

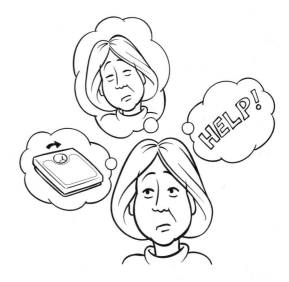

If you are not careful this can lead to substantial weight gain of around 3–6 kg after starting insulin. You can control this by reducing your portion size and being sensible

---

Key concerns people have about insulin treatment

- How will I cope with the injections?
- Will I gain weight on insulin treatment, why does this happen, and how can I limit it if possible?
- What about hypoglycaemia and insulin treatment?
- Why do people with Type 2 diabetes need more insulin than those with Type 1 diabetes?
- How do I avoid problems with injection sites?

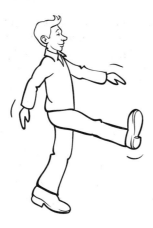

You will need to be careful about keeping your weight under control when you start on insulin. Making sure you get enough exercise will help.

about trying to exercise where you can. If you are on a twice a day regime, you could plan to exercise during the day, for example spending a couple of hours working in the garden – enough to make you slightly short of breath. This allows you to continue working without needing to snack to prevent low blood sugars. The work you have done will then be translated into weight loss.

A basal bolus insulin regime, where you take one long-acting insulin injection per day and three mealtime short-acting ones, may be associated with less weight gain. This is because the insulin that you take mimics the natural insulin response to meals much more closely and you don't need to snack to feed your insulin. Of course, four injections per day doesn't suit every-

one, and if you choose a two injections per day regime, this should lead to a substantial improvement in your long-term blood glucose control.

There is some evidence that the new long-acting insulin analogues, Lantus (glargine) and Levemir (detemir) may be associated with less weight gain. Various theories have been put forward to explain this observation. Levemir, in particular, binds to human albumin, a protein found in the blood. This may mean it is less likely to cause hunger and may have slightly different effects on the liver compared with other insulins.

Sometimes glitazones (rosiglitazone or pioglitazone) are used in combination with insulin treatment. Studies have shown that the combination improves control of blood glucose. But the risk of fluid retention and weight gain must be taken into account when deciding on this combination.

In contrast, combining metformin with insulin leads to less weight gain and better control than using insulin alone. If you had minor stomach upsets on metformin, you may find the slow-release preparation suits you better.

Hypoglycaemia

People who take tablets for diabetes are only at risk of hypos if they take sulphonyureas or repaglinide, both of which work by stimulating insulin production by the pancreas. The risk of hypos from these tablets is highest when they are first being used, or in older people who may not eat properly after taking these tablets. In such cases, hypos can be prolonged and dangerous. However, none of the other tablets used to control diabetes can cause troublesome hypos.

People with Type 2 diabetes treated with insulin are at risk of hypos, though the problem is usually less challenging than in Type 1 diabetes.

In one population-based study, patients with Type 2 diabetes taking insulin suffered around 16 hypoglycaemia events per year. This would translate into one event about every 23 days.

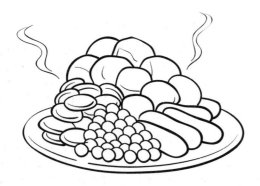

Think carefully about portion size at mealtimes.

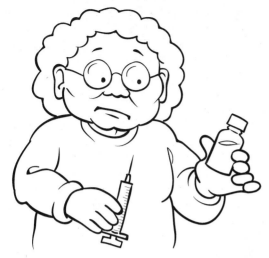

Don't put up with frequent hypos. Consult your diabetes team to suggest how to avoid hypos while keeping your blood glucose under good control.

Severe events which required the patient to have help from another person were much more rare, with a rate of 0.35 per year. In other words, a patient could expect one event about every 3 years.

While this may seem a relatively minor problem to most people, if you are working as a commercial driver, for example in a minicab, this may be significant. (See the section on driving and diabetes, page 180.)

If you live alone or are elderly, then the prospect of having a hypoglycaemic attack may seem very scary. As a consequence, some people do not to take quite as much insulin as they need to avoid hypoglycaemia. Thus, sugars begin to rise and overall control is not as good as it should be. With the right support from your diabetes team, you should be able to work through these problems and reduce the likelihood of hypoglycaemia, while preserving good glucose control.

Long-acting insulin analogues, Lantus and Levemir, may cause less hypoglycaemia as well as reduced weight gain. A number of studies have shown that neither Lantus nor Levemir has peaks of action. This reduces the chance of having too much long-acting insulin, which prevents blood glucose levels from falling too low.

If you take a twice a day mixed insulin preparation and you have troublesome hypoglycaemia without reaching your target HbA_{1c}, the likelihood is that your diabetes nurse or doctor will recommend switching to three injections of short- or rapid-acting insulin and one injection of long-acting insulin per day. Depending on the policy in your local area the long-acting insulin may be an older or newer analogue type. If it is one of the older long-acting insulins and you still suffer from hypos, switching to an analogue insulin would be the next option.

Why do patients with Type 2 diabetes have to take such large amounts of insulin?

As we discussed earlier in the book, one of the primary defects associated with Type 2 diabetes is insulin resistance. Put very simply, this means that you need more insulin to reduce your blood glucose to a given level than someone who is insulin sensitive.

Developing insulin resistance lies at the heart of the pathway to developing Type 2 diabetes itself. You are partly genetically predisposed to developing diabetes, and the remainder of your risk of becoming insulin resistant comes from a sedentary lifestyle and over-eating.

This leads to an over-accumulation of fats in the body, particularly in the liver and muscles. They may also interfere with the ability of the pancreas to produce insulin.

Insulin resistance syndrome

People with Type 2 diabetes develop the insulin resistance syndrome, which is characterized by obesity, particularly an accumulation of fat around the abdomen, raised blood sugar levels, raised levels of fats or triglycerides, and raised blood pressure.

In essence, where glucose is concerned, being insulin resistant means that your raised blood sugar levels may be overcome but, in order to achieve this, you may need many times more

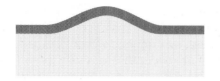

Insulin causes the subcutaneous tissue to grow if you inject frequently into the same spot. You will get a 'fatty lump' (lipohypertrophy) in the skin that feels and looks like a soft bump.

insulin than a person with Type 1 diabetes who is the same weight. This is because Type 1 diabetes is caused by a failure of the beta cells, not by insulin resistance.

Reducing the insulin dose

You can do something to reduce your insulin dose. There is some evidence that drugs which increase insulin sensitivity, namely metformin and the glitazones, should reduce your insulin requirements. Metformin is less good at doing this but has the advantage of reducing the weight gain associated with insulin therapy.

The glitazones may spectacularly reduce the amount of insulin you need to control your blood sugar, but this is at the expense of increasing weight gain. Glitazones are not licensed for use in every country in conjunction with insulin because of the risk of fluid retention, so this may not be an option depending on where you live.

Problems at the injection sites

Two conditions are associated with injecting insulin that you need to be aware of: lipoatrophy and lipohypertrophy. Some people also experience redness at the injection site.

Lipoatrophy

Lipoatrophy is related to shrinkage and disappearance of subcutaneous fat in the area where you have injected insulin. One of the causes is thought to be the formation of antibodies to the insulin injected into the subcutaneous tissue.

The use of pork or beef insulin was associated with a much higher rate of antibody formation. Of course, most people now take human insulin or a modified 'insulin analogue'. Lipoatrophy is virtually never seen with these insulins.

Lipohypertrophy

Lipohypertrophy is seen much more commonly. If insulin is injected repeatedly in the same area, fat is laid down at this site and can interfere with insulin absorption. This can then lead to great unpredictability in the speed with which the insulin is released, but it usually slows it down and causes hyperglycaemia.

Lipohypertrophy seems to occur less frequently in Type 2 diabetes than in Type 1 diabetes. This is possibly because lipohyper-

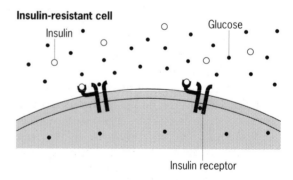

The diagram on the left shows the surface of a normal cell, which contains around 20,000 receptor sites. The receptors attract the molecules of insulin and glucose, containing them. The diagram on the right shows an insulin-resistant cell. This contains only about a quarter of the number of receptor sites to that in a normal cell. As a result, only around 25% of the glucose and insulin molecules can be contained, leading to a lot of free-floating (unstable) glucose and insulin.

trophy is less easy to identify in people who are overweight. In Type 1 diabetes, lipohypertrophy occurs in up to 20–30% of patients, though the incidence in people with Type 2 diabetes is thought to be only around 4%.

A group of patients with lipohypertrophy who had poor glycaemic control were followed in one study after a period of education about rotating injection sites and not injecting into lipohypertrophied tissue. In this study, within only three months HbA_{1c} declined from 7.9% to 7% and total insulin requirements were significantly reduced.

If you aren't sure about which sites you can use for injecting insulin, or about how you rotate them, talk to your healthcare professional about this.

Redness at injection sites

Redness, sometimes with itching, that occurs immediately or within hours of an insulin injection can be due to an allergy towards the insulin or a preservative. This type of reaction will usually subside after some years as you continue with insulin treatment. Tell your doctor if you have problems with redness after injections. A special skin test is available to find out whether you are allergic to the insulin or the preservative. There is often an increased level of insulin antibodies in the blood as well (see below). If problems with redness continue, so-called antihistamine tablets can be helpful. Adding a small amount of corticosteroids to the insulin may also help. Switching to rapid-acting insulin (NovoRapid or Humalog) has reduced the problem with redness after injections in some cases.

It is important to make sure your insulin has not passed its use-by date and that it is store correctly (see page 106). Inappropriate storage conditions can result in the insulin breaking down and give rise to harmful substances that can cause local allergic reactions. A generalized allergic reaction after insulin injection is very rare.

Allergy to the nickel in pen and syringe needles can cause redness after injections. The needles are covered with a layer of silicone lubricant. If you are allergic to nickel you should not use the needles more than once as the silicone layer wears off and the nickel will come in closer contact with the skin. Needles on syringes have a thicker silicone layer since they need to penetrate the membrane of the bottle when drawing up insulin. For this reason, they will be more appropriate if you are allergic to nickel. You can have a skin test to see whether this is the case. If you are allergic to nickel, you will usually react to it in other items as well, for example earrings, belt buckles or wrist watches.

Insulin antibodies

Your body will produce antibodies to 'defend' itself against foreign substances. Insulin antibodies were common with pork and beef insulin. With the use of human insulin, it is not common to have sufficiently high levels of antibodies to cause problems. In Type 2 diabetes, insulin antibodies do not appear to affect the action of insulin.

Anticipating the problems

Common problems associated with insulin therapy such as weight gain or hypoglycaemia can be managed with appropriate intervention. The amount of insulin you take is not important, and you should not compare notes with your friend who has Type 1 diabetes. If you happen to need large doses of insulin to control blood glucose, this is not because your diabetes is particularly severe but simply reflects a high level of insulin resistance which is part of the cause of Type 2 diabetes. Side effects associated with insulin therapy, such as lipohypertrophy, can be avoided with some basic measures around injection technique. As always, if there is something you are not sure about with respect to your insulin therapy, do ask.

Hypoglycaemia

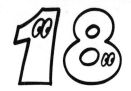

Hypoglycaemia means 'low blood glucose'. A number of different symptoms can be experienced when the blood glucose is low, and some of these may occur with other conditions or as a response to other problems in the body. Most people, particularly those in the first few years of diabetes, get 'sensations' warning of hypoglycaemia before their blood glucose falls to dangerously low levels.

In addition, hypoglycaemia is rare in Type 2 diabetes unless people are treated with suphonylurea tablets or insulin. Many patients may not experience a severe attack of hypoglycaemia for many, many years. With the use of modern insulin regimes and shorter-acting sulphonylureas, significant hypoglycaemia is becoming rarer still. Patients on metformin or glitazones suffer hypoglycaemic attacks very infrequently and, even when these do occur, they tend to be mild in nature. For this reason, a number of problems and solutions described in this chapter may never apply to you.

The glucose level can be measured as whole-blood glucose or plasma glucose. Most patient meters now display plasma glucose, and for the purposes of this book the numbers refer to plasma blood glucose levels. If you have books or references which refer to whole-blood glucose levels, corresponding plasma levels are around 11% higher.

Not everyone will have the same symptoms when they develop hypoglycaemia. However, the symptoms usually follow the same pattern for each person. In the early stages of drug treatment for Type 2 diabetes, particularly if you are prescribed metformin, it is very unlikely you will suffer hypoglycaemia at all. Indeed, many healthcare professionals think that home monitoring of glucose levels probably isn't necessary in the early stages of Type 2 diabetes. Patients with Type 2 diabetes who are most at risk of attacks of hypoglycaemia are those patients taking sulphonyl-

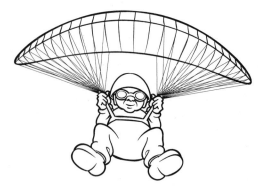

Avoid situations where hypoglycaemia could have catastrophic consequences. This does not mean that it is impossible for people with Type 2 diabetes who are taking sulphonylurea combination therapies or insulin to engage in risky sports such as mountain climbing, paragliding or scuba diving. What it does mean, however, is that they should prepare carefully, thinking about the sorts of adverse situations that could arise, tailoring their food intake and medication towards the expected activity.

ureas or on insulin treatment. When you start either of these two treatments, your doctor or nurse will explain about the symptoms of hypoglycaemia and will encourage you to test your glucose at home. This will help you learn how to recognize the way your body reacts to hypoglycaemia. When you start insulin treatment, it is worth explaining to partners or other close family members what they need to do to treat hypoglycaemia in a safe and effective manner.

Usually, symptoms of hypoglycaemia are divided into two categories:

- symptoms caused by the body attempting to raise the blood glucose level, by adrenaline for example (known as 'autonomic' or 'adrenergic' symptoms);
- symptoms originating in the brain as a result of a deficiency of glucose in the central nervous system ('neuroglycopenic' symptoms).

See the key fact boxes overleaf.

When a person with diabetes starts to become hypoglycaemic, it is bodily symptoms (e.g. shakiness, heart pounding) he or she is likely to notice first. However, observers are more likely to be aware of symptoms such as irritability, and behavioural changes, which indicate the brain is being affected. The brain's reaction to hypoglycaemia is usually triggered at a slightly lower blood glucose level than the symptoms from the body.

The brain is very sensitive to hypoglycaemia so the body automatically reacts to try and avoid this. Adults seem to cope a little better than children with low blood glucose concentrations as they experience neuroglycopenic symptoms (i.e. symptoms from the brain; see above) at lower blood glucose concentrations of 2.8–3.0 mmol/L, 50–55 mg/dl).

Hypoglycaemia is usually an unpleasant experience, involving loss of control over your body. This is indeed what happens as the brain does not function well without glucose. Some people become unusually irritable, while others may look pale, sick or sleepy. Occasionally, people something uncharacteristically dangerous or stupid that may damage themselves or someone else. Traffic accidents on a bicycle or in a car can sometimes be caused by hypoglycaemia (see page 131). Sometimes people do really strange things, so it is very important for your family and friends to understand that you are not quite in control of yourself when you are having a hypo, and you cannot help what you are doing.

Even if individuals with diabetes are aware of having symptoms of hypoglycaemia, they may find it difficult to eat or drink. This can still be a problem if food is right in front of them. Observers find this difficult to understand, but patients describe the feeling as: 'You know you should drink the juice, but your body just does not obey the orders from the brain'.

If the blood glucose is lowered quickly, even if it stays within the normal range, some people will continue to feel hypoglycaemic. This type of reaction is more common in people with a high HbA$_{1c}$ (see page 135) and can occur people with Type 2 diabetes starting insulin. In one study, in a group of adults with diabetes with an HbA$_{1c}$ of 11%, the blood glucose was lowered from 20 to 10 mmol/L (360–180 mg/dl) using intravenous insulin. These subjects showed the same type of increased blood flow to the brain that both people in good control and people without diabetes had at a blood glucose of 2.2 mmol/L (40 mg/dl).

Blood glucose levels and symptoms of hypoglycaemia

Symptoms of hypoglycaemia may not be recognized by a person with diabetes, particularly when the focus of his or her attention is

---

Stages of hypoglycaemia

1 Mild hypoglycaemia
Minor symptoms. Self-treatment is possible, and blood glucose levels are easily restored.

2 Moderate hypoglycaemia
Your body reacts with warning symptoms of hypoglycaemia (autonomic symptoms) and you can take appropriate action. Self-treatment is possible.

3 Hypoglycaemia unawareness
You experience symptoms from the brain (neuroglycopenic symptoms) without having had any bodily (autonomic) warning symptoms beforehand. However, it is obvious to people observing you that something is wrong.

4 Severe hypoglycaemia
Severe symptoms of hypoglycaemia disable you temporarily, requiring the assistance of another person to give you something to eat or a glucagon injection. Severe hypoglycaemia can cause you to lose consciousness and have seizures.

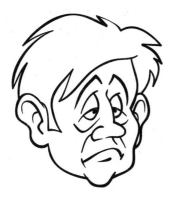

Symptoms of hypoglycaemia from the brain

The blood glucose concentration at which your brain begins to show symptoms of dysfunction (neuroglycopenic symptoms) is lower than that for bodily symptoms, and largely independent of your recent blood glucose levels. The last two bullet points occur in extreme cases only.

- Weakness, dizziness.

- Difficulty concentrating.

- Double or blurred vision.

- Disturbed colour vision (especially red-green colours).

- Difficulties with hearing.

- Feeling warm or hot.

- Headache.

- Drowsiness.

- Odd behaviour, poor judgement.

- Confusion.

- Poor short-term memory.

- Slurred speech.

- Unsteady walking, lack of coordination.

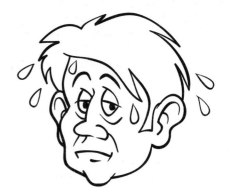

Symptoms of hypoglycaemia from the body

Bodily symptoms (autonomic and adrenergic symptoms) are the result of both adrenaline secretion and the autonomic nervous system. They usually start when the blood glucose concentration dips below 3.5–4 mmol/L (65–70 mg/dl). The threshold for triggering these symptoms will change depending on the person's recent blood glucose concentrations (the 'blood glucose thermostat').

- Irritability.

- Hunger, feeling sick.

- Trembling.

- Anxiety.

- Heart palpitations.

- Throbbing pulse in the chest and abdomen.

- Numbness in the lips, fingers and tongue.

- Looking pale.

- Cold sweats.

elsewhere. For example, some people report that they are less likely to recognize symptoms of hypoglycaemia at work than when relaxing at home.

Your brain contains a kind of blood glucose meter that triggers defence reactions in your body and raises a low blood glucose level. It works in a similar way to a thermostat ('gluco-stat') and is triggered at a certain blood glucose level. This reaction depends very much on where your blood glucose level has been during the last few days. If your blood sugar has been high for some time, symptoms of hypoglycaemia and the release of counter-regulating hormones will appear at a higher blood glucose level than usual. If your HbA$_{1c}$ is high, you may start having symptoms of hypoglycaemia when your blood glucose level is 4–5 mmol/L (70–90 mg/dl) or even a little higher.

For some unknown reason, caffeine can increase your awareness of the symptoms of hypoglycaemia.

Severe hypoglycaemia

Severe hypoglycaemia is defined as a hypo-glycaemic reaction with documented low blood glucose (3.5 mmol/L, 62 mg/dl) or reversal of symptoms after intake of glucose, with symptoms sufficiently severe for the person to need help from another person or even admission to hospital. In some cases, the person with diabetes will lose consciousness (either fully or partially)

> ### Research findings: effects of low blood glucose
>
> - In one study, tests involving associative learning, attention and mental flexibility were the ones most affected at a blood glucose level of 2.2 mmol/L (40 mg/dl).
>
> - Women were less affected than men in this study. This may be explained by women having lower levels of adrenaline and less pronounced symptoms of hypoglycaemia than men.
>
> - Changes in EEG (brain wave) activity will occur when the blood glucose falls below 2.2 mmol/L (40 mg/dl) in adults.
>
> - Unconsciousness occurs when the blood glucose level drops to approximately 1 mmol/L (20 mg/dl).
>
> - Symptoms of hypoglycaemia can change over time, depending on your average blood glucose levels (see text).

and may have seizures. Insulin coma results from severe hypoglycaemia with loss of consciousness. Approximately 10–25% of individuals with Type 1 diabetes experience a severe

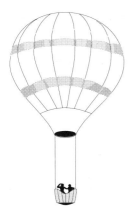

The level at which you start experiencing symptoms of hypoglycaemia will change depending on how often your blood glucose level has been low in the last few days. Make it part of your routine to measure blood glucose as soon as you notice symptoms. If you usually become hypoglycaemic when the level is 3.7 mmol/L (67 mg/dl, 'normal-level hypoglycaemia') and now have no symptoms until it falls to 3.2 mmol/L (58 mg/dl, 'low-level hypoglycaemia'), you have probably had too many low blood glucose values recently. On the other hand, if you start experiencing symptoms of hypoglycaemia with a blood glucose level of 4.0–4.5 mmol/L or higher (72–81 mg/dl 'high-level hypoglycaemia'), you have had too many high blood glucose values and your HbA$_{1c}$ is probably rising.

What caused your hypoglycaemia?

➡ Too little to eat or delayed meal.

➡ Skipped a meal?

➡ Neglecting to eat despite symptoms of hypoglycaemia.

➡ Physical exercise?
  ➡ The risk of hypoglycaemia is increased for up to 4 hours after heavy physical exercise.

➡ Too large a dose of insulin?

➡ Too large an increase in your dose of sulphonylurea?

➡ New site for your insulin injections? e.g. from thigh to abdomen or to a site free of fatty lumps (lipohypertrophy).

➡ Recent hypoglycaemia?
  ➡ Glucose stores in the liver may be depleted. This can lead to more hypoglycaemia and fewer warning symptoms of hypoglycaemia (hypoglycaemic unawareness).

➡ Very low HbA$_{1c}$
  ➡ Increased risk of hypoglycaemic unawareness as low blood glucose can lead to reduced warning signs.

➡ Drinking alcohol?

➡ Variable insulin absorption (see 'How accurate is your insulin dose?' on page 98). Rates of insulin absorption can vary if you have recently moved to a new injecting area which may have more or less subcutaneous fat.

➡ Gastroenteritis or tummy upset.

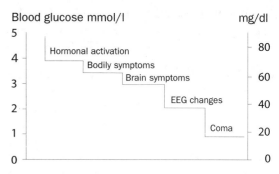

When your blood glucose is lowered, the reactions in your body and brain take place at different levels. These levels are in turn dependent on your recent blood glucose levels, i.e. if you recently have had higher blood glucose readings, the symptoms will occur at a slightly higher blood glucose level and if you recently have had lower blood glucose readings and hypoglycaemia, the symptoms will occur at a slightly lower blood glucose level. The graph is taken from work by Amiel (1998).

hypoglycaemia of less than 1% in the majority of patients with Type 2 diabetes. Sulphonylureas may sometimes cause low blood sugar, particularly when used in combination with insulin. Other factors that will increase your risk of severe hypoglycaemia include taking the wrong dose of insulin, missing a meal, and drinking alcohol after an unusual amount of activity such as energetic dancing at a party. Even planned activity, such as digging over the vegetable patch, can cause hypoglycaemia when you are taking insulin, unless you take steps to avoid it by eating extra food or taking less insulin before and after exercise.

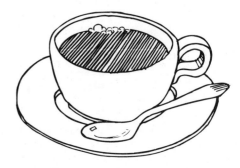

Caffeine in coffee and cola can increase your awareness of hypoglycaemic symptoms.

hypoglycaemic episode during a period of one year. The incidence of severe hypoglycaemia is much less in Type 2 diabetes. Even insulin analogues such as Lantus have rates of severe

Seizures

Seizures can be very alarming for those who witness them. The person having the seizure should be turned onto his or her side (the recovery position), after making sure that the airway is free. This is the safest position for someone who might be sick. Call an ambulance immediately if you can. You should not leave the person alone so delegate this task to someone else if at all possible, especially if you do not have a mobile phone with you.

If the person is carrying a glucagon injection, this should be given as soon as possible. People with Type 2 diabetes do not usually carry glucagon, however, so you may not be in a position to help in this way. If some sugar is available, you could rub this onto the person's lips.

After recovery, the insulin doses should always be reviewed, and the dose should be reduced if the cause of the low blood glucose cannot be identified.

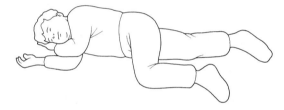

The recovery position, with the patient lying on his or her side, is the safest position for someone who is unconscious.

Hypoglycaemia unawareness

Hypoglycaemia unawareness is defined as a hypoglycaemic episode that comes on without the usual warning symptoms associated with decreasing blood glucose. If you have frequent hypoglycaemic episodes, the threshold at which you recognize symptoms will occur at a lower blood glucose level. If the threshold for secreting counter-regulatory hormones falls below the blood glucose level that provokes a reaction in the brain, you will not have any physical warning symptoms. Because of this, you will not react

in time (by eating, for example) so your hypoglycaemia can rapidly become severe. Sometimes you will not even remember afterwards that you had hypoglycaemia.

Hypoglycaemic unawareness will increase the risk of severe hypoglycaemia and is more common among those prone to severe hypoglycaemia. It should be part of your routine to check your blood glucose as soon as you start getting symptoms that might indicate hypoglycaemia. If your readings are below 3.5 mmol/L (65 mg/dl), this is a warning sign that your risk of becoming severely hypoglycaemic may increase considerably.

If you have hypoglycaemia unawareness, you should aim for a slightly higher average blood glucose. Above all, you should avoid a blood glucose level that is lower than 5.0 mmol/L (90 mg/dl). Within a fortnight, you are likely to find you can recognize symptoms of hypoglycaemia more easily. By training yourself to recognize subtle symptoms as your blood glucose is decreasing, you will increase your chances of treating your hypoglycaemia in time.

Many people with long-standing diabetes will have a reduced adrenaline response to low blood glucose, which reduces the warning symptoms they receive from their autonomic nervous system. Thus, these people have less effective counter-regulation when their blood glucose is falling. A number of people report a loss of their hypo warnings when changing from pork or beef insulin to human insulin. Several studies have looked at this issue, and there is no scientific proof of a relationship between human insulin and hypoglycaemia unawareness.

Driving and insulin

Driving is the most widely-practised activity that can be seriously affected by hypoglycaemia. Each year a number of people with diabetes, treated with insulin, are involved in road accidents. It is often clear that these took place while the driver's blood glucose was below normal. In some cases, the driver or an innocent third party may be seriously injured.

The Driving and Vehicle Licensing Authority (DVLA) is aware of this and people using insulin have to renew their driving licence every year and declare that they are not subject to hypos without warning.

Tips for safe driving:

- Have glucose, sweets or Lucozade to hand – not in the glove compartment.

- Test your blood glucose before driving and at intervals on long journeys.

- If you feel you could be hypo, pull off the road, get out of the car or move into the back seat. This is so that you are obviously seen not to be driving the car if the police should come along.

- Take concentrated sugar to correct the hypo immediately and prove that your sugar is above 4 mmol/L.

- Consider running your blood glucose levels a little high while driving.

- Following a hypo your judgement may be impaired for up to an hour afterwards, even though you feel normal and your blood glucose levels are above 4mmol/L.

Rebound phenomenon

Your body will try to reverse hypoglycaemia by using counter-regulatory responses (see Chapter 6 on Regulation of blood glucose). Sometimes this counter-regulation will be too effective and the blood glucose will rise to high levels during the hours following hypoglycaemia. This is called the 'rebound phenomenon'. People who live alone may be unaware of nocturnal hypoglycaemia and may misinterpret a high morning glucose, believing it to be due to insufficient insulin, when it is actually a result of a rebound from a night time hypo. Where HbA_{1c} is near to target and the morning blood glucose levels are very high, rebound phenomenon should be considered.

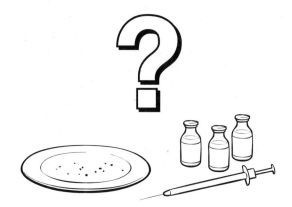

Too little food or too much insulin?

Both can result in a low blood glucose level, but the body's way of handling the situation is different. The effect of glucagon in breaking down the stored glucose (glycogen) is counteracted by insulin. Insulin acts in the opposite direction, by transporting glucose into the liver cells to be stored as glycogen. From this, it follows that the more insulin you have injected (resulting in a higher insulin level in the blood), the more difficult it will be to release glucose from the liver. This means that a low blood glucose caused by a large insulin dose (e.g. if you have taken extra insulin) will be more difficult to reverse than a low blood glucose due to inadequate food intake.

Night time hypoglycaemia

Although uncommon in Type 2 diabetes, night time hypoglycaemia may occur in association with escalating insulin doses to help achieve target blood sugar levels. Adrenaline responses are reduced during deep sleep, which may contribute to the failure to wake up. Symptoms of hypoglycaemia may also be more difficult to recognize when you are lying down than when you are standing up.

Night time hypoglycaemia can be caused by too large a dose of bedtime insulin. Another cause can be too high a dose of short-acting insulin just before your evening snack, which will result in hypoglycaemia early in the night.

There are several studies with NovoRapid and Humalog insulins which suggest that reducing the action time of the short-acting insulin (by the use of rapid-acting insulin) helps to decrease night time hypoglycaemia. Evidence is also accumulating that use of long-acting insulin analogues (Lantus/glargine and Levemir/detemir) may also be associated with a reduced incidence of night time hypoglycaemia in Type 2 diabetes. Attacks of night time hypoglycaemia can also be caused by vigorous afternoon or evening exercise.

If you are injecting short-acting insulin into your thigh before the evening snack, the slow absorption of insulin can result in night time hypoglycaemia. If you inject your bedtime insulin holding the needle at right angles to the skin, or without lifting a skin fold, you might be

---

Symptoms indicating night time hypoglycaemia

➠ Nightmares.

➠ Sweating (damp sheets).

➠ Headache in the morning.

➠ Tiredness on waking.

➠ Bed-wetting (can also be caused by high blood glucose during the night).

---

injecting intramuscularly. The insulin will then be absorbed more quickly, putting you at risk of low blood glucose early in the night.

A good basic rule for avoiding night time hypoglycaemia is always to have something extra to eat if your blood glucose is below approximately 7 mmol/L (120–130 mg/dl) before going to bed. See also 'Bedtime insulin' on page 97. Taking extra food before going to bed reduces the risk of night hypoglycaemia but does not abolish it completely. If in doubt, it is worth doing one or two 2 am blood checks, which will answer the question. If you are tak-

---

Night time hypoglycaemia may be caused by:

➠ The dose of short-acting insulin before the evening snack being too high (hypoglycaemia early in the night).

➠ The dose of bedtime insulin being too high (hypoglycaemia around 2 am or later with NPH insulin).

➠ Short-acting insulin before dinner/tea or the evening snack being given into the thigh (hypoglycaemia early in the night is being caused by a slower absorption from the thigh).

➠ Not enough to eat in the evening, or an evening snack containing mostly 'short-acting' foods being absorbed too quickly.

➠ Exercise in the afternoon or evening without decreasing the dose of bedtime insulin.

➠ Alcohol consumption in the evening.

Taking the wrong type of insulin

☞ Be careful not to mix up different bottles or types of insulin when using syringes.

☞ Make sure that the pens you use for daytime and night time insulin are so different that you cannot accidentally use the wrong pen, even if it is completely dark.

☞ Often only the colour coding will differ between pens from the same company. You may want to consider using disposable pens for one type of insulin and a regular pen for the other or use pens from two different manufacturers.

ing twice a day mixed insulins for your Type 2 diabetes and can't reach your target without being at risk of night time hypoglycaemia, it might be sensible to consider changing to a three times per day short-acting insulin-based regime. Remember, taking extra calories because of the inflexibility of a twice a day insulin regime and needing to snack may contribute to further weight gain.

Can you die from hypoglycaemia?

Major hypoglycaemia associated with Type 2 diabetes is very rare. Modern insulin therapy regimes are associated with episodes of severe hypoglycaemia with an incidence of 1% or less per year. Long-acting sulphonylureas such as chlorpropamide, previously known to cause problem low blood sugars, are no longer used in routine clinical practice. People with Type 2 diabetes are extremely unlikely to fall victim to the 'dead in bed' syndrome. This is a rare phenomenon, occasionally found in association with Type 1 diabetes, which may be due to electrolyte imbalance, cardiac arrythmia or diminished response in association with an episode of hypoglycaemia.

Some potentially dangerous activities put people in danger if they are hypo at the time. The most important of these is driving (see pages 131–2).

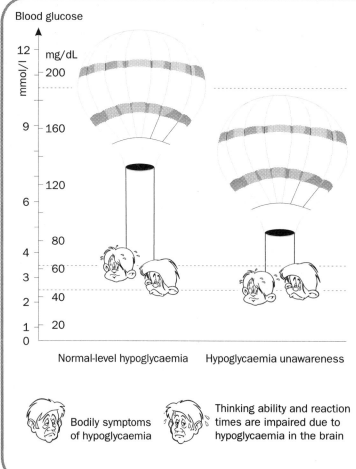

Normal-level hypoglycaemia

Hypoglycaemia unawareness

Bodily symptoms of hypoglycaemia

Thinking ability and reaction times are impaired due to hypoglycaemia in the brain

Normally, you will notice bodily symptoms (such as shaking and cold sweats) at slightly higher blood glucose levels than symptoms from the brain (such as difficulty in concentrating). This enables you to continue to think clearly and to take appropriate action promptly.

If you have many low blood glucose readings (less than 2.5–3.0 mmol/L, 45–55 mg/dl) you will risk having hypoglycaemia unawareness (see page 131). The hypoglycaemia may then go unnoticed until the blood glucose level is so low that it affects the brain. By then, you will find it difficult to think clearly, and your reaction times will have slowed down. Bodily symptoms begin to occur when your blood glucose level drops even lower, but by this time you will have problems taking appropriate action.

It would be much better if your bodily symptoms could appear before the symptoms from the brain, warning you in time to do something about your low blood glucose level in an effective way.

Why does the blood glucose level at which hypoglycaemia is noticed vary?

The hot air balloon

A hot air balloon can be used to illustrate the variations in the level at which hypoglycaemia is first noticed. The height of the balloon corresponds to your average blood glucose level during the day. The basket under the balloon corresponds to the blood glucose level where you first notice symptoms of hypoglycaemia. With an average glucose level of 10 mmol/L (180 mg/dl), symptoms are usually noticed when the level is around 3.5 mmol/L (65 mg/dl).

The HbA$_{1c}$ scale on the right of the graph corresponds to the average blood glucose level over a 2–3-month period, which is presented on the left side of the scale. An average blood glucose of 10 mmol/L (180 mg/dl) will give an HbA$_{1c}$ of approximately 8% (DCCT equivalent numbers; see page 76).

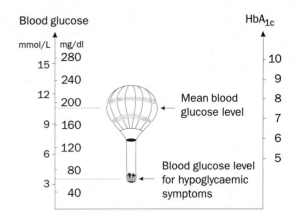

Treating hypoglycaemia

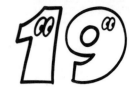

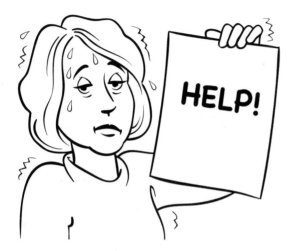

Although giving pure glucose may be the preferred treatment for hypoglycaemia, any form of carbohydrate that contains glucose will raise blood glucose levels. Ten grams of glucose will raise the blood glucose of an adult by about 2 mmol/L (35 mg/dl) after 15 minutes. The blood glucose will rise over 45–60 minutes and then start to fall. It is important not to take too much glucose 'just to be on the safe side' since the blood glucose will then rise too steeply. If you tend to eat too much when your blood sugar is low, you will put on weight.

Which dose of insulin contributed to your hypoglycaemia?

Practical instructions

1. Test your blood glucose. The sensations of a hypoglycaemic reaction do not necessarily imply that your blood glucose is actually low. If your symptoms are so intense that it is difficult to measure the blood glucose, you should of course eat something containing glucose or sugar as soon as possible. This will prevent your hypoglycaemia becoming more severe during the time it takes you to test. If your blood glucose happens to be high, a little extra glucose will not make much difference.

2. If your blood glucose is low (less than 4.0 mmol/L, 70 mg/dl), have some glucose tablets or something sweet to drink. Start with a lower dose according to the table on next page and wait 10–15 minutes for the glucose to take effect. If you don't feel better after 15–20 minutes and your blood glucose has not risen, you can take a repeat dose of the same amount of glucose.

3. Glucose will give a quicker rise in blood glucose than other types of carbohydrate. Avoid food and drink containing fat (e.g. chocolate, biscuits, milk or chocolate milk) if you want a quick increase in blood glucose. Fat causes the stomach to empty more slowly, so that the glucose reaches the bloodstream later (see page 37). If your blood glucose is only slightly low (3.5–4.5 mmol/l 65–80 mg/dl), you may need to make a decision about eating some carbohydrate, postponing exercise or changing your insulin dose. In this situation, a glass of juice may be appropriate.

4. Don't take any physical exercise until all symptoms of hypoglycaemia have vanished. Wait at least 15 minutes before you do anything that demands your full attention or quick understanding, such as driving, operating a machine or taking a meeting at work.

5 If eating something containing glucose or sugar doesn't bring the blood glucose level back to normal, it may be because the stomach isn't emptying its contents into the intestine (where the glucose is absorbed). If your blood glucose doesn't increase sufficiently within 15 minutes, try drinking some carbonated lemonade to encourage the relaxation of the muscle (pyloric sphincter) that controls the exit of food from the stomach to the intestines.

6 Occasionally, there may be additional problems, and hypoglycaemia will carry on for hours unless some other measure is taken (for example, if you have

---

Treatment of hypoglycaemia (*as recommended by the DAFNE study*)

ALWAYS TREAT HYPOS IMMEDIATELY!

When you feel the symptoms of a hypo coming on, take some quick-acting carbohydrate as soon as you can. This will stop the symptoms and prevent your needing help from anyone else. Even if you do not have symptoms, if your blood glucose level is below 4 you must treat it with quick-acting carbohydrate.

The best treatment is fruit juice or a sugary drink, equivalent to 20 g of carbohydrate, for example:

- Lucozade (100–130 ml/half a teacup).
- Fruit juice (150–200 ml/one small carton).
- Lemonade or cola (150–200 ml; approximately one teacup full).
- Glucose tablets can be useful too, but some people find chewing and swallowing them difficult when they are hypo.

How many glucose tablets are needed to treat hypoglycaemia?

'RULE OF THUMB'

20 g (six tablets of glucose) will raise your blood glucose approximately 4–6 mmol/L (70–110 mg/dl) i.e. your blood glucose will be approximately 4 mmol/L (70 mg) higher after 15–30 minutes than it would be without extra glucose. Usually, an increase of 2 mmol/L (35 mg/dl) will be enough, but if you have recently taken insulin and your blood glucose level is falling, you may need more glucose. Check the type of glucose tablets you use as they are likely to contain 3–4 g of glucose.

---

gastroenteritis). The most effective measure is likely to be injecting a small dose of glucagon, which may need to be repeated.

7 If there is no apparent explanation for why the hypoglycaemia occurred, you should decrease the 'responsible' dose of insulin the next day. For more information, see Chapter 16 on Changing insulin doses.

8 If the person is conscious but has difficulty in chewing, give glucose gel (e.g. HypoStop) or honey.

9 If the person is unconscious or has seizures, give a glucagon injection. Never give an unconscious person food or drink because it might be accidentally inhaled and cause suffocation or subsequent pneumonia.

Timing and hypoglycaemia

The time interval between the bout of hypoglycaemia and your next meal will determine how you should treat the hypo.

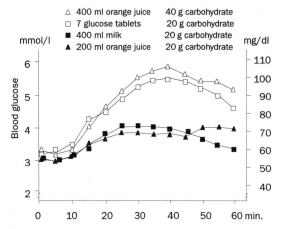

The graph shows results from a study where 13 adults with diabetes were given different types of sugar to reverse hypoglycaemia. Four hundred ml (2/3 pint) of water was given with the glucose tablets. Milk contains fat and gives a slower rise in blood glucose as fat leads to a slower emptying of the stomach.

Hypoglycaemia just before you eat

Take glucose and wait 10–15 minutes before starting to eat. If you eat straight away, your food will mix with the glucose in your stomach. Since it normally takes about 20 minutes for solid food to be digested (sufficiently to be emptied into the intestines), an increase in your blood glucose will take at least this long. Remember that glucose from the food must reach the intestines before it can be absorbed into the blood.

Hypoglycaemia 45–60 minutes before your next meal

The same advice applies as in the example above for a rapid reversal of your hypoglycaemia. Afterwards, you will need something to eat (a piece of fruit, for example) to keep your blood glucose level up until the next meal.

Hypoglycaemia 1–2 hours before your next meal

Take glucose and wait 10–15 minutes before you eat anything else in order to reverse your hypoglycaemia quickly. Since it will be a while until your next meal, it is important to eat something that contains more 'long-acting' carbohydrates. If the hypoglycaemia develops slowly, you can skip the glucose and have a glass of milk and/or a sandwich instead. An alternative approach is to take fast-acting sugar only, and

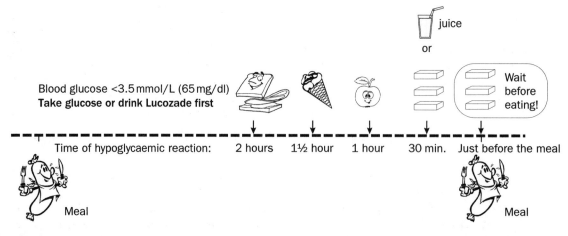

It is important to consider how much time there is before your next meal when you have hypoglycaemia. Don't eat more than you will need to get you through to your next meal. It is all too easy to have too much to eat since it takes a while before the blood glucose rises and makes you feel better. If your blood glucose is below 3.5 mmol/L (65 mg/dl) or the symptoms of hypoglycaemia are troublesome, it is best to take only glucose and then wait 10–15 minutes before eating anything else to cure the hypoglycaemia as soon as possible. If you become hypoglycaemic while sitting with a meal in front of you, it may be quite a while before you feel better again if you eat immediately. It is better to eat something with a higher sugar/glucose content (e.g. glucose tablets), wait 10–15 minutes or until you feel better, and then enjoy your meal.

repeat if necessary. This has the advantage of helping to avoid unwanted weight gain. Try to find out what works best for you and discuss this with your diabetes team.

Helping someone with diabetes who is not feeling well

If you find yourself in the situation of helping someone else with hypoglycaemia, it is very unlikely you will know what the person's blood glucose level is, and you may lose precious time trying to measure it. The best course of action is to give something containing sugar as quickly as possible and then call for help. Make sure that people who may need to help know this simple advice.

Remember that the little packets of sugar available in cafes and fast food restaurants will be very effective in this situation, as will fruit juice or fizzy drinks such as lemonade or cola (as long as they are not the 'diet' variety).

If a high blood glucose is making someone feel ill, taking extra glucose will not make them feel any worse. But they DO need to take insulin.

Glucose

Pure glucose has the quickest effect when correcting hypoglycaemia. Emergency glucose is available in tablets and gel form (for example Glucogel). It is important to think of glucose as a medicine for hypoglycaemia and not as a

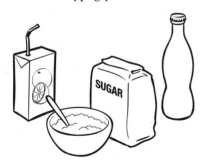

If someone you are with develops hypoglycaemia, the best thing you can do is give them something containing sugar, and fast!

Should you always eat when you feel hypoglycaemic?

1 Measure your blood glucose.

2 If it is 3.5 mmol/L (65 mg/dl), eat something sweet, preferably glucose.

3 If it is greater than 3.5–4 mmol/L (65–70 mg/dl), eat something if your next meal is more than ½–1 hour off or if you know that your blood glucose is decreasing, e.g. after physical exercise.

4 If it is 4.0–4.5 mmol/L (70–80 mg/dl), you may be having hypoglycaemic symptoms at too high a blood glucose level. Wait a short while and test yourself again. Don't eat until the blood glucose has fallen below 4.5 mmol/L (80 mg/dl, see point 3). See also page 134.

But beware!

● This advice must be taken in context.

● Blood glucose meters are not always accurate, especially at low levels, so a measured 4.5 may well already be below 4.

● Blood glucose levels can fall particularly fast if you are doing something active like running or swimming.

● You CANNOT afford a low blood glucose if you are driving, for example.

'sweet'. Everyone with Type 2 diabetes who is taking insulin should always have glucose handy and must know when they need to take it. Friends must also know in which pocket the glucose tablets are kept. If you are taking acarbose, particularly in combination with other drugs, hypoglycaemia may rarely occur. If it does, acarbose blocks the metabolism of complex sugars, so you will need to take glucose tablets, not ordinary sugar, to reverse hypoglycaemia.

Sports drinks contain different mixtures of sugars and give a quick increase in blood glucose. Pure fruit juice contains mostly fructose, which gives a slower increase in blood glucose. A glass of juice containing 20 g (⅔ ounce) of carbohydrate gives a slower increase in blood glucose than glucose tablets containing the same amount of carbohydrate. Ordinary sugar is sucrose (also called saccharose) which is composed of both glucose and fructose. It will therefore not give the same increase in blood glucose as an equal amount of pure glucose, but it is useful if glucose is not available.

Fructose

Fructose has a sweeter taste than ordinary sugar. It is absorbed more slowly from the intestine and is not as effective as glucose in

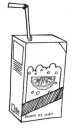

A carton of juice can come in handy if your blood glucose drops. It is easy and discreet to carry with you. If you don't feel like eating, or are in a public place, it is often easier to sip from a carton than to take glucose tablets or gel.

raising the blood glucose level. This is because it does not affect the blood glucose directly. It is mainly taken up by the liver cells (without the help of insulin) where it is converted into glucose or triglycerides. A high intake of fructose will increase the body fat. Fructose can also raise the blood glucose by stimulating glucose production in the liver. Honey contains 35–40% glucose and the same amount of fructose. Sorbitol, found in many sweets, is converted in the liver to fructose.

Sweets containing chocolate and chocolate bars raise the blood glucose very slowly and should not be used to treat hypoglycaemia (see graph on page 138). This is particularly important when blood glucose levels are below 3.5 mmol/L (65 mg/dl) as you need to raise your level rapidly.

After hypoglycaemia

You will usually feel better within 10–15 minutes after you have eaten something containing glucose. However, it will often take 1–2 hours after the blood glucose has normalized before you find yourself returning to a level of maximum performance again.

Headaches are common after recovering from hypoglycaemia, particularly if your blood glucose level was very low. If the hypo is very severe, you may also experience symptoms in the nervous system, though this is less common. These may include temporary weakness or difficulties in speaking and are caused by swelling in part of the brain following hypoglycaemia. If you find yourself experiencing any symptoms like these, you should contact your doctor.

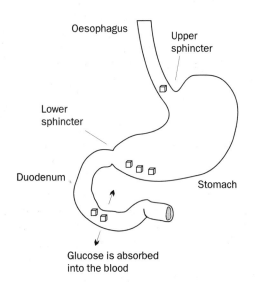

Sugar must reach the intestine to be able to be absorbed into the bloodstream so that it can raise the blood glucose level. Glucose cannot be absorbed through the lining of the mouth (oral mucosa), or from the stomach. The lower sphincter (pylorus) regulates the emptying of the stomach. Different factors influence how quickly the stomach empties, and this will have a direct effect on the speed with which glucose can be absorbed into the blood to correct hypoglycaemia.

Sometimes people feel sick or vomit after hypoglycaemia, especially if the blood glucose has been low for some time. This may be associated with raised levels of ketones in the blood and urine. Both ketones and nausea are caused by the hormone glucagon, which is secreted from the pancreas during hypoglycaemia. This is the same type of side effect that can be experienced after a glucagon injection. If the vomiting continues, you should tell the hospital.

Learning to recognize the symptoms of hypoglycaemia

Every time your blood glucose measures less than 4.0 mmol/L (70 mg/dl), you should ask yourself: 'Exactly what symptoms caused me to take the blood test now? Did I experience any symptoms 10 or 20 minutes earlier that might have warned me my blood glucose was falling?' If your blood glucose is below 3.5 mmol/L (65 mg/dl) and you have not experienced any symptoms, you should always ask yourself: 'Were there really no symptoms at all warning me that my blood glucose was low?' Ask your friends if they have noticed any change in your behaviour that could have been caused by a drop in your blood glucose.

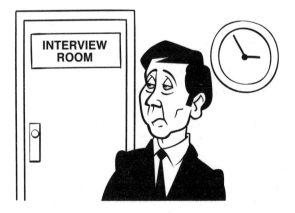

It will be difficult to be as impressive as you should be in a job interview if you have hypoglycaemia, or have had it recently. Usually it will take a couple of hours after a difficult hypoglycaemic episode before you are back on top form.

> ### Research findings: recovery from hypoglycaemia
>
> - In a study of adults without diabetes, insulin was used to induce hypoglycaemia (blood glucose 2.7 mmol/L, 50 mg/dl, for 70 minutes). The reaction time was decreased for 1½ hours and only returned to normal 4 hours after the blood glucose had normalized.
>
> - Another study of adults with Type 1 diabetes found cognitive functions (short-term memory, attention and concentration) to be normal the morning after a night with hypoglycaemia (blood glucose 2.2 mmol/L, 40 mg/dl, for 1 hour).
>
> - A British study of adults showed their capacity for exercise was unchanged after an episode of night time hypoglycaemia (2.6–3.0 mmol/L, 45–55 mg/dl, for 1 hour) even though participants complained of more fatigue and less wellbeing, and felt that they had experienced a bad night's sleep.

There are now programmes that train people with diabetes to recognize subtle and variable changes in their behaviour and how they feel while hypoglycaemia is developing. Such programmes include the use of simple cognitive tests, and their success has been demonstrated. To test for bodily symptoms, stand up and walk around. Move your outstretched arm in a circle or hold a pen between your fingers to test for shakiness. To test for symptoms from your brain, repeat your mother's or brother's age and birthday, your friends' phone numbers or the combination for your briefcase key. Whatever test you set yourself should be sufficiently difficult when your blood glucose level is normal for you to notice the difference when doing the same thing while your blood glucose is low.

Stress

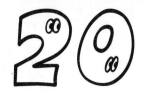

Stress and psychological strain affect your body and will, at times, increase the blood glucose levels as a result of the way different hormones respond to stress. This may vary from individual to individual.

When your body is exposed to stress, the adrenal glands secrete the hormone adrenaline (the 'fight and flight' hormone) which increases the output of glucose from the liver. To explain this, you must understand our Stone Age legacy. During this far-off period, stress was usually associated with danger, for example an attacking bear. The alternatives were to stay and fight or to run away as quickly as possible. Extra fuel in the form of increased glucose in the blood is needed for both these responses.

Today, the same stress reaction can occur in front of the TV if you are watching something exciting, but you will not benefit from the increased blood glucose level. People who do not have diabetes will automatically release insulin from their pancreas to restore the glucose balance. In theory, it is possible for someone who is taking insulin for their diabetes to take extra insulin in this situation. In practice, this is often hard to accomplish since it is difficult to evaluate one's stress level, and stress (by its very nature) tends to vary from day to day.

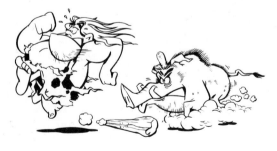

Your body is built to withstand the strenuous life of a Stone Age man or woman. In a stress situation, large amounts of adrenaline are secreted to help prepare the body for fight against, or flight away from, the danger.

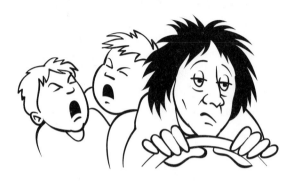

In one study, adults with diabetes performed a mental stress test for 20 minutes, causing the blood glucose level to rise after an hour. It continued to be raised by about 2 mmol/L (35 mg/dl) for another 5 hours. The blood pressure was increased as well, and the stress induced a resistance to insulin (see page 209) via increased levels of the hormones adrenaline, cortisol and growth hormone. Individuals who were able to produce some of their own insulin found the stress had less influence on their blood glucose level. Another study used a stress test composed of a 5-minute preparation task, a 5-minute speech task where subjects had to introduce themselves and apply for a job, and a 5-minute mental arithmetic task. Blood glucose levels were raised by approximately 1.0–1.4 mmol/L (18–25 mg/dl) with a delay of 30 minutes after the test and lasted for approximately 2 hours. However, the effect of stress on blood glucose was only seen after a meal, and not if the test was performed in a fasting state.

After the earthquake in Kobe, Japan, HbA_{1c} levels rose in people living in the affected area. The highest increase was found in those who had experienced the death or injury of a close relative, and those whose homes had been severely damaged.

Studies of heart attack victims have shown that so-called positive stress is not as dangerous as other forms of stress. Positive stress is defined

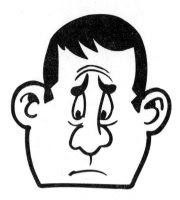

'Negative stress' is experienced when a person cannot change a stressful situation. Insurmountable problems at work, or at home within the family, may contribute to a raised blood glucose level.

as the kind of tension that is produced when you have a lot to do, but you choose to do it yourself and you are in control of the situation.

The type of negative stress that increases the risk for heart attack occurs when the person cannot influence the situation, for example if they are having problems at work or at home within the family, such as relationship break-up or divorce. Similar situations may contribute to an increased blood glucose level as well. For example, blood glucose readings taken at the hospital are often higher than those taken at home. Raised blood glucose levels have been observed in people with diabetes, in both outpatient and inpatient settings. This is also the case for blood pressure measurements, so called 'white coat hypertension'.

Stress in daily life

Everyday stress factors can cause a higher HbA_{1c}. For example, people who are going for interviews or changing jobs often find the stress makes their blood sugar levels go up. Any change to routine will also make you more likely to forget to take your medication.

Stress reactions have an effect on everyone within a family. So even if the family member experiencing the primary stress is not the one with diabetes, everyone else will be affected to some degree. Distress and anxiety can make

Stress

➧ Stress that cannot be influenced (such as problems in the family or at work) will have the greatest effect on your health.

➧ Stress can also affect your blood glucose for the simple reason that you will not have as much time to care for your diabetes when life becomes busy and stressful.

➧ Adrenaline (stress hormone) gives

1 Increased blood glucose level by:
(A) Release of glucose from the liver.
(B) Decreased uptake of glucose into the cells.

2 Ketones by:
Breakdown of fat into fatty acids that are transformed into ketones in the liver.

adapting to stressful situations more difficult, so it is better (wherever possible) to focus on finding practical ways of dealing with, or addressing, the stressful situation. If practical solutions can be shared with partners and other family members, everyone is likely to benefit.

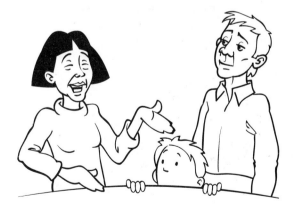

Families who talk to each other, and focus their emotional upset on practical aspects and use problem-solving strategies, are more likely to be better able to deal with stress.

Research findings: stress and HbA$_{1c}$ levels

- One study found that individuals with higher HbA$_{1c}$ levels reported poorer quality of life and more anxiety and depression.

- When the HbA$_{1c}$ value was increased or decreased during the scope of the study, the scores for quality of life, anxiety and depression changed accordingly.

- These results suggest that you will feel better with a lower HbA$_{1c}$. However, another interpretation is that it is easier to obtain a good HbA$_{1c}$ when you feel well.

- Individuals who had experienced many severe stress factors (unpleasant life events, ongoing long-term problems, conflicts with other people) within the previous 3 months had higher HbA$_{1c}$ in one study.

- Another study showed that stress causes a higher HbA$_{1c}$ but only in individuals who handle the stress in an ineffective way. Anger, impatience and anxiety were examples of ineffective coping mechanisms. Stoicism (not reacting emotionally in stressful situations), pragmatism (handling stress in a problem-oriented way) and denial (disregarding the stress and thereby not letting it affect you) were effective coping mechanisms.

- Denial has also been shown to have a correlation with impaired blood glucose control. This might be explained by the fact that a problem must first be recognized before being solved. Appearing to accept a chronic disease initially, but then refusing to let it affect your daily life negatively, may be an effective form of denial.

- In an analysis of 24 studies (known as a meta-analysis), depression in people with diabetes was associated with a higher HbA$_{1c}$. However, it is difficult to conclude whether an elevated HbA$_{1c}$ is the result of depression or the other way around.

- Some data indicate that anti-depressive medication can improve HbA$_{1c}$ in people with depression.

Learned helplessness is a phenomenon that can occur when you feel unable to control a situation and the reason for this is unrealistic expectations rather than insufficient ability on the part of the individual. One example is when you follow every piece of advice given by the diabetes team and your blood glucose is still much too unstable. This 'teaches' you that it is not possible to control your blood glucose and, after a while, you will stop trying. The reason for this is the unrealistic expectation that you can achieve a stable blood glucose level simply by 'trying hard'. This has also been called 'diabetes burnout'. An example of a realistic expectation is that your blood glucose will swing between high and low values and that you will have at least one reading above 10 mmol/L (180 mg/dl) every day. It can be realistic to try to achieve a lower average blood glucose (HbA$_{1c}$) without laying yourself open to an increase in hypoglycaemia-related problems. Realistic expectations for the long term might include being able to manage work or a normal social life, for example, without being inconvenienced to any great extent by your diabetes.

For more information on psychological aspects of diabetes, see Chapter 29.

Coping with sickness

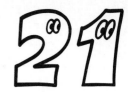

If you have an infection, especially if you are running a temperature with it, the secretion of blood glucose-raising hormones (particularly cortisol and glucagon) is increased. So at a time when you are not feeling hungry and eating less, you may be surprised to find your blood sugar rising. If you are treated with diet or tablets, there is not much you can do to correct the high sugar levels. If possible, continue to take your normal tablets and test your blood four times a day if you have the means. You should drink as much fluid as you can when you are ill – up to 3 litres (6 pints) a day, and even more if you have a high temperature and are sweating profusely.

If you are taking insulin, you can deal with the problem of high sugars by taking more insulin than usual. However, it is common to eat less and rest more when you are ill, so these factors usually balance each other out. Start by taking your usual dose. Measure your blood glucose level before each meal and adjust the dose before eating. Correct the high blood sugar using the rule of thumb that 1 unit of insulin reduces the blood glucose by 3 mmol/L.

If your temperature is above 38° C (100° F) you may need to increase your insulin dose by as much as 25%. Indeed, you might even need an increase of up to 50% of your total dose over a 24 hour period if your temperature is above 39° C (102° F). If you use a two-dose treatment, it can be difficult to meet the changing needs of insulin when you are ill. If you are worried about finding it difficult to control your blood

> ### Feeling ill or well on insulin
>
> **1** If you feel well
>   - Decide what you want to eat.
>   - Work out your insulin dose in relation to the size of the meal.
>   - If your sugar is high, correct it by giving extra insulin.
>   - Use the formula that 1 unit of insulin will reduce blood glucose by 3 mmol/L.
>
> **2** If you feel ill and don't want to eat
>   - Remember, you still need insulin.
>   - Take your usual insulin dose to begin with (unless your blood glucose is low) and try to eat enough to supply the insulin with carbohydrates 'to work with'.
>   - Aim at preventing your blood glucose level from falling too low by drinking something sugary when necessary.

sugar levels, contact your diabetes nurse to discuss a plan of action.

Good glucose control increases the body's defence against infections. Document your blood glucose readings (as well as insulin doses) in your logbook and contact your diabetes

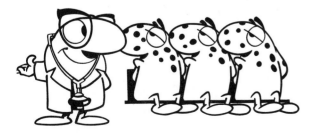

> ### IMPORTANT RULE
>
> **IF YOU START VOMITING, SUMMON MEDICAL HELP AND BE PREPARED FOR HOSPITAL ADMISSION. YOU WILL NEED INTRAVENOUS FLUIDS IN A DRIP.**

Illness and need for insulin

➟ Fever increases the need for insulin.

➟ But – decreased appetite and food intake decrease the need for insulin.

➟ Thus – you will probably have at least the same need for insulin per 24 hours as usual.

➟ You are likely to need up to 25–50% more insulin when you are feverish.

➟ It is unusual for people with Type 2 diabetes to develop ketoacidosis. If you are vomiting and unable to keep fluids down, contact your doctor as you will probably need fluids into a vein (a drip).

➟ But – you may need less insulin if you have gastroenteritis with vomiting and diarrhoea.

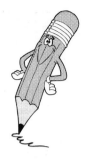

Write down all insulin doses and test results in your notebook. You will find it easier to adjust insulin doses and food intake next time you are faced with the same situation. Make a note of how many units you have taken over 24 hours. This is the best way of measuring how the illness has affected your diabetes.

(ORS), available at the pharmacy, is very useful in this situation, particularly if you are elderly or frail.

Many people don't like the taste of ORS, which is quite salty. Try adding some juice to improve its taste. Sports drinks such as Lucozade can be helpful in this situation as they already contain both glucose and salts, thus helping to prevent dehydration and salt imbalance. A small dose of metoclopramide (Maxolon) can be helpful for preventing vomiting.

If you normally take tablets for your diabetes, it is obviously impossible for them to work if you are vomiting. You may need insulin instead, and for this reason people on tablets for diabetes may need admission to hospital if they are unable to keep fluids or tablets down.

healthcare team or the hospital if you are in the least unsure about your condition or how to handle the situation.

The increased insulin requirements during illness (e.g. a cold with fever) usually last for a few days, but sometimes they can last up to a week after recovery. This is due to the increased blood glucose level which, in turn, gives rise to increased insulin resistance (see page 209). Sometimes there are increased insulin requirements during the incubation period for a few days before the onset of the illness.

Nausea and vomiting

If you feel sick while you are running a temperature, and if you eat less, it is important that the food you do eat contains sugar and carbohydrates, both to give your body nourishment and to lessen the risk of hypoglycaemia. Any nausea will usually get worse if you drink large amounts of liquid at one sitting. It is better to drink small amounts frequently, for example a couple of sips every 10 minutes. Oral rehydration solution

Insulin treatment while you are ill (excluding gastroenteritis)

➟ Monitor your blood glucose before each meal and in between when needed.

➟ Adjust insulin doses according to the results of the blood tests. Increase the pre-meal doses by 1 unit for every 3 mmol/L of glucose above 10.

➟ Always start out by taking your usual dose (except when you have gastroenteritis, i.e. vomiting with diarrhoea).

➟ Contact your diabetes healthcare team or the hospital if you start vomiting or if your general condition is affected.

How do different illnesses affect blood glucose?

1 Not much influence at all
Illnesses that do not make you feel significantly unwell do not usually affect your insulin requirements either.

2 Low blood glucose levels
These illnesses are characterized by difficulties in retaining nutrients due to nausea, vomiting and/or diarrhoea. Examples are gastroenteritis or a viral infection with abdominal pain.

3 High blood glucose levels
Most illnesses that give obvious distress and fever will increase the blood glucose levels, thereby increasing the need for insulin. Examples are any illness with fever, such as a cold, otitis (inflammation of the ear), urinary infection or pneumonia. A genital herpes infection may also result in a substantial increase in insulin requirements.

The signs that tell you when to go to hospital

➡ It is unclear what the underlying problem might be.

➡ Repeated vomiting.

➡ Too unwell to check your blood glucose.

➡ Exhaustion on the part of the person or their carer, for example due to repeated night time waking.

➡ Blood glucose levels remaining high despite extra insulin.

➡ Severe or unusual abdominal pain.

➡ Confusion, or a deterioration of general wellbeing.

Always call if you are in the least bit unsure about how to manage the situation.

If you are on insulin, it is *very* important that you keep taking it, even if you cannot eat regular meals. Have something sweet to drink so that your blood glucose level will not fall. Make sure that the drink contains real sugar rather than artificial sweeteners. You could try fruit juice, fruit smoothies or ice cream. Once you have had enough sugary drink to bring your blood glucose level up to a reasonably normal level, do take extra water if you need it, especially if you are running a temperature.

Gastroenteritis

Gastroenteritis is an infection of the intestinal tract, which usually causes both vomiting and diarrhoea. Very little nourishment will stay in the body and there are generally problems with low blood glucose levels. You may need to lower your insulin doses considerably. Gastroenteritis

and food poisoning are therefore exceptions to the rule that the need for insulin will increase during illness. This reduction in need for insulin may go on for some time (possibly 1–2 weeks) after the gastroenteritis has been cured, as the low blood glucose levels cause a drop in insulin resistance (increased insulin sensitivity.

A slower emptying of the stomach contributes to a low blood glucose level when a person has

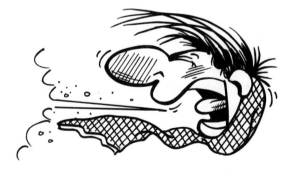

A cold with fever increases your insulin requirements, often up to 25% and sometimes even up to 50%. Begin by increasing your doses if your blood glucose levels are high. Use the rule of an extra unit of insulin for every 3 mmol/L of blood glucose above 10. Increase further if needed, depending on results from blood glucose tests.

gastroenteritis. You may need to lower the insulin doses by 20–50% in order to avoid hypoglycaemia. For prolonged problems with low blood glucose, repeated mini-doses of glucagon may be helpful.

Remember to drink plenty of fluids containing sugar, but take small sips at a time as long as you are being or feeling sick. When you are ready to eat, take food with rapidly absorbed carbohydrate as this is easier to digest.

Vomiting without diarrhoea can be a sign that your diabetes is out of control. If it continues, seek medical advice.

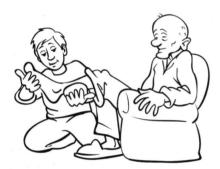

Wound healing

It is commonly believed that when people with diabetes injure their feet, they will heal more slowly. This is certainly true for individuals who have had diabetes for many years, and who are beginning to suffer from complications in the form of reduced circulation and loss of feeling in the feet and toes (see also Chapter 32, Problems with feet). If you have any worries at all about your feet, try to see a State Registered podiatrist on a regular basis.

The body's defence system will not work as well as it should if the diabetes is uncontrolled and the blood glucose level high. This will increase everyone's susceptibility to infection.

Surgery

People with diabetes should be taken care of in hospital if they need surgery, even if the operation is only a minor one. The operation should

---

Take care of small wounds and poor friends . . . (Swedish saying)

☛ Wash the wound with soap and water.

☛ Apply a clean, dry dressing.

☛ Signs of infection? See a doctor!

1 Pain/throbbing from the wound after the first 1–2 days.

2 Increasing redness of the skin.

3 A red streak in the skin going from the wound towards the body (infection of the lymph vessels).

4 A painful nodule in the groin or armpit (infected or inflamed lymph node).

5 High temperature.

---

be scheduled for as early in the day as possible. If you take tablets for diabetes and the surgery is minor, you can delay the tablets until you are ready to eat. If the surgery is more major and you are likely to miss more than one meal, you should have intravenous insulin. This is very easy to adjust and ensures that you receive the correct dose of insulin throughout the operation and during the recovery phase. If you take

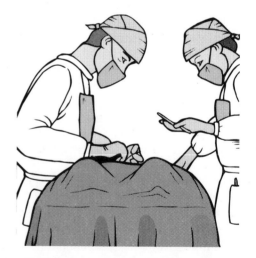

During surgery, it is advisable to administer insulin intravenously. This is a convenient and safe way to obtain a stable blood glucose level without risking hypoglycaemia.

insulin, you should omit insulin and have intravenous insulin for any except the most minor operations.

You should let your diabetes team know if you have to go to hospital for surgery. If you are admitted to hospital in an emergency, you or whoever is with you should try to make sure all staff know about your diabetes.

Drugs that affect blood glucose

Drugs that contain sugar can sometimes affect blood glucose. However, the sugar content is often low enough not to raise the blood glucose appreciably. If a medication is given with a meal, 5 g (⅙ ounce) of extra sugar is unlikely to make a noticeable difference to the blood glucose level. If it does rise, however, you can give a small extra dose of insulin (½–1 unit/10 g of sugar).

Some drugs which do not contain sugar can still cause a rise in blood glucose. Treatment with cortisol or other steroids (e.g. prednisolone, dexamethasone) causes a marked increase in the blood glucose level, often to above 20 mmol/L (360 mg/dl). This can happen even when the steroid is given as a single dose, for example to treat asthma. When taking cortisol medication for several days or longer, the insulin doses need to be increased considerably. The total dose for a 24-hour period often needs to be doubled, increasing both the pre-meal doses and the intermediate or long-acting insulin. Steroids for inhalation affect glucose levels far less. At times, a slight increase in glucose levels is seen as a small amount of the given drug is absorbed into the bloodstream. You should try to find the lowest possible dose that is effective to control the asthma. This will make it easier for you to increase your insulin if necessary to counteract the effect of the steroids. On the other hand, many people find that taking a dose of prednisolone before they go to bed prevents them from sleeping. In acute severe asthma, the combination of beta-sympathomimetics, such as salbutamol, with prednisolone often raises the blood glucose level considerably.

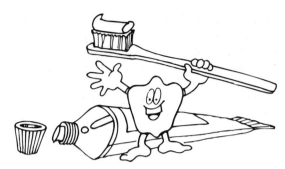

Even if you do not eat too many sweet things, you are at risk of tooth decay. This is caused by glucose in the saliva when your blood glucose level is high. Don't forget to brush your teeth at least twice a day.

Teeth

It is a good idea to see your dentist regularly, and ask for advice about your dental hygiene so that you can minimize any risk of damage. Be sure to tell your dentist that you have diabetes!

Glucose is excreted into the saliva when the blood glucose level is high, and this may contribute further to cavities. The saliva would not normally contain glucose but, if the blood glucose level is above a certain threshold, increased amounts of glucose will be found in the saliva. In this sense, a person with very high or variable blood glucose level has a higher risk of tooth decay. Unfortunately, the agreement between the glucose level, in blood and saliva is not very good, so it not possible to use tests on saliva to estimate the blood glucose level.

A study on adults with diabetes found that they had the same amount of caries as those in the control group who did not have diabetes. This may be because they tended to be more careful about their diet than members of the control group. It may also be that they paid better attention to oral hygiene than the group without diabetes. Either way, it is encouraging for anyone with diabetes to know that they can be proactive in looking after their teeth.

Gingivitis

Gingivitis is an inflammation of the gums caused by bacteria accumulating in the tooth sockets. The bacterial deposits on the teeth harden into tartar. The gums go red and bleed when you brush your teeth. Gingivitis and periodontal disease are slightly more common in people who have diabetes than in people who don't, even in young people. They are also more common when the blood glucose level is high. People with diabetes may also find their gingivitis progresses more rapidly and causes more damage than it does in people who don't have diabetes. Periodontal disease is also more common in smokers.

Having a tooth out

Dental extraction is a common procedure, particularly as people get older. If the person concerned has diabetes, however, the dentist will need to take special precautions. The procedure is usually carried out on a 'walk in' outpatient basis or 'in the dentist's chair'. The dentist or oral surgeon should have a formal protocol to follow when treating a person with diabetes. However, if you are likely to need intravenous insulin, your dentist will refer you to hospital so that this can be carried out safely. If you need to have a tooth extracted, it is essential that you ensure everyone involved in treating you knows well in advance that you have diabetes.

Vaccinations

Just because you have diabetes, this does not mean you shouldn't have the same vaccinations as other other people if you are travelling, for example. See page 185 for more information about vaccinations when travelling abroad.

In addition, everyone with diabetes is entitled to receive an annual influenza vaccination from their GP or health centre free of charge. This is because people with diabetes (along with certain other groups such as people with asthma or people over the age of 65) are more likely to develop complications as a result of a bout of 'flu. Do be sure to take up your opportunity for regular 'flu vaccinations and remind your surgery if you are not called to the 'flu clinic.

Type 2 diabetes and younger people

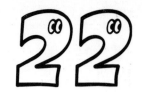

In recent years Type 2 diabetes, traditionally a problem for people later in life, has started to appear in younger age groups. You may be a teenager picking up this book, or the parent of a younger child seeking answers about Type 2 diabetes. Lots of questions are probably filling your mind. This chapter attempts to answer some of the most obvious ones.

Why me?

If you have family members with Type 2 diabetes, being overweight may bring on the dis-

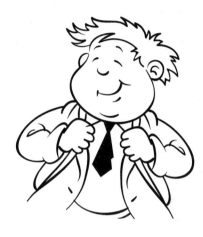

An increasing number of teenagers, and even children, are being diagnosed with Type 2 diabetes.

Type 2 diabetes: why me?

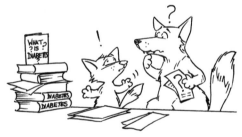

* Was it because I ate too much, or because I'm overweight?
* Are the symptoms different because I'm younger?
* What can I do about having diabetes?
* Will I need insulin eventually?
* What does the future hold?
* Are you always overweight when you develop Type 2 diabetes at a young age?

ease, particularly if you carry excess fat around the abdomen (central obesity). This stops insulin from lowering the blood sugar effectively, a condition known as 'insulin resistance', which is the underlying cause of Type 2 diabetes. With the worldwide increase in obesity, Type 2 diabetes is becoming increasingly common. In the past, it usually affected the middle-aged and elderly, but it is now being seen in a younger age group and is even appearing in children's clinics. In some American centres, half the children have Type 2 rather than Type 1 diabetes at diagnosis. You might feel as if you're completely alone and that no-one else in the world could possibly have Type 2 diabetes at your age. Try asking the nurses at your clinic if there are other people with the same problem who might like to meet up so you can help and support each other. In the UK, young people who originate from South-Asian countries like India, Pakistan and Bangladesh are at particular risk of having Type 2 diabetes.

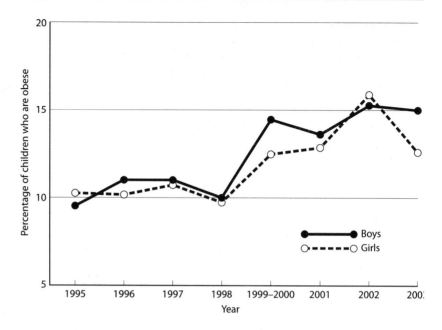

Obesity trends among children aged 2–15, England, by sex, 1995–2003.

Type 2 diabetes and overweight

Unfortunately, the rates of Type 2 diabetes in younger people are increasing very rapidly. Ultimately over the past few years, less sport is played in schools, and other activities like football after school are being replaced with Playstation games or the cartoon channel. Coupled with fast food that is cheap, easily available and very high in calories, everyone is taking in more food than they need. Cheap and poor quality school meals have made the problem worse. (See also Chapter 9, Weight control.)

If you have put on excess weight, you will become resistant to insulin and have to produce more insulin to keep your blood sugar normal.

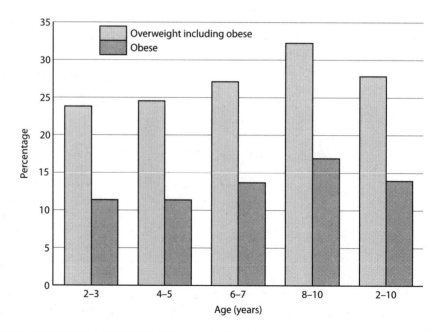

Prevalence of overweight and obesity among children, by age, England, 2003.

Over the course of a few years, your pancreas will be unable to keep up with the excess requirements and your sugar levels will rise. At this stage, you will become aware of symptoms such as thirst and frequent passing of urine.

Are the symptoms any different in younger people?

Like adults, young people with Type 2 diabetes can develop symptoms slowly over a long period. These might include thirst and tiredness, frequent trips to the bathroom, blurred vision and recurring infections. Other symptoms can include vaginal or penile thrush (yeast) infections of the vagina or penis, which cause itching or burning, particularly when passing urine. On the other hand, you may have no symptoms at all; your diabetes may be picked up by chance when you visit the doctor or nurse about something completely unrelated.

What can be done?

Type 2 diabetes in teenagers is treated in the same way as in adults. The mainstay of therapy is education, where you and your parents, brothers and sisters can talk about your fears and worries, learn about what diabetes means and what you can do about it. It is important to involve the whole family as, if you have all been overeating a little, you may not be the only one at risk of developing diabetes. This also allows the whole family to make the healthy changes in your eating habits and the exercise you take. It would be good to choose something you can do as a group activity, which will help you keep going and reach your goal. Your GP should refer you to a specialist dietitian who is expert at working with young people. You may find it useful to measure your blood sugar and discover for yourself the effect of exercise, and of particular foods. You can confirm that the information from the dietitian actually applies to you.

As well as changes in your diet and exercise, you may need a medicine to help you lose

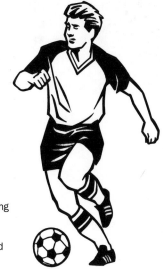

Many people enjoy playing football. It is also an activity involving lots of people so you may be able to persuade brothers and sisters to join in too.

weight. You will probably be asked to take metformin, which has the advantage of causing a little bit of weight loss as well as lowering the glucose levels. Metformin may cause gastric side effects, such as wind, diarrhoea and indigestion. If so, you should start with a very small dose and increase it gradually. There is also a slow-release form which you may be able to take without problems. There are other tablets you can take as an alternative to metformin, however they are not approved for use in people under the age of 18. (For more information about tablet treatment for Type 2 diabetes, see Chapter 13.)

Is treatment with insulin inevitable in time?

Unfortunately, your blood sugar levels are likely to rise over time, even if you stick to a good diet, take exercise and take all the recommended tablets. Over the course of a number of years, the pancreas finds it more and more difficult to keep up with insulin production. There are ways of slowing the failure of the pancreas. A particular tablet, called a glitazone, appears to protect the cells that produce insulin. The best thing you can do, which may be the most difficult, is to lose weight. People who are able to continue to reduce their weight will also reduce insulin resistance and make the insulin they produce more effective. However, it is likely that you will need insulin at some stage in the future.

What does the future hold?

Unfortunately, all the complications which occur in adult Type 2 diabetes may also occur in young people. Eye problems due to diabetes are extremely rare in young people. The American Diabetes Association plays safe and recommends screening at 10 years old and every year after that. Photographs of the back of the eye (retina) are taken with a special camera. (See also page 198 for more information about eye problems.)

Nephropathy or kidney disease can also occur in young people, and you should make sure that your urine is tested for any leaks of protein (microalbuminuria). You should have your blood pressure measured, and some people need a tablet to control blood pressure and protect their kidneys.

Many people with Type 2 diabetes have problems with control of blood fats, and your doctor may want to start tablets to reduce them. High cholesterol, coupled with high blood pressure and insulin resistance, increases the risk of heart disease so it's important to keep this under control even if you think you're too young to run into any problems. Your treatment, though, may be different from that recommended for an older person.

One American study looked at how frequently risk factors for heart disease occurred in groups of young people aged 12–19 years. These included high cholesterol, triglycerides, blood pressure and increased waist circumference. In the general population of American children, 6.4% in this age range had two or more of these risk factors. In young people with Type 1 diabetes, the frequency was 14%, while in those with Type 2 diabetes it was greater than 90%.

Some tablets used to treat diabetes, blood pressure and blood fats shouldn't be used in pregnancy. If pregnancy is a possibility, it is vital that you do not take a statin (for cholesterol) or

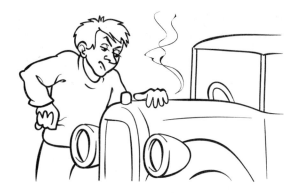

Like an old car, the pancreas will wear out in time and find it increasingly hard to do what it is designed to do. This tends to happen through no fault of the owner. However, you can make your pancreas, like your car, function better for longer if you treat it with care and respect.

an ACE inhibitor (for blood pressure). Indeed, if there is any possibility at all of an unplanned pregnancy, it is probably better not to take this type of medication at all. You should also take folic acid in the run up to pregnancy. The dose is 5 mg a day and it can be prescribed by your GP. Folic acid taken in the first 3 months of pregnancy reduces the risk of the baby developing spina bifida.

Eventually, you may meet a partner who you want to settle down and have children with. You may worry about the chances of your children developing diabetes. If your partner also has diabetes, the chances of the children developing diabetes is increased, but the degree of increased risk isn't entirely clear. Many researchers have tried to study the inheritance of diabetes but have still not discovered how much is caused by genes and how much by environment. The best way to reduce the risk of Type 2 diabetes for your children is to work as hard as you can at a healthy lifestyle for the whole family.

Type 2 diabetes in young people who are not overweight

One special form of diabetes in the young is called maturity onset diabetes of the young or MODY ('maturity-onset diabetes' is an earlier name for Type 2 diabetes). In the 1970s, it was noticed that, in a handful of families, several members developed diabetes in their teens or 20s (about 50% of family members were affected). These young people developing diabetes were usually not overweight, and the pattern of diabetes suggested a certain sort of inheritance (autosomal dominant). Family members with diabetes have a specific defect in their insulin-producing cells. Research into these patients has increased our understanding of the causes of diabetes. Individuals with MODY can be accurately identified by special genetic blood tests, and the condition turns out to be more common than was originally believed.

There are several distinct types of MODY. One type (MODY 2) involves a modest increase in blood glucose levels, and often does not need any treatment at all apart from care with the diet. People with MODY 2 seldom get complications from their diabetes. Some forms of MODY can be treated successfully with drugs (sulphonylureas) while others may need insulin.

MODY is inherited so if you or your partner have MODY there is a strong chance that your children will be affected. Ask your doctor whether you should be referred for genetic counselling and testing genetic test if diabetes has occured in several generations of your family.

Finding out more

Developing Type 2 diabetes at such a young age might seem very daunting with your whole life ahead of you. You can make giant strides in reducing your blood sugar by making simple changes to your diet and exercise regime. If you continue to lose weight, you should be able to put off treatment with insulin for several years. By controlling your sugar, blood pressure and blood fats, you can effectively reduce the risk of any complications from your diabetes. You should try to meet the targets set by your healthcare team, and not turn your back on their advice. This will enable you to enjoy a happy and healthy life. (See also the box on right).

Useful resources if you are a young person with Type 2 diabetes, or the parent of a young person with Type 2 diabetes

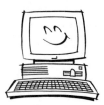

1 MODY websites
To find out more about this unusual form of diabetes, visit these websites:
www.projects.ex.ac.uk/diabetesgenes/mody/index.htm
www.rch.bham.ac.uk/PCH/Diabetes/Diabetes1.htm
You will find these useful for gaining information about the condition. They also provide support and advice.

2 National diabetes education program (NDEP)
www.ndep.nih.gov
This website deals with education for patients and carers of those with Type 2 diabetes and is run by the American government. It is an excellent resource and has a number of downloadable fact sheets which you can refer to.

3 Royal Children's Hospital, Melbourne
www.rch.org.au/diabetesmanual
This is another useful information website from Australia.

4 American Diabetes Association
www.diabetes.org
The ADA website has a user-friendly Youth Zone, which contains downloadable fact sheets, advice and recipes for foods you might like to try at home.

Smoking

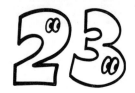

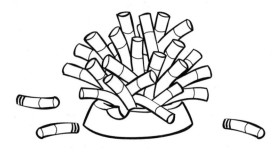

Everyone knows that smoking is bad for you, and the majority of long-term smokers want to stop because the increased risk of death from smoking is well publicised. Out of 1000 people who smoke for 20 years, around 50% will die from smoking-related disease. The problem is that by the time most people are first diagnosed with Type 2 diabetes, the habit has become a part of their life. This chapter examines the risks presented by smoking in diabetes and what you might be able to do to 'kick the habit'. Your chances of succeeding can be affected by many different factors and some of these are explored.

The risks

The combination of smoking in conjunction with Type 2 diabetes speeds up the rate at which complications may develop, especially complications affecting your macrovascular and microvascular systems (involving the blood supply to all your body's organs). If you have diabetes, your life expectancy is less than that of someone who doesn't have diabetes. If you smoke, you can expect to die earlier than someone who doesn't smoke. So if you have diabetes and you smoke, you are going to reduce your chances of a long life.

There is plenty of evidence that smoking in conjunction with diabetes is linked to increased risk of stroke, heart attack, peripheral vascular disease, kidney failure and diabetic eye disease.

Smoking also leads to narrowing of the blood vessels, and damages blood vessel walls. Nicotine causes constriction of the blood vessels and the release of hormones such as catecholamines which increase blood pressure. Research shows that blood pressure in Type 2 diabetes is particularly hard to control because of accelerated blood vessel damage. Smoking places additional strain on the body's ability to control blood pressure. Evidence from long-term studies also shows that smoking increases insulin resistance, leading to impaired glucose tolerance or pre-diabetes. This insulin resistance may also make it more difficult to control your diabetes after it has been diagnosed, although this is more difficult to demonstrate in a clinical study. Quite apart from the blood vessel damage, high blood pressure and contribution to raised blood glucose, smoking affects the lungs. All smokers, whether or not they have diabetes, put themselves at at high risk of chronic lung damage which will limit the capacity to exercise and lose weight. It also makes people more likely to develop cancer – lung cancer of course, but a range of other cancers as well.

Some people think that if they switch from smoking cigarettes to smoking a pipe, they will get rid of the problem. But evidence suggests that even though pipe smoking may be marginally less dangerous than cigarette smoking, this

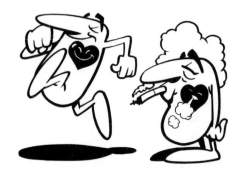

You will stay much more healthy if you give up smoking!

Effects of smoking related to diabetes

- Increased heart rate.
- Raised blood pressure.
- Increased LDL (bad) cholesterol.
- Reduced HDL (good) cholesterol.
- Increased platelets – blood is more viscous and likely to clot.
- Atherosclerosis – narrowing of the arteries.
- Increased insulin resistance.

is really only for people who have never smoked cigarettes. Switching your method of smoking will not make the outlook any better for you.

Some people feel that there is no point in stopping smoking because they have been smoking for so long already that the damage must have been done. But in fact, if you stop smoking, your body will gradually repair some of the damage that has been done, and your health is likely to improve. So if you smoke, and can possibly stop, then do! It is a really positive way you can increase your chances of good health and a longer life.

How do I stop?

Willpower

It is important to face facts. The chances of giving up smoking by willpower alone are tiny. Over the course of a year, fewer than 5% of people attempting to quit without help actually manage it. If you know someone who has, they are most definitely the exception rather than the rule.

Counselling services

Your GP will be happy to help by referring you to a 'quit smoking' service. In the UK, as in most developed countries, the health service offers its own smoking cessation service. This is usually managed by a mixture of nurses and counsellors, and sessions are often conducted in a group setting to encourage people to support each other and thus increase their chances of quitting. Without the addition of nicotine replacement or other medication, counselling probably doubles the chances of giving up smoking at one year, but the chances are still probably less than 10%.

Complementary therapies

Although we can offer you little or no scientific evidence that complementary therapies such as hypnotherapy and acupuncture are effective in helping smoking cessation, we know a few people who state that these methods were highly effective for them. The idea of treating you as a whole person, rather than as someone who has diabetes or even just someone who is trying to stop smoking, is an important part of any complementary therapy. This is a view we strongly support. Hypnosis in particular may help by improving relaxation and reducing stress. It is very important though that you seek a qualified, registered practitioner. Some NHS smoking cessation services offer these therapies free of charge. Others may be able to recommend a trusted therapist.

Nicotine replacement therapy

Nicotine, the major habit-forming component of cigarette smoke, is highly addictive. It causes

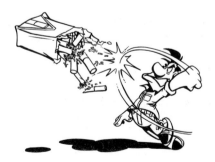

It is never too late to give up smoking. For every day without a cigarette, the damaging effects of tobacco in your body are reduced.

physiological symptoms (changes in body function) which stimulate cravings during the first few days after stopping smoking. Later on, there is a psychological addiction to overcome where you still feel a compulsion to smoke during stressful situations – at work for instance or during a social occasion like a party or going out to the pub.

Replacing nicotine from cigarettes using another method of delivery helps with both immediate physiological addiction and later psychological addiction to cigarettes. A number of methods of delivering nicotine have been developed by the pharmaceutical companies. They all increase your chance of being able to give up cigarettes. Methods available from the pharmacy now include gum, patches, lozenges and a nicotine inhaler. Consult your doctor first before trying these products. It is best to use them under supervision if you have diabetes because they may increase risks from low blood glucose (hypoglycaemia).

Nicotine replacement therapy works best when used in conjunction with support, usually from the NHS Stop Smoking service or similar groups. It is encouraging to see that, depending on which study you look at, people who make use of counselling at the same time as using a nicotine replacement raise their chances of giving up successfully to between 15 and 35%.

Buproprion

Buproprion (trade name Zyban) was originally developed as an anti-depressant medication, but quite soon doctors began to notice that patients who were using it for depressive illnesses began to give up smoking.

Studies using special techniques in animals showed that buproprion affects the addiction and reward centres in the brain. For this reason it can help people to stop a number of forms of addictive behaviour, including cigarette smoking, pathological gambling and excessive eating. In total, the quit rates for studies involving buproprion are around 30–40% at the one-year stage. It appears that buproprion is the most effective add-in to

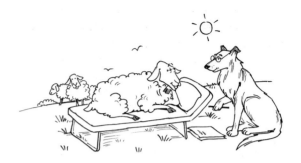

Counselling can help motivate you to give up smoking completely, especially if it used in conjunction with nicotine replacement therapy.

counselling for helping patients to stop using cigarettes.

Buproprion is not totally without problems, however. Like all anti-depressant type drugs, it does increase your chances of suffering a seizure or epileptic fit. The chance of suffering a fit if you take bupropion is around 1%. This is increased if you suffer from frequent low blood sugars or if you have a lifestyle which itself increases the chance of epileptic fits (e.g. if you drink too much alcohol).

A number of drugs also interfere with the way in which bupropion is broken down by the body. This can lead to increased levels of the drug in the blood, which can increase the risk of fits. This problem has led to a number of cases of problems with bupropion being featured in the press where patients have used it and been taking drugs such as anti-malarials which interfere with the way the body can rid of it.

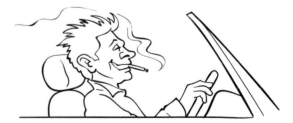

Stopping smoking is difficult but crucial if you are to do your best to avoid future problems and complications associated with your diabetes. Type 2 diabetes accelerates the passage of your life, prematurely shortening it. Smoking also presses harder on the accelerator and cuts further years off your life expectancy.

This means that it is crucial, particularly when you have Type 2 diabetes, that if your GP is considering prescribing bupropion, he or she makes a thorough examination of the other drugs that you are taking, and looks for any which might lead to increased levels of bupropion. You can look for any drugs that may interfere yourself – on the Internet (see the links on page 226). Your doctor will also want to hear about your lifestyle, particularly with regard to such aspects as your consumption of alcohol.

New drugs

A number of promising new drugs to help with stopping smoking are currently in clinical trials. Two in particular, rimonabant from Sanofi-Aventis, which is likely to be licensed soon for weight loss, and an anti-depressant type drug from Pfizer, look as though they may be particularly useful.

Passive smoking

Even passive smoking can damage your prospects with respect to diabetes complications. Whilst the increased risks are not as great as

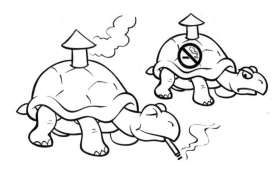
If your partner smokes, encourage them to stop.

when you are smoking yourself, they are still considerable. If your partner smokes, do try to encourage him or her to stop.

Snuff

While snuff is no longer in general use in the UK, it is still quite popular in other countries, particularly in Northern Europe and Scandinavia. Although using snuff doesn't result in long-term respiratory damage, nicotine is absorbed in a highly effective way through the buccal mucosa, is just as addictive and still causes hypertension and damage to the arterial wall.

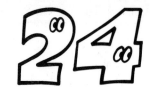

Alcohol
and other substances

We do not recommend a total ban on drinking alcohol if you have diabetes. However, it is important to know how alcohol works and that you take it easy, making sure you stop drinking before you get drunk. Your diabetes team can neither allow you to do something, nor forbid it. They can only tell you how things work and where and why you should be particularly careful.

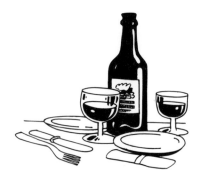

Alcohol and the liver

Alcohol counteracts the ability of the liver to produce new glucose (a process called gluconeogenesis) by keeping the enzymes occupied with the breakdown of alcohol. The liver can still release glucose from the glycogen store (see page 17). But when this store is depleted you will experience hypoglycaemia. The concentration of cortisol and growth hormone in the blood will decrease after alcohol intake. Both hormones lead to a rise in the blood glucose level, and reduced levels will contribute to an increased risk of hypoglycaemia many hours after alcohol intake. These biological factors come together, making the risk of hypoglycaemia much greater after drinking alcohol. This effect of alcohol will last the entire time it takes the liver to break down the alcohol in your body. The liver will break down 0.1 g (1.5 grains) of pure alcohol/kg body weight per hour. For example, if you weigh 70 kg (155 lb) it will take 1 hour to break down the alcohol in a bottle of light beer, 2 hours for 40 ml of liqueur and 10 hours to break down the alcohol in a bottle of wine. Therefore, if you drink during the evening you will be at risk of hypoglycaemia all night as well as part of the next day.

Why is it dangerous to drink too much if you have diabetes?

When you have diabetes, you must be able to think clearly in many situations so you can take corrective action, for example if you feel yourself becoming hypoglycaemic. You won't be able to do this if you have had too much to drink, in exactly the same way as you cannot drive a car safely after taking more than a small amount of alcohol. Severe hypoglycaemia after drinking alcohol has occasionally caused death in people with diabetes. Scientific studies show the role of alcohol in causing hypoglycaemia has more to do with losing the ability to recognize the signs of impending hypoglycaemia than with reducing the liver's ability to produce glucose. However, some medications (metformin in particular) interact with alcohol to cause additional problems.

In one study, people with diabetes drank either white wine (approximately 600 ml, three average-sized glasses) or water 2–3 hours after the evening snack. The morning blood glucose was 3–4 mmol/L (55–70 mg/dl) lower after drinking wine, and five of the six individuals experienced symptomatic hypoglycaemia

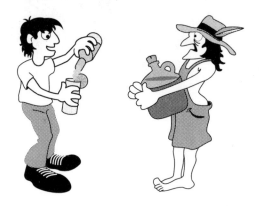

Drinking too much can impede your judgement and cause you to think less clearly.

2–4 hours after breakfast. This suggests it is advisable to be prepared for late-morning hypoglycaemia after an evening spent drinking. If you are on insulin, you would do well to lower your insulin dose both at bedtime and before breakfast.

Alcohol and calories

Drink	Alcohol content %	Kcal	Carb. g
1 bottle, 300 ml:			
Non-alcoholic beer	0.5	~60	~16
Low alcohol beer	0.5–1.2	~40	~7
Light beer	~3–5	~90	~5
Beer	4	~160	~13
1 glass, 150 ml:			
Red wine	9.9	114	3.5
White wine, dry	9.5	99	0.7
White wine, sweet	10.7	147	8.9
60 ml:			
Sherry	16	91	6
45 ml:			
Vodka	32	100	0
Whisky	32	100	0
Punch	20	132	14
Liqueur	19	150	24

Basic rules

If you have Type 2 diabetes, you should limit your alcohol intake to 2 units of alcohol for women and 3 units for men in one day. Make sure that your friends know you have diabetes and wear some type of diabetes ID (necklace or Medic-Alert bracelet) when you are socializing. If you are drinking alcohol containing no carbohydrate (e.g. spirits with low-calorie mixers), you should eat something while drinking this sort of alcohol. But if there is carbohydrate in your drink – beer or lager – you do not need to take extra food. Because alcohol prevents your liver from producing glucose, it often leads to hypoglycaemia, which occurs several hours after drinking. It may also make glucagon less effective, should you need this to correct a severe hypo. Research has shown that the glucose-lowering effect of alcohol is often delayed till the following morning. So, if possible, you should have a good breakfast the next morning and perhaps reduce your morning dose of insulin.

It takes a long time for your liver to break down alcohol, which increases the risk of severe hypoglycaemia. Because of this, sleeping late is particularly dangerous the morning after you have been drinking. If you have also been especially active, playing team games or dancing at a club for example, the combined risks of extra activity with alcohol intake put you at much greater risk than usual of severe hypoglycaemia. In such circumstances, preventing hypoglycaemia becomes imperative.

What if you have had too much to drink?

Eat extra food immediately before going to bed. You can eat potato crisps in this situation as they give a slow increase in blood glucose over several hours (see page 45). The blood glucose level should not be less than 10 mmol/L (180 mg/dl) when you go to bed. If you are taking insulin, decrease the dose of bedtime insulin by 2–4 units to avoid hypoglycaemia. Don't go to bed alone if you have an alternative; if you have severe

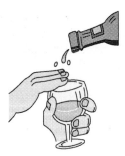

Your doctor and diabetes nurse can tell you how alcohol affects your body, and what the risks might be of drinking too much if you have diabetes. But it is down to you to decide how much alcohol you have, and when it is appropriate to refuse another drink.

hypoglycaemia during the night you will need someone to help you. If you come home very late, make sure to wake a family member or partner and let them know about your condition. Your life may actually depend upon it, even if you find the situation embarrassing. Set your alarm clock. Don't sleep in late! Be sure to eat a proper breakfast as soon as you wake up the next morning. If you feel sick, check your blood glucose level, as your nausea may be caused by high glucose levels rather than a hangover.

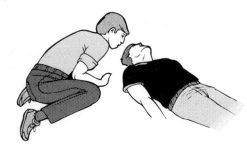

If you develop severe hypoglycaemia after drinking alcohol, the person finding you is likely to assume that you are simply drunk. It is essential that you wear a Medic-Alert necklace/bracelet. (You can also carry an ID card, but this may not be found as readily.)

Dieting and weight loss

As discussed above, alcohol contains a significant number of calories and may lead to weight increase. (See also Chapter 9 on Weight control.)

Illegal drugs

Drugs affect the brain and nervous system, and will make it much more difficult to maintain

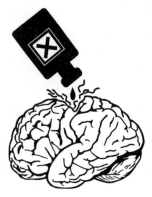

Illegal drugs act as poisons on your brain and are likely to be extremely addictive.

motivation to control your diabetes carefully. Drugs make you forgetful and can lead to missed meals or medication, leading to high or low blood sugars. Wear a diabetes ID, which may help you receive the right sort of help if you become confused.

The whole problem with recreational drugs is the obvious fact that they are addictive, and having experimented with them in a casual way, some people soon become dependent to the extent that drugs begin to control their lives.

Certain drugs may have specific extra risks associated with the blood vessels. These include amphetamines, which are known to damage the linings of blood vessels, thereby increasing the risks of diabetes complications in both the short and the longer term. Many people who are drug users would find it extremely difficult to take good care of themselves and their diabetes while continuing their drug use, because of the behavioural aspects of drug use. Casual drug users would have the same problems as those of other medications that interfere with rational self-care at the time.

'Uppers'

Uppers like amphetamine (speed, whizz, sulph), ecstasy (E, eckies, doves) and cocaine (coke, charlie, snow) are used to give more energy and confidence and have been popular at rave parties. There is a risk of dehydration when the body loses fluid through continuous dancing or

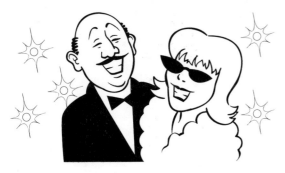

Cocaine was once a drug for the rich and famous. But falling prices mean it is much more widely available now.

other strenuous activity. Uppers can suppress appetite, and combined with dancing, there is a risk of experiencing severe hypoglycaemia. In this sense, these drugs can be extremely dangerous for a person with diabetes, especially if not enough extra fluid is taken or the extra bedtime snack is forgotten.

Cocaine (coke, Charlie, snow) is also used to produce 'highs' and increase confidence. The price of these drugs has come right down in recent years, meaning that they are available as street drugs rather than just for the rich and famous. Cocaine is a Class A drug and, particularly in the form of crack, can be very addictive. Cocaine is known to cause sudden heart attacks in young users at an age when normally serious heart disease would not occur.

Benzodiazepines

These are a group of drugs that are used in a controlled way by doctors, prescribing them to people who have difficulty sleeping or suffer from anxiety. But there is a 'black market' for them too, and they are used illegally as 'recreational' drugs.

The best known drug in this group is temazepam. This can make you feel relaxed and sleepy, but if you take a larger dose it can have similar effects to a large amount of alcohol. It can make you talkative or over excited and sometimes aggressive. It also gives you a false sense of confidence and undermines your judgement. It would certainly be very

difficult for you to be aware that your blood glucose level was too high or too low, and it may well cause you to forget to take your medication, including insulin.

Cannabis

Use of cannabis (marijuana, hash, blow, weed) is often viewed as less harmful than the use of 'hard drugs' such as heroin, cocaine or amphetamines. In terms of making rational decisions about complex activities such as driving or diabetes self-management, marijuana is likely to be at least as risky as alcohol. Combining cannabis with alcohol (as often happens) adds special risks for making diabetes-related decisions about, for example, when to wake up the next day. Many people who take cannabis find themselves becoming especially hungry and want to eat everything in sight, especially junk food (the 'munchies') which will raise the blood glucose level considerably and lead to weight gain.

Smoking cannabis has also been shown to be associated both with accelerated cardiovascular disease and increased risk of lung cancer. In addition, studies have shown increased risk of psychological disorders such as schizophrena.

Hallucinogenics

Hallucinogenic drugs alter your perception of the outside world. Perhaps the best known, lysergic acid or LSD (acid), was widely used in

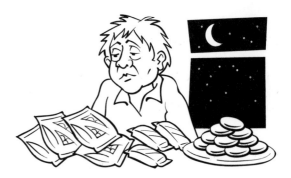

Cannabis can give you the 'munchies', making you want to eat everything you can lay your hands on.

the 1960s and 70s. Taking an acid tablet or 'tab' can take you on a bizarre and dream-like journey, or one that is a nightmare beyond your wildest imaginings. Even if you have taken acid before, the effects are unpredictable, and trips usually last between 7 and 12 hours.

Another common hallucinogenic drug, ketamine hydrochloride (ketamine, K), was originally developed for use in hospital anaesthetics, but it is no longer used this way in humans. Much of the ketamine that is sold on the street now was originally intended for veterinary use. As the drug was originally developed as an anaesthetic, it can lead to loss of physical sensation and even ability to move, as well as hallucinations and out of body experiences. The effects can be particularly alarming when mixed with alcohol, and anecdotal evidence suggests that it has been used as a 'date rape' drug. The combination of such effects with hypoglycaemia could well be life-threatening.

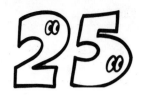

Sexual problems and Type 2 diabetes

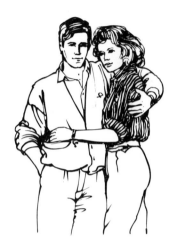

Sexual problems are very common, and are often associated with Type 2 diabetes. However, it is important to be aware that they affect many other people too, both men and women, especially as we get older. Don't panic if you are having problems with your sex life, as many others are in the same position whether or not they have diabetes. Both men and women frequently consult their doctor about problems with their libido and sexual performance.

This chapter examines the impact of mood and depression on sexual difficulties, some of the symptoms that men and women with Type 2 diabetes might suffer because of microvascular problems (see also Chapter 31), and a number of strategies to solve these.

Problems with your erection

Many men both with and without diabetes suffer erectile dysfunction. The severity may range from minor softening which makes penetration of your partner difficult, to problems with ejac-

ulation or complete failure to rise at all. The underlying cause may not be physical but could be related to depression or problems with your relationship. It can also relate to underlying cardiovascular disease, anatomical problems with the penis itself, or a range of other disorders.

Depression

Many people with diabetes are depressed about their diagnosis, changes in their life, alterations they have to make to their routine to keep good glucose control, disagreements with their partner, problems at work and implications for the future, to name a handful of possible reasons. Whatever the cause, depression is strongly associated with erectile dysfunction. If you have issues in your life which need to be sorted out, medical treatments for erectile dysfunction are less likely to be successful. It is important to talk to your doctor and be properly assessed so that treatment can be tailored to your individual needs. Your GP will be able to direct you to an appropriate person for counselling or advice, whether it be specifically about your diabetes or about your relationship. A number of the tablet treatments for depression can make erection problems worse, so it is worth persevering with counselling advice rather than taking medication. Try to persuade your partner to come with you to counselling sessions, but if this isn't practical, share your problems with your partner if at all possible.

Adequate investigation of any medical problems

Erectile dysfunction can be a symptom of disease of the blood vessels (see page 193). Achieving an erection depends on two things:

1 Adequate function of the nerves which can be damaged by microvascular disease (See Chapter 31).

2 A circulation which is sufficiently well-functioning to be able to carry enough blood to the penis.

A proportion of men with erectile dysfunction also have cardiovascular disease. It is important to identify this because the most widely-used treatment for erectile dysfunction (Viagra) cannot be used by men who take a certain treatment for angina, namely nitrates. If you have cardiovascular disease, it is important to make sure that any risk factors are identified and treated. Your GP will be alerted to look for signs of cardiovascular disease if your blood pressure is difficult to control, if you are overweight, if your lipid (blood fat) levels are too high or if you have microalbuminuria (traces of protein in your urine; see page 200). There are a number of ways that health professionals can examine your condition in more detail. These might include a resting ECG, an exercise ECG or specialist referral to a heart doctor to do an ultrasound of your heart under conditions mimicking exercise (a stress ECHO).

You may also have other problems associated with disease of the nerves (neuropathy), these might include a drop in blood pressure when you stand up (postural hypotension), or prob-

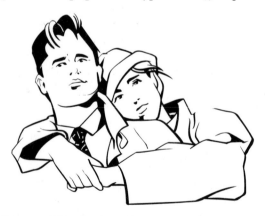

It is a good thing if your partner can come along to counselling sessions with you, as this will help you approach the problem as a shared one.

lems with the passage of food through the gut, where the transit can be too rapid or to slow.

Medical treatment of erectile dysfunction

Seeking specialist advice is really important. There are a number of nurse specialists with a particular interest in erectile dysfunction. Your GP will be able to refer you to one at your local hospital. Before you visit your GP, it is a good idea to read about potential treatment options. Websites are a good source of information: the Sexual Dysfunction Association (www.sda.uk. net) contains question and answer sections and a range of downloadable pieces of information about diseases and treatments associated with erection problems.

A specialist nurse should be able to help you choose the most suitable approach for managing your needs, and talk to you about all options and their implications.

Tablets

Four products are available at the moment. Three belong to the same class of drugs, known as PDE-5 inhibitors, and go by the brand names of Viagra, Cialis and Levitra. The first drug to be developed, Viagra, was originally intended to be used for treating angina, but it soon became apparent in male users that the main effect was on the arteries supplying blood to the penis, not the arteries of the heart. PDE-5 inhibitors work by dilating the smooth muscle which lines small arteries, leading to increased blood flow. Each of the three drugs has a slightly different profile in terms of how long it takes to work and how long the effects last. They are also available at varying strengths. People with diabetes often require the higher dose, so don't despair if you don't respond adequately at the starting dose. Side effects of these drugs are mainly headache and a fall in blood pressure; sometimes nausea and indigestion can also occur. The fall in blood pressure can be particularly noticeable in individuals taking nitrate tablets for angina. For these reasons,

PDE-5 inhibitors should be not be used by people who are taking nitrate tablets.

The other oral treatment is Uprima, containing apomorphine. Apomorphine was originally developed as a treatment for Parkinson's disease but can also be useful as a treatment for erection problems. It is given by a tablet under the tongue and takes around 20 minutes to work. Side effects include nausea, indigestion, headache and dizziness.

Local agents

There are three local agents that you may encounter. These are described in the table below.

Mechanical devices

Various pump or constriction devices can also help you to achieve an erection. They can be very effective but require a sense of humour in both partners.

A rigid prosthesis can be inserted by a surgical operation but this is a last resort.

What happens if nothing works?

Of course it is very reassuring to discover a range of possible treatments. It is possible, however, that none of them will work for you. In this case, you can still achieve physical intimacy with your partner in many other ways. A good source of information is the Sexual Dysfunction Association website – see previous page.

What about women?

Sexual problems in women are similar to those in men with diabetes. Just because there isn't a visible sign which requires intervention, doesn't mean that troubles don't exist. The same problems which lead to depression in men with diabetes also affect women, and this can lead to reduced libido

Name	What does it involve?	Disadvantages	Side effects
Caverject (prostaglandin E)	Caverject involves an injection into the penis which encourages local changes in the blood vessels to promote an erection.	The dose needs to be adjusted, depending on individual response.	Can lead to a persistent erection (priapism) which may need hospital treatment if it persists. Other side effects include pain in the penis or a haematoma (collection of blood).
MUSE (prostaglandin E)	Muse is another preparation of prostaglandin E, administered by pushing the tablet using an applicator down the middle of the penis via the urethra.	This requires some degree of dexterity to administer.	Can be associated with persistent erection, as for Caverject.
Papaverine	In rare cases, this drug can also be used as a local injection for erection problems.	This can also be associated with persistent erection.	If the erection lasts longer than 4 hours, it is important to consult your doctor urgently.

and decreased arousal during the times when love-making is attempted. Counselling and advice about specific problems can help.

Neuropathy in women may cause decreased lubrication on intercourse and make it more difficult to reach orgasm. Adequate lubrication with a suitable water-based personal lubricant can help with this difficulty. A range of water-based lubricants exist, from the standard KY jelly, to exotic varieties that you can have fun choosing with your partner! It isn't an admission of failure to use additional lubrication; many couples with no sexual problems at all find the extra slipperiness adds to their sense of enjoyment.

High levels of sugar in the urine may also lead to increased risk of infection, particularly with Candida ('thrush', a yeast infection) which may lead to problems with vaginal soreness and irritation. Thrush can usually be treated by an antifungal cream or pessary, or a tablet to act upon your entire body. These treatments are available with a prescription from your doctor.

For acute infection, topical treatments such as clotrimoxazole exist. These can be given as a cream pessary to treat infection deep in the vagina, with additional cream to treat itching and soreness of the labia. These local treatments are normally used in conjunction with oral therapy such as fluconazole, 'Canesten oral'.

The best way of eliminating Candida permanently is to maintain good blood glucose control. Apart from this a number of effective treatments exist. Regular washing with a lactic acid based feminine wash such as Lactacyd may reduce recurrent Candida.

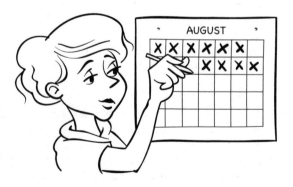

Menstruation

Many women who take insulin find that their blood sugar levels increase in the days before their period starts. In a Hungarian study, the premenstrual doses were approximately 3 units higher than they were mid-cycle. However, during the first couple of days of menstruation, the insulin requirements may fall, increasing the risk of hypoglycaemia. If you notice that you have this type of problem, check your blood glucose level especially carefully on the days close to your period. This will enable you to adjust your insulin doses upwards just before it starts and lower them just after it finishes. If your HbA_{1c} is high, this may make your periods irregular or cause you to miss periods altogether.

Fertility

Men with diabetes do not appear to be any less fertile than men who do not have diabetes. In addition, women with average diabetes control have much the same chances of getting pregnant as women without diabetes. However, it does appear that women with consistently high blood glucose readings may find it difficult to conceive. This may be a good thing as high blood glucose levels can harm a developing baby and lead to developmental abnormalities. It does make it particularly important, however, to plan your pregnancy and talk to your doctor or diabetes nurse about the best way to ensure you have a consistently low HbA_{1c} before you start trying for a baby.

Contraception

The Pill

In the past, the 'minipill', containing only progesterone, was usually recommended to all women with diabetes. However, this increases the risk of 'spotting' between periods and has a narrower time margin for taking the pills (not

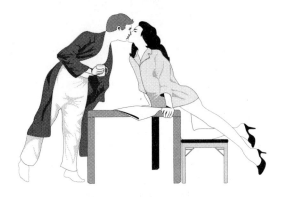

Contraceptive methods

Condom	The only contraceptive that protects against sexually transmitted diseases.
Diaphragm and spermicidal jelly	Not easy to use. Risk of itching as side effect.
Combined Pill	Sometimes result in a slight increase in blood glucose levels.
Minipill	Risk of spotting. Smaller margin for error if a tablet is missed. Carries a higher risk of pregnancy than the combined Pill.
Intrauterine device (IUD, coil)	Risk of pelvic infection is low, but an IUD is not recommended for use before the first pregnancy.
Depot injection	Can affect metabolic control. Sometimes troublesome side effects.
Implant	Same as depot injection but easy to remove if side effects are not acceptable.
'Morning-after' pills	For 'emergency' situations. Needs to be taken within 72 hours of unprotected intercourse.

more than 30 hours between pills in most cases, though new versions such as Cerazette, which suppress ovulation, have a slightly longer potential 'window' between pills.

Combined contraceptives ('ordinary' pills) are more effective in preventing pregnancy, especially in younger women. Combined pills contain two types of female sex hormone. Oestrogen prevents the egg from developing and being released from the ovary. Progesterone prevents the sperm from passing through the mucus at the neck of the womb (cervix). The use of oral contraceptives does not appear to increase the risk of later complications with the eyes or kidneys.

At one time, combined contraceptive pills were thought to raise the blood glucose levels slightly, but more recent studies show no adverse effects on glucose control. If you find it difficult to adjust your glucose control in the week without pills, it might be appropriate to wait longer before having a break, for example taking 3 months-worth of pills without interruption. Today, combined pills are recommended for younger women who have no other complicating factors (such as migraine). In addition, combined pills are not recommended if you smoke (due to an increased risk of thrombosis and heart attack), or if you have high blood pressure or complications with your eyes or kidneys.

Intrauterine devices and implants

An intrauterine device (IUD, coil) is a safe contraceptive for women with diabetes according to recent studies. Problems with infections or spotting are no more common than they are in women without diabetes. However, they are not recommended for women who have heavy or irregular menstrual periods. As there is a small risk of infection of the womb or ovary (and thus a risk of becoming infertile), intrauterine devices are not recommended for women who have never been pregnant. However, for a woman who has diabetes complications affecting the eyes or kidneys, intrauterine devices may be a good alternative to contraceptive pills.

Depot injections or implants contain the same hormone (progesterone) as minipills. However, they will give a higher hormone concentration and affect the blood glucose level more than minipills. Common side effects include nausea, increased appetite and irritability, all of which make it more difficult to control the blood glucose levels. The contraceptive depot injection is not considered suitable for women with diabetes as the effects of one injection last for many months. A contraceptive implant contains the same hormone as a depot injection. It is implanted under the skill using local anaesthesia. The advantage is that it can be removed if the woman experiences side effects. This makes it more suitable for a woman with diabetes than the depot injection.

Staying healthy

Remember that most contraceptive methods only prevent unwanted pregnancy. It is as important to protect yourself against sexually transmitted diseases. Some of these diseases can be life-threatening; others can have a serious effect on a woman's fertility. A condom is the only contraceptive that offers full protection from sexually transmitted diseases. Talk to your GP, family planning nurse or pregnancy advice service about which type of contraceptive would be best for you. Women using oral contraceptive pills should have regular blood pressure monitoring and gynaecological check-ups.

Pregnancy and diabetes

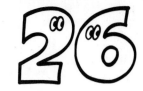

Pregnancy used to be unusual in women with Type 2 diabetes, but now that many younger people are developing the condition, it now accounts for around 30% of pregnancies involving diabetes in the UK (according to CEMACH).

One of the first questions a younger woman who is diagnosed with Type 2 diabetes is likely to ask, is whether she will still be able to have babies. Being pregnant exerts a certain strain on every woman, but there is no reason to discourage women with diabetes from having children. The mother's risk of developing diabetes complications in later life is not affected by pregnancy.

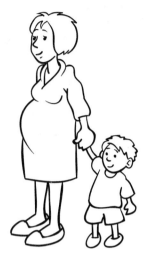

Preparing for pregnancy

If you are hoping to start a family, it is really important that you talk it through with your doctor first so that you can learn about and discuss the issues involved. Really good management of blood pressure and blood glucose is crucial to ensure that the strain that having a baby places on your body systems doesn't worsen the complications associated with your

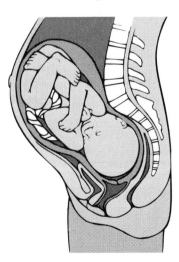

If you make up your mind to sort out your general health and nutrition, as well as your diabetes control, before you get pregnant, you will give your developing baby a better start in life.

diabetes. In addition, the insulin resistance associated with Type 2 diabetes can both make it difficult to get pregnant and increase the chances of suffering a miscarriage.

All women trying for a baby, no matter what their state of health, need to be careful about their diet in the weeks before conception. Folic acid is an essential vitamin supplement, and you should take a daily supplement of 5 mg. This has been shown to reduce the risk of nervous system abnormalities such as spina bifida. Try to eat balanced meals containing a good range of nutrients (see Chapter 8 for more information about a good diet).

Pre-existing complications like renal failure can put you at risk during pregnancy, so you must discuss any significant health problems with your doctor before deciding to become pregnant. If you are taken by surprise by an unplanned pregnancy, you should see your doctor as soon as is possible.

It is important that your cholesterol (blood fat) levels are under control (see page 200) before you become pregnant. It is also advisable to have your eyes checked carefully (see page 196).

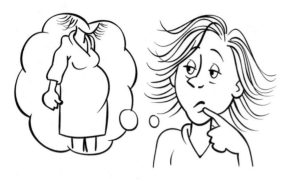

If you have diabetes, it is particularly important that your pregnancy be planned. You must discuss contraception with your doctor.

Research findings: diabetes and pregnancy

- Women with long-standing diabetes have around a 44% chance of miscarriage. This can be reduced to the general population level by good glycaemic control.

- Birth defects are between 4 and 8 times more likely to occur in patients with diabetes mellitus but the risk is reduced if control is good.

- Most developmental abnormalities occur 3–6 weeks after conception, meaning that good control in the run up to pregnancy is crucial.

- Babies born to mothers with diabetes are at significantly increased risk of excessive size (macrosomia). This may lead to birth trauma to mother and baby. Caesarean section may be advised if the baby is large.

- Good blood glucose control helps to reduce macrosomia.

- Serial ultrasound may be useful in determining timing of intervention for early delivery.

Glucose control

A number of drugs used in the treatment of Type 2 diabetes are not recommended for use in pregnancy and may have to be stopped before conception takes place. Glibenclamide, a sulphonylurea, can be used to manage Type 2 diabetes in pregnancy, but is not usually recommended. Insulin treatment is the best way of controlling blood glucose levels, and your diabetes team will encourage you to start insulin treatment. Metformin may be helpful in some circumstances, particularly if you have insulin resistance and polycystic ovary syndrome (PCOS; see page 210). Glitazones should not be used in pregnancy. However, metformin and glitazones may increase your chances of getting pregnant so, if you are taking either of these, you should use reliable contraception. If you become pregnant while taking a glitazone, you should stop taking it immediately and consult your doctor as soon as possible. Throughout pregnancy it is crucial that glucose control is perfect. You should use insulin injections to respond to your food intake as closely as possible.

Poor blood sugar control in the first 3 months may increase the chance of miscarriage and also the chance of the baby suffering from a malformation. The most common malformations occur in the heart, nervous system and skeleton.

Blood pressure control

Many of the commonly used drugs for blood pressure in diabetes, such as the ACE inhibitors, must not be used in pregnancy as they may harm the growing fetus. For this reason you may need to change your blood pressure medication before you get pregnant. You should remind your GP about changing your blood pressure tablets prior to getting pregnant.

If you have significant kidney problems, you should speak to your diabetes specialist before attempting to become pregnant. Women with kidney failure are at a higher risk of miscarriage, pregnancy-induced hypertension and premature delivery. Kidney function may worsen during pregnancy but usually returns to the previous level afterwards.

During the pregnancy

Most centres have a combined clinic where you can be seen by both the obstetric team and the diabetes specialists, both nurses and doctor. This means that, at the same visit, you can discuss your blood sugar results and also receive detailed care of your pregnancy. It is important that your baby's development and growth are carefully monitored by ultrasound.

Perfect blood glucose control is essential for your own and your baby's health. As well as the risk of abnormalities in your baby, raised blood sugar levels can cause your baby to grow too large. Other problems you may encounter as a result of diabetes include worsening of retinopathy, and increased risk of pre-eclampsia. Although women with kidney complications can have successful pregnancies, they need close monitoring and it is important to discuss all the issues before deciding whether to go ahead.

Gestational diabetes

A woman who develops diabetes during pregnancy has a condition known as 'gestational diabetes' or diabetes of pregnancy. This condition is related to the fact that a hormone produced by the placenta has made you more resistant to insulin. Before becoming pregnant, the insulin you produced was just enough to satisfy your requirements, and your body was able to use it effectively. But as the pregnancy progresses, your body is no longer able to use the insulin effectively, which leads to a rise in blood glucose and the diagnosis of diabetes.

In this condition, the blood glucose is raised and the extra blood glucose crosses the placenta to the unborn baby. The baby has its own pancreas, which responds by producing extra insulin. The combination of excess glucose and excess insulin makes the unborn baby grow fat and bloated, so he or she is likely to have a high birth weight. After the birth, the baby is cut off from the high glucose input and then runs the risk of a low blood glucose level (hypoglycaemia) for a day or so after delivery.

Most women who develop gestational diabetes find the condition goes away after the baby's birth, but a small number continue to have diabetes. Once gestational diabetes has been identified, it is likely to recur during subsequent pregnancies. Provided that glucose levels are kept within normal limits (insulin may be needed to achieve this), the baby will be a normal weight and will not be at risk.

Women who have had gestational diabetes have a 40–60% chance of developing Type 2 diabetes later in life. This is because, although the pancreas can produce enough insulin to cope with everyday life, its reserves are low. The extra demands of pregnancy are more then it can manage, hence the need for insulin injections during pregnancy and the increased risk of 'running out' of insulin in the future.

You can reduce your long-term risk of diabetes by making changes to your lifestyle. If you can lose weight so that you are in the ideal weight range, this will help, as will a regular programme of exercise such as swimming, walking or jogging. Both losing weight and regular exercise will reduce your insulin resistance, and this in turn reduces the extra strain on your pancreas to produce insulin.

Drug treatments that reduce insulin resistance may also have a role to play in reducing future risk of Type 2 diabetes. Three agents, metformin, troglitazone and rosiglitazone, all have robust study evidence that they do reduce risk of future diabetes in those who are insulin resistant. The TRIPOD study with troglitazone (now no longer available) looked specifically at reducing future Type 2 diabetes in women with previous diabetes in pregnancy. All three drugs reduce the incidence of future diabetes by around 50–70%. At present, none of these agents is licensed for use in people at risk of developing diabetes.

Delivery

The raised levels of sugar in your blood are likely to lead to an increase in your baby's size and weight. For many women, larger babies are more difficult to deliver, and carrying a big fetus can lead to other problems toward the end of your pregnancy. This means that the majority of maternity units in the UK will now recommend strongly that you come in a week or two before your due date to have your labour induced, or arrange for you to have a planned caesarean section. Full-term, large babies born to mothers with Type 2 diabetes are at increased risk of birth trauma, such as damage to the shoulders, during the later stages of delivery.

Feeding your baby

Breastfeeding is a good idea for mothers with diabetes mellitus. It is very beneficial for babies and has been shown to reduce their risk of future diabetes. In addition, studies have shown significant improvements in both glucose and lipid profiles in mothers who choose to breastfeed. Unfortunately, most of the oral treatments for diabetes are secreted in breast milk and may cause levels of blood sugar to drop in the baby. For this reason, you may well have to stay on insulin therapy while breastfeeding.

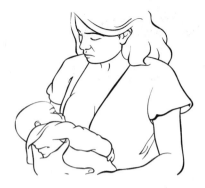

Breast milk contains a significant amount of calories. Coupled with the birth of the baby, breastfeeding will be associated with a significant decrease in your insulin requirements. During your inpatient stay it is worth discussing with one of the diabetes specialist nurses how much you should reduce your insulin by.

Eventually, when the baby is weaned, you may be able to restart tablet treatment for your diabetes. If you have breastfed for a number of months, you may well be lighter and have less body fat than when you became pregnant. For this reason, you might need less diabetes treatment as you will be less insulin resistant.

Do not try to breastfeed while hypo: feed yourself first so that you can feed and look after your baby safely. Always seek medical advice if you are in any doubt. If you find breastfeeding too difficult, it is perfectly all right to bottle-feed.

Social and employment issues

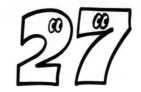

If you have been diagnosed with Type 2 diabetes recently, you may fear that life as you know it is about to end. It isn't. Rest assured that many people who have been living with diabetes for years lead full and rewarding lives with every bit as much variety and enjoyment as those of people who don't have diabetes. Diabetes will bring an end to a normal life *only* if you choose to let it.

Another aspect of having diabetes is that 'official' people may start asking you for all sorts of information. Ever-increasing numbers of employers and government authorities who deal with the public are asking for information about any medical condition individuals might have. In the case of employers, this may be in relation to their fitness to perform tasks connected with the job in hand. In the case of government agencies, some understanding of how the medical condition impacts on daily living activities will have a bearing on the provision of facilities and (if and when it becomes appropriate) any financial benefits to which you or your relatives may be entitled. This is usually less of a problem if your diabetes is controlled with diet and / or tablets. When you need treatment with insulin, outside bodies such as the DVLA become more intrusive.

You need to be aware, however, that your doctor cannot communicate anything about your diabetes, or any other aspect of your health, to a third party without your permission.

Social life

There is absolutely no reason why a diagnosis of Type 2 diabetes should signal an end to your social life. With a bit of careful planning and some good communication, you can carry on

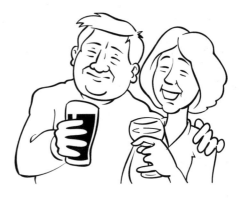

seeing your friends, eating out and generally enjoying yourself. It is important to remember that you have your diabetes – your diabetes doesn't have you!

Eating out

Eating with friends is an important part of many people's social life, and there is no reason why you should feel you need to give it up. As an appropriate diet for someone with diabetes is, to all intents and purposes, a really healthy diet, there should be no problem preparing food for

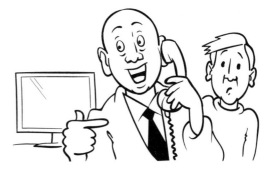

It is important to understand that your doctor cannot talk to anyone else about your health problems without you giving your permission first.

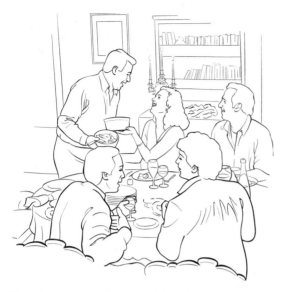

There is no reason why your diabetes should stop you enjoying meals with friends.

others. Chapter 8 gives you more information on a healthy diet. If you are invited to a meal at someone's house, it would be a good idea to talk to them first. You should explain that, because of diabetes, you have to be careful about the amount of sugar and fat you eat. If you are on insulin, you would also like to know if there is going to be a major delay in the timing of the meal. Most people would far rather know your situation and be involved in helping you manage it for an evening than find themselves entertaining a guest with a low blood sugar!

Eating in a restaurant or having a take-away should be less of a problem as you can choose from a range of dishes. Many people using a basal bolus regime choose to take extra short-acting insulin to cover the additional food they are eating. Estimating the amount of carbohydrates in the food and deciding how much insulin you need is a skill that develops with experience, but you will find some guidelines in Chapter 8 on Nutrition. If you are not sure how large a portion you will be given (in a restaurant, for example), you should wait until you see the plate before deciding what dose of insulin to take. Modern insulin pens allow people to give themselves their insulin discreetly at the table if necessary, without anyone noticing. Do not take

your insulin dose before leaving home in case the meal is delayed.

If you are not on insulin but taking tablets, you will find the advice on page 71 more helpful.

Diabetes ID

It is a good idea always to carry something on your person showing that you have diabetes, such as a special necklace or bracelet (Medic-Alert or something similar). It is not uncommon for a person with diabetes to be mistaken for being drunk when in fact he or she is hypoglycaemic. Even if you have had only a small amount to drink, people noticing the smell of alcohol are likely to pass by without helping you.

If you take insulin and are travelling abroad, it is a good idea to have some kind of identification stating that you have diabetes and need to carry insulin and accessories. Insulin companies and diabetes associations often have special cards with text in different languages explaining what help you will need if you become hypoglycaemic.

Being a parent with diabetes

Many people worry about how their diabetes will affect their children, especially if those children are still young. After all, parenting is both an important part of a person's social role and a job of work in itself (and a very important one). For many people, their role as 'parent' is the most important role they fill. In general, maintaining a balanced, healthy lifestyle, and taking as good care of your diabetes as you possibly can, will benefit your children. Do be honest and 'up-front' with your children about the fact that you have diabetes. If you can have a positive attitude, they will learn positive thinking from you, and that may stand them in good stead in all sorts of circumstances. They are also likely to benefit from a healthy eating plan aimed at the whole family.

Explain to your child how your diabetes functions and especially what to do in case of hypoglycaemia. A young child may have difficulties understanding why Mum or Dad suddenly behaves strangely because of hypoglycaemia, and may think this is their fault.

Whatever age they are, your children will probably want to know (at some stage) whether they are likely to develop Type 2 diabetes too. The honest answer to this will be that no one knows for sure, but they do have a higher risk than someone with no Type 2 diabetes in their immediate family. However, there are things they can do to make diabetes less likely to develop: eat well, take regular exercise and keep their weight at a healthy level. If they do go on to develop diabetes at some stage, however, they will benefit from the example you give to them now.

Adoption

Some countries have restrictions on adoption by a parent with diabetes. Such restrictions are usually due to outdated information about life with diabetes, but you may be required to get medical clearance indicating your ability to manage your diabetes and provide appropriate self-care.

Diabetes and work

In general, people with Type 2 diabetes can do whatever work they want. Those treated with diet and tablets with no risk of hypoglycaemia do not have any restrictions on their employment. Sulphonylureas carry a theoretical risk of causing hypoglycaemia, but this is much more likely in a frail elderly person than someone who is holding down a job. Once people start insulin therapy, there are some restrictions, particularly regarding licences to drive Large Goods and

Public Service vehicles (i.e. HGVs and buses).

In a survey of employment among a sample of 200 people attending a hospital diabetic clinic in London, the rate of unemployment was 12% compared with an average rate in Greater London of 4%. However, those individuals attending hospital clinic were more likely to have significant problems which might prevent work. Of those not working, 50% had retired on medical grounds and were receiving disability allowances, while 37% were in receipt of a Disability Living Allowance.

The Disability Discrimination Act

Describes 'discrimination' as occurring when:

➡ A disabled person is treated less favourably than someone else.

➡ The treatment is for a reason relating to the person's disability.

➡ There is a failure to make a reasonable adjustment for a disabled person.

The Disability Discrimination Act was passed in 1995 and revised in 2005. It aims to prevent discrimination against people who are disabled, specifically mentioning diabetes as being covered by the Act.

Diabetes UK offers sensible advice on what to tell a (prospective) employer. The organization points out that while there is no legal requirement to tell your employer or potential employer that you have diabetes, by doing so it will make it easier to look after your diabetes and you will, for instance, be able to arrange clinic appointments without embarrassment. Diabetes UK advises you to be honest about your condition and if diabetes is brought up at interview, try to accentuate the positive: having diabetes means that you lead a healthy lifestyle and will have a thorough medical check-up every year.

So while an employer, or potential employer, cannot demand to know facts about your health without your consent, it is often in your interest to be as open as possible. This will be easier if you are in a stable position, where your colleagues and managers know and trust you already. It is understandable that you might feel more vulnerable when applying for a new job. If an employer needs information, you should provide this as fully as possible at the beginning, so you won't need to go back to answer more questions later.

Whether you are employable in a particular job is based on two key questions, regardless of whether or not you have diabetes:

1 Are you fit to carry out tasks with an acceptable level of risk?

2 Will doing the job make your health worse?

3 Will this job mean you are likely to be a risk to people you come into contact with (particularly hypoglycaemia risk)?

What is an occupational role that involves significant risk? Most people whose work falls into this category would be involved with driving (e.g. buses, trains, taxis, heavy goods

> ### Fitness for employment
>
> The following points should be considered when assessing a person's suitability for employment, where there is a risk of injury to self or to others connected with the work in question:
>
> ⇒ Where the job involves driving or any other particular hazard, such as operating dangerous machinery, potential employees should be evaluated according to the same criteria as a person without diabetes.
>
> ⇒ The Disability Discrimination Act will apply and is in place to protect the rights of people with diabetes.
>
> ⇒ The person's health should be under regular review by their GP and nurse or hospital clinic.
>
> ⇒ Control of blood glucose should be reasonably stable.
>
> ⇒ If the potential employee is on insulin therapy, he or she should be confident in self-monitoring blood glucose levels.
>
> ⇒ The person should have a normal awareness of approaching hypoglycaemia, and not be subject to disabling attacks of hypoglycaemia.
>
> ⇒ Annual reviews should be carried out by an appropriate diabetes specialist.

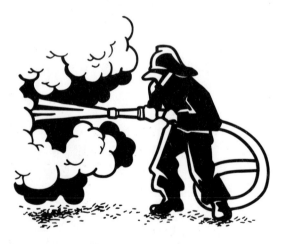

Policemen, firefighters and pilots are examples of professionals who might be putting their own or other people's lives at risk if they develop severe hypoglycaemia. In most countries, you are not allowed to work as a pilot or policeman if you have diabetes. But being a firefighter or driving an ambulance may be possible if you do not have problems with hypoglycaemia.

vehicles), with operating machinery, with climbing ladders, or with taking responsibility for others. More unusual and exotic occupations such as deep-sea diving would also come under this definition.

If your job doesn't involve significant hazard, and your performance in a particular role is satisfactory, your employer can't penalise you for having time off to attend review appointments for your diabetes. Indeed, a responsible employer should welcome the fact that you are proactive in looking after yourself.

Telling your colleagues

A common reaction when someone is first diagnosed with Type 2 diabetes is, 'Do I really have to tell the people I work with?' It is never easy to give personal information to colleagues, but unfortunately hypos do happen, especially when someone is just starting on insulin treatment. You should warn the people you work with on a daily basis that if you start behaving in a peculiar way they should persuade you to take some sugar. Warn them too that you are likely to be pretty uncooperative if this happens and may even resist their attempts to help you – but could they please persevere anyway.

It can be difficult to admit to your workmates that you have diabetes but, if you keep it secret once you have started insulin treatment, you run the risk of causing a scare by having a bad hypo. The natural response of anyone who doesn't know what is going on will be to dial 999 and if this happens you are likely to be taken to hospital by ambulance for treatment. If you get your colleagues onside before a problem arises, however, it is very likely they will be able to help you avoid getting into such a situation.

Discrimination, and what to do about it

Unfortunately, there is still too much ignorant prejudice against people with diabetes and you can come up against this when you are looking for work, changing job, or at a point where you are vulnerable (such as a contract coming up for renewal). Unfortunately, this sort of discrimination does happen, especially in large organizations, although it an be difficult to prove. The Disability Discrimination Act covers people with diabetes, but taking a company to court can be difficult. You will need the support of your own diabetes team if you wish to take proceedings against an employer under the Disability Discrimination Act.

Diabetes UK has had discussions with medical officers responsible for occupational health in several large organizations. There is useful information on the Diabetes UK website, although it does date back to 2001.

The IRFD (International Register of Firefighters with Diabetes) is a UK organization that works to prevent diabetes discrimination in employment.

Shift work

People whose diabetes is controlled with diet and tablets should not be faced with difficult decisions if they have to work shifts. It should be easy to take once a day tablets around the same time each day and fit other tablets in with meals, which may of course be eaten in the middle of the night.

Many people taking insulin are able to combine shift work with good control of their blood glucose. They do have to be organized about it, however, as most insulin regimens are designed

---

Guidelines for safe shift-working for people on insulin

➡ Aim for an injection of short- and intermediate-acting insulin every 12–16 hours, or use a basal bolus regimen. This way of giving insulin makes it much simpler to plan for shift work.

➡ Try to eat a good meal after each injection.

➡ If there is a gap of 6–8 hours when you are changing from one shift to another, take some short-acting insulin followed by a meal.

➡ Because your pattern of insulin and food intake is constantly changing, you will have to test your blood glucose more frequently than usual. You cannot assume that one day is just like another.

➡ If your blood glucose results are not good, be prepared to make changes in your dose of insulin. You will soon become an expert in managing your own diabetes.

around a 24-hour day. Shift workers often find that just as they are settling into one routine, everything changes and they have to start again. It is hard to generalize about shift work as there are so many different possible patterns, but the box gives some basic rules which should be helpful for anyone in this situation.

Many people work irregular hours, even if they are not doing shift work, and many of the same principles apply here too. People with an erratic lifestyle often find that a basal bolus regime gives them more freedom and flexibility. A basal bolus regime is usually easier to deliver using an insulin pen (see page 108).

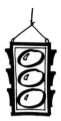

Diabetes and the Armed Forces

Although military service is no longer compulsory in the UK, it is still obligatory in many other countries. However, young people in many parts of the world will automatically be exempt from mandatory service if they have diabetes.

If you have Type 2 diabetes and want to become a soldier, sailor or airman, you will find that the Armed Forces are exempt from the Disability Discrimination Act and, therefore, they are able to refuse you entry. Diabetes UK is working to try and reverse this situation and are looking for examples of discrimination, which they can use to fight for this cause. It is likely that if you take tablets which carry no risk of hypoglycaemia, you should be able to argue for admission. However, they may turn you down on the grounds that, in the course of time, you are likely to need insulin treatment.

If you are already in the Forces and develop Type 2 diabetes, you may be asked to take on a desk job on the grounds that you may come to harm if you have a hypo while engaged in active soldiering.

To consider while driving

1 Check your blood glucose level before you drive and every 2 hours when on a long journey. It should not be below 4.5 mmol/L (80 mg/dl) when you set out. Your driving performance will be impaired if your blood glucose level falls below 4 mmol/L.

2 Eat before driving or riding a bicycle Keep dextrose tablets or rapid acting glucose drinks in the glove compartment of your car.

3 Pull over and stop the car if you have hypoglycaemia. Wait until your glucose is >5.5 mmol/L before continuing. Remember that your thinking and judgement may take up to an hour to return to normal.

4 Be extra careful when the risk of hypoglycaemia is increased – for example, after playing sport or when you have recently adjusted your insulin doses.

5 Alcohol in the previous 12 or more hours increases the risk of hypoglycaemia.

6 Changes in your blood glucose level can cause blurred vision.

7 Try to avoid driving if you make major changes in your insulin regime. Wait until you are confident about the effects of the change.

8 If you have hypoglycaemic unawareness (no warning signs when your blood glucose is low), it is always risky to drive. See page 131 for advice on how to treat this problem.

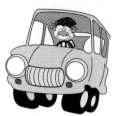

Driving and diabetes

Diabetes can have an impact on your ability to drive safely in two ways. Firstly, it puts you at risk of hypoglycaemia, which will affect your concentration, may impair your judgement and, in severe cases, it may even lead to loss of consciousness. Secondly, diabetes can affect your eyesight, either because of high blood glucose levels leading to lens distortion and blurred vision, or because of damage to the retina or cataracts, which can be longer-term complications of diabetes. When actuaries calculate the increased risk that diabetes brings to driving, it is similar to that of epilepsy, at around 25%.

For the purposes of advice about driving and diabetes, the Driver and Vehicle Licencing Authority (DVLA) makes specific recommendations as to whether the licence you carry is a Group 1 or Group 2 licence. A Group 1 licence is a standard car or motorcycle licence that also allows you to drive a private minibus. A Group 2 licence is for passenger carrying vehicles like coaches, and heavy goods vehicles.

If you hold a Group 2 licence, you need to inform the DVLA that you have diabetes whatever treatment you are taking.

If you have a Group 1 licence and your diabetes is being treated by diet alone, you don't need to inform the DVLA unless your ability to drive is impaired by complications or you change treatment and begin drug therapy. The rules are slightly different in Northern Ireland, where you do have to inform the authorities.

If you take insulin, you must inform the DVLA, and your licence will be renewed every 1–3 years. At renewal, you must demonstrate a satisfactory record with no significant daytime hypoglycaemia. You must also be able to show that your control of the vehicle is adequate, and that you have not suffered any significant deterioration in your eyesight.

If you take tablets, you can usually keep your driving licence until the age of 70 and continue to hold one for Group 2 vehicles. This will change, however, if you suffer significant hypoglycaemia, find yourself in need of treatment by insulin or suffer significant new complications resulting in, for example, deterioration of your eyesight.

If you hold a licence to drive LGV (large goods vehicle) or PCV (passenger carrying vehicle), you will be banned when and if you need treatment with insulin. There seems to be no way round this.

Diabetes UK managed to win a concession for C1 vehicles (between 3.5 and 7.5 tonnes). These can now be granted provided there has been a full medical assessment, which confirms that certain criteria have been fulfilled.

Travelling with diabetes

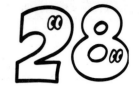

Travelling is an important part of life for many people, and you should not avoid this activity just because you have diabetes. If you think things over and plan ahead, no destination or means of travel is impossible. However, travel across time zones, unaccustomed periods of heavy exercise and risk of infections all mean you need to be prepared when you go on holiday.

Travelling with insulin

If you take insulin to control your diabetes, travel needs a bit of extra planning. Ask your doctor for additional insulin supplies, in case some equipment gets lost or damaged. If you need insulin from a doctor in a foreign country, you should be aware that the number of units per ml may be different (40 or 80 units/ml) from the 100 units/ml used in the UK. Read the label carefully and check with the doctor or pharmacist if you are uncertain.

If you are going through airport security, it is worth taking an open letter from your doctor confirming that you have diabetes and need to carry insulin, needles and blood testing equipment. An official letter is worth a thousand words when you are stopped at customs! Bring along the box of insulin from the pharmacy where your name is printed (especially important if you flying to the US).

While you are away, you should test your blood glucose more frequently than usual as changes in food and activity levels may lead to unexpectedly high or low readings.

Always take spare insulin, at least twice the amount you expect to use. Keep insulin and pens/syringes in your hand-luggage but make sure that you have an extra supply in another bag in case you lose one bag. Don't put insulin in the check-in luggage as there is a risk of it

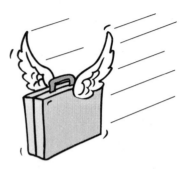

freezing in the aeroplane luggage hold at high altitudes. Besides, there is always the risk of your luggage being lost or arriving late.

You should have no problem obtaining insulin from a pharmacy abroad if you can prove that you have diabetes. Take a card on which your doses, concentration and brand of insulin are documented, or bring the original box with the pharmacy's label. It may be difficult to store your insulin in a refrigerator all the time, but it will usually not be wasted during a short trip, as long as you avoid temperatures above 25–30°C (77–86°F). Remember that it can be extremely hot (up to 50°C, 122°F) in a closed car on a sunny day. Bring a thermos flask or similar with you, containing cold water (cool it with ice before putting insulin into it) on hot days. Cool storage bags suitable for carrying insulin are available (try Amazon.com or www.frio.co.uk). Insulin is

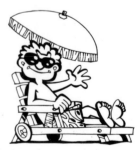

Remember that insulin cannot withstand heat and sunshine as well as you can. The boot of a car or bus will be too hot for insulin in the summer and too cold during the winter.

absorbed more quickly from the injection site if you are very warm and that this can result in unexpected hypoglycaemia (see also page 130).

Insulin that has been frozen loses its effect. Don't leave it in the car on a skiing trip, for example. Keep your insulin bottles or pen injector in an inner pocket if it is below freezing outside. Damaged insulin will often turn cloudy or clumpy, sometimes with a brownish colour. Some blood glucose strips can give too high a

Names of insulin abroad

Type	UK	US
Rapid-acting analogue	NovoRapid Humalog	NovoLog Humalog
Regular insulin	Actrapid Humulin S Insuman Rapid	Novolin R Humulin R
NPH insulin	Insulatard Humulin I	Novolin Humulin N
Basal analogue	Lantus Levemir	Lantus Levemir
Lente insulin	Humulin L Novolin L	Humulin L
Ultralente	Humulin Zn	Humulin U
Mixed insulin (70% NPH)	Mixtard 30 Humulin M3	Novolin 70/30 Humulin 70/30
Mixed analogue (75% basal)	NovoMix 30 Humalog Mix 25	NovoLog 70/30 Humalog Mix 75/25

Most insulins can be found under different names in different parts of the world. If you plan a longer trip, have the insulin vial and box available or ask your doctor to write down what types of insulin you use so that you can get them from the local pharmacy if you lose your supplies. Be aware that in the US, pre-mixed insulins have their proportions stated in the **opposite** ways from the UK!

reading when it is very hot outside and too low a reading when it is very cold. Many glucose meters will give you a warning if the temperature is too high or too low.

Remember that some countries use other concentrations of insulin, mostly 40 units/ml. If you use insulin of 100 units/ml in syringes designed for 40 units/ml or vice versa, you will be in trouble. The insulin concentration appropriate for each syringe is clearly printed on the side of the syringe. If you run out of insulin, it is probably better to buy both insulin and syringes for 40 units/ml if 100 units/ml is not available. You can continue taking your usual doses when counting in units. The units are the same and will give just about the same insulin effect with both 40 units/ml and 100 units/ml. The only difference is that insulin of 40 units/ml may give a slightly quicker onset of action. (See also 'Units and insulin concentrations' on page 93.)

Blood glucose is measured in mmol/L in some countries and mg/dl in others.

$$1\,mmol/L = 18\,mg/dl$$
$$100\,mg/dl = 5.6\,mmol/L$$

Make sure that you have dextrose and glucagon when travelling, sailing or hiking. With glucagon you can treat a serious hypoglycaemia even if you are a long way from emergency care. Make sure that your friends know how and when dextrose and glucagon should be used.

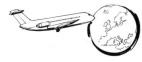

Passing through time zones when on insulin

Multiple injection treatment

When you travel to other continents, there will be a time difference. If you go westwards, the day will be longer, and if you go eastwards, it will be shorter. If you are taking short-acting insulin before food and background insulin once or twice a day, it is often simpler while in the air to rely mainly on taking insulin before meals

Passing through time zones

(Adapted from the work of Kassianos, 1992)

Multiple daily injections

✈ Going west (longer day):

➠ Take mealtime insulin as usual.

➠ Usual doses of basal and bedtime insulin are adjusted to the 'new' day and night.

✈ Going east (shorter day):

➠ Decreased number of meals.

➠ Take bedtime dose of insulin as usual.

Two-dose treatment

✈ Going west (longer day):

➠ Extra doses of mealtime insulin with meals.

➠ Usual dose of pre-mixed insulin before evening meal at destination.

✈ Going east (shorter day):

Night time flight:

➠ Take the ordinary mealtime insulin with dinner/tea.

➠ If the night on the plane is shorter than 4–5 hours, miss the second dose of pre-mixed insulin and take instead short-acting insulin before you eat.

Daytime flight:

➠ Usual insulin dose with breakfast.

➠ Reduce pre-mixed insulin at dinner/tea time on the plane by 5% for each time shift hour.

time of travel. On arrival at your destination, you can take background insulin before you go to bed (and the following morning if you have this twice in 24 hours). Some people leave their watches on UK time and continue their normal doses of background insulin at the same time until they get back in synch on their return. This may work well if you are abroad for only a day or two. It does carry a theoretical risk as the dose of background insulin will be designed to control sugars during sleep, and insulin requirements may be different when people are up and about. If you are travelling eastwards, the night may be shorter and you may need to reduce the dose of bedtime background insulin on arrival.

Two-dose treatment

If you take twice daily injections of mixed insulin, it is best to stick with the ordinary in-flight menu. Due to the pressure differences in the cabin, air bubbles may accumulate in the pen

Safety rules for flying within the US

✈ Syringes or insulin delivery systems should be accompanied by the insulin in its original pharmaceutically labelled box.

✈ Capped lancets should be accompanied by a glucose meter that has the manufacturer's name embossed on the meter.

✈ An intact glucagon kit should be kept in its original preprinted, pharmaceutically labelled container.

✈ No exceptions will be made. Prescriptions and letters of medical necessity will not be accepted.

✈ A passenger encountering any diabetes-related difficulty because of security measures should ask to speak with a Complaints Resolution Officer (CRO) for the airline.

every 4–6 hours. However, there are no hard and fast rules, and it depends largely on the number of time zones you are crossing and the cartridges. To avoid this, remove the needle immediately after each injection. If you notice air bubbles in the insulin, get rid of them before taking an injection (see page 111). Jet lag may make you feel a bit weary before adjusting to the new time zone, and it will usually take a couple of days before your energy levels and sleeping pattern are back to normal.

Travelling if you are taking blood glucose-lowering tablets

Long-distance travel usually causes no problems to people whose diabetes is normally controlled by tablets. If you cross time zones, the day will become longer or shorter, and you may have to decide when and if to take extra tablets. As a general rule, if the 'day' is an extra 12 hours longer, take one and a half times the normal dose. If the day is significantly shorter, you may want to reduce the dose of anti-diabetic tablets.

If you have blood glucose monitoring equipment, it is worth taking this with you. If anything should go wrong with your blood glucose levels while you are away, you will at least have some useful information about the problem.

Vaccinations

You should have the same immunization and malaria prophylaxis as travellers without diabetes. Indeed, it is particularly important that you do this, as illness can lead to difficult consequences which make your blood glucose more difficult than usual to control. Vaccination for

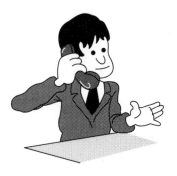

Remember that you are never more than a phone call away from your diabetes healthcare team when on holiday or a business trip.

hepatitis A, typhoid and other diarrhoeal diseases is a sensible precaution if you travel to areas where these may be a problem. It is sensible to have the vaccinations well ahead of the trip, as some cause an episode of fever that can affect the blood glucose for a few days.

Ill while abroad?

When you buy travel insurance, check the small print on the policy to find out whether it only covers acute illness, or whether it also covers any problem related to your diabetes. If you are a citizen of the UK or another EU country, you should acquire a European Health Insurance Card (EHIC). Apply online at www.dh.gov.uk/travellers – it is a very efficient service.

Always say that you have diabetes if you need to see a doctor abroad. In some third world countries, precautions against cross infection are not as stringent as we expect in the UK. You may need to be wary of injections and blood transfusions. If you are travelling to less developed parts of the world, you will presumably take advice about the standard of medical care before you set off.

Diarrhoea

Prophylactic antibiotic treatment aimed at avoiding diarrhoeal diseases while on holiday is a controversial issue. Since you may have difficulty with blood glucose levels and insulin adjustments if you are ill, you should take some antibiotics with you in case of need. Ciproflaxacin 500 mg twice daily, for 5–10 days, is recommended only if you have severe or prolonged symptoms. In cases of resistance, you may be offered a single (1000 mg) dose of azithromycin or a three-day course of 500 mg per day. Sulphametazol or trimethoprim are recommended as alternatives for women who are or might be pregnant.

Since this is not really covered under the NHS, you should be prepared to pay for this.

Problems with travel sickness?

➡ Take medication: depot adhesives (e.g. scopolamine) or travel pills.

➡ You will be less likely to feel sick if you eat 'little and often' rather than large helpings several hours apart.

➡ Avoid fizzy drinks.

➡ If possible, sit in the front if you are in a car or bus, so you can see the road.

This is safer than waiting till you develop diarrhoea while abroad, when you may have difficulty obtaining reliable supplies of the correct antibiotic.

Considering the risks of gastroenteritis, you should avoid drinking water in some countries if you cannot be sure it is entirely clean. Avoid all tap water (even frozen, i.e. ice cubes!) Bottled water and fizzy drinks (cola, fizzy lemonade or similar) are usually safe. Oral rehydration solution (e.g. Dioralyte) is a good alternative if you feel sick or are vomiting (see 'Nausea and vomiting' on page 146).

If you travel in primitive conditions, water should be disinfected by boiling it briefly or by using purifying tablets (Chlorine, Puritabs, Aqua

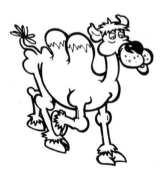

A camel can survive many days in the desert without drinking on account of its hump. Diabetes makes you more sensitive to dehydration. Be sure always to drink plenty of fluid when you are in a hot country, especially if you have problems with diarrhoea or vomiting. If you find yourself feeling or being sick, you should drink often, but only a few sips at a time.

Diabetes equipment you may need on the trip

✈ ID and necklace or bracelet indicating that you have diabetes.

✈ Any tablets you are taking to control your diabetes, with spares in case some get lost or you are delayed.

✈ Finger-pricking device, and lancets if you want to test your blood sugar.

✈ Test strips for blood glucose, and meter.

✈ Extra insulin pen and/or syringes if you are being treated with insulin (pre-filled pens are handy for this).

✈ Dextrose/glucose tablets and gel.

✈ Glucagon, if you are taking insulin.

✈ Anti-diarrhoeal medication (such as Immodium).

✈ Oral rehydration solution (such as Dioralyte).

✈ Travel sickness medication.

✈ Paracetamol or aspirin (whichever suits you best) for suppressing fever.

✈ Clinical thermometer.

✈ Telephone and fax numbers for your diabetes healthcare team at home.

✈ Insurance documents and EHIC card.

Care or similar). If you do not drink enough while you are outdoors in the heat, you will risk dehydration, which causes insulin to be absorbed more slowly. Later, when, you drink properly, more insulin will be absorbed and you will risk becoming hypoglycaemic. A high blood glucose level above the renal threshold (see page 244) will also cause you to lose extra fluid as you will be passing more urine.

Psychological aspects of Type 2 diabetes

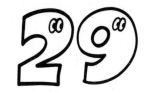

This account of the psychological consequences of Type 2 diabetes starts with practical observations which should apply to most people with the condition. At the end of the chapter, there is a description of some research findings in greater detail.

No two people respond in the same way on being told that they have Type 2 diabetes. Responses range from quiet acceptance to intense anger. If you are lucky, your health professionals will take time to discover what perceptions about diabetes you had at the outset and take a detailed family history about diabetes and cardiovascular disease. You may find you have a great deal to 'unlearn' before you can move on.

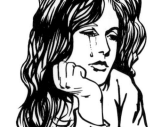

'You cannot stop the birds of sorrow from flying over your head – but you can stop them from building a nest there.'

Chinese saying

Common responses to the diagnosis of Type 2 diabetes

- Relief that symptoms are not due to a more serious condition.
- Anxiety about future complications.
- Early lack of concern followed by indignation, when the need for lifestyle changes becomes apparent.
- Demands for detailed information about the next move.
- Self-blame about body weight, lifestyle, etc.
- Anger about the loss of health, impact on occupation (e.g HGV drivers) or delayed diagnosis.
- Bewilderment about the lifestyle changes required.

The different ways people respond to being told they have diabetes will be due in part to differences in personality. But the way they are told, and the extent to which their health professionals give them time to take in the information, will also be factors. So, too, will the extent to which individuals feel supported by their doctor and diabetes nurses. If you leave the clinic feeling that your fears have not been addressed and your questions have not been answered, you may find yourself becoming angry and upset. These negative emotions can lead to depression and a (false) belief that you can do nothing to help yourself, so it is really important to try to ensure this situation does not develop. You can ask to see a different doctor or nurse if one is available. If not, you do have a perfect right to say that you feel you are not being listened to properly. Your health professional may not realize the extent to which his or her communication skills are falling short.

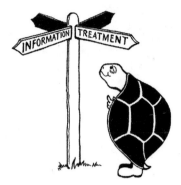

Need for information

Not only do people vary in their response to hearing the diagnosis of diabetes, they also vary in how and when they need to be given information about the condition. Some people want to be told all the details about the causes of diabetes and the likely treatment, while others are too numbed by the diagnosis to take on board anything but the basics. Just because your response is different from someone else's, doesn't make it any the less 'normal'.

If you find you have a strong emotional reaction, it is important you are given the time to deal with this before starting to learn about your diabetes and how to manage it. If you are not given a chance to adjust, you will simply not be able to absorb much, or even any, of the information you are given. Don't forget, your partner and other family members may also be in a state of shock, particularly if they too know little about diabetes. As a family, you may find it takes quite a long time for you all to get to grips with the implications of this complex condition.

Your doctor or diabetes nurse may approach the whole subject of information by asking you directly how much you want to be told. People often complain later that they were told too much, too quickly. A lot of time and effort goes into producing information leaflets, but these are not an effective way of providing education about diabetes unless a sympathetic health professional takes the time to talk you through the contents. It is all too easy never to get around to reading something that is simply handed to you when you are upset.

Handling the diagnosis of diabetes: what your health professional should do

➡ Tell you that you have diabetes, after first asking whether you would like a partner or other close companion present.

➡ Ask you what you already know about diabetes.

➡ Take a detailed family history from you, paying particular attention to whether either of your parents or other close relatives have/had diabetes or cardiovascular disease (e.g. high blood pressure, stroke).

➡ Ask whether you have any friends or workmates with diabetes.

➡ Ask whether you know anything about how they reacted to their diagnosis.

➡ Give you basic information, including a brief explanation of the differences between Type 1 and Type 2 diabetes.

➡ Arrange further education sessions for you with the practice nurse.

➡ Arrange for you to take part in group sessions (e.g. as part of the DESMOND programme) if possible.

➡ Make all necessary medical and screening appointments, e.g. for retinal screening or biochemistry tests, and teach you how to test your own blood and urine for glucose levels.

Psychological support

Anyone attending a diabetes clinic run by a GP or practice nurse will have an expectation of receiving some degree of psychological support. At the very least, this should include an acknowledgement of the emotional response to the diagnosis and an exploration of any fears they may have about diabetes. This process should be repeated at subsequent consultations, when people have had time to consider the problem and feel ready to express deep-seated anxieties. Some people are unable to accept the diagnosis and need specialized psychological help.

Group/peer support

The most effective and least complicated form of psychological support comes from other people with diabetes, preferably those with a similar experience of Type 2 diabetes. This is incorporated into most structured group education packages, and several programmes are in place in the UK. One such programme, called DESMOND, is based on recognized principles of adult learning and is promoted by the Department of Health. For more information, see the section on patient support programmes in Chapter 35.

Support from partners and other family members

Diabetes is a condition that is with you for 24 hours of every day, so those who live with you will also be living with your diabetes. You will make life easier for those you love if you talk to them about how you are feeling and, wherever possible, encourage them to come with you to clinic appointments. If there is diabetes in your family, you may already have been through the experience of watching a parent or a sibling come to terms with the diagnosis. What can you learn from what they have already shown you? Will you react the way they did, or will you try to behave differently?

It is also important that anyone you spend time with on a regular basis (friends, colleagues, etc.) knows that you have diabetes so that if you have a hypo, for example, they are not taken by surprise. Enlist their help rather than risk embarrassing yourself by putting them in a situation where they don't understand what is happening to you.

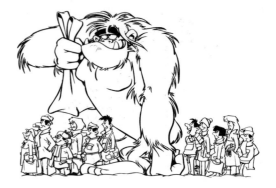

Diabetes is an invisible handicap and can't be seen from the outside. You may sometimes feel better if nobody knows. However, both you and your friends will find it easier in the long run if you let everyone know. If, for instance, you become hypoglycaemic, everyone will understand what is going on and what to do if you have informed them beforehand. Many people have described how embarrassing and troublesome they found it, having to explain their diabetes for the first time when they became hypoglycaemic and needed help.

Anxiety and Type 2 diabetes

One might assume that people with Type 2 diabetes would be less anxious about their condition than those with Type 1 diabetes. The onset of their disease is less dramatic, and their life is not turned upside down by the immediate need for insulin accompanied by other major lifestyle disturbances. However, there are many changes that people with both forms of diabetes have to come to terms with, as indicated in the box overleaf.

Sadly, many young people with Type 1 diabetes are still threatened by parents, relatives and even healthcare professionals that they risk blindness, kidney failure and loss of limbs if they fail to meet the intrusive demands of diabetes and keep their blood sugar under control. In contrast, the onset of Type 2 diabetes is often a gradual process which at the beginning involves changing to a healthy eating pattern. The menace of insulin injections is several years ahead, and the main health risks of Type 2 diabetes, namely heart attacks and strokes, are faced by all individuals in an affluent middle-aged population, whether or not they have diabetes. Given these

Issues to come to terms with following a diagnosis of diabetes

➥ Frequent blood testing.

➥ Dietary changes.

➥ Driving regulations.

➥ Embarrassment about hypos.

➥ Feeling socially different.

➥ Impact on employment.

➥ Fear of complications.

➥ Realization that it is for life.

observations, it is perhaps surprising that most formal research studies suggest that anxiety is at least as common in Type 2 as in Type 1 diabetes.

Depression and Type 2 diabetes

Once you have been diagnosed with diabetes, it will be with you for life. This is a situation which many people will find upsetting. However, many research studies have shown that the majority of people with diabetes have a normal quality of life unless they are affected by complications which interfere with daily living.

On the other hand, depression is a very common problem and so is diabetes. So there are many people with a tendency to suffer from depression or anxiety, who go on to develop diabetes quite independently. Whatever the cause of their depression, people who feel negative about themselves find it difficult to summon up the energy to look after their diabetes properly. This makes it more difficult for them to maintain good control.

Diabetes and underlying psychiatric illness

Diabetes is more common in patients with psychoses, such as schizophrenia. An analysis of medical insurance claims in people with

Research findings: anxiety and Type 2 diabetes

● A research group from Germany studied 420 people with diabetes using a questionnaire to screen for anxiety. Those who screened positive were invited to a diagnostic interview. In this group, minor anxiety was more common in Type 2 diabetes (21%) than in Type 1 diabetes (15%). However, the risk of severe anxiety was only increased in patients with Type 2 diabetes on insulin (6.7%), while patients with either Type 1 or Type 2 diabetes not on insulin had the same risk of severe anxiety as the non-diabetic population (5.2–5.7%).

● Similar results were reported in an American study, which investigated emotional distress in 815 primary care patients with Type 2 diabetes. Using a 20-item self-report measure of diabetes-related emotional distress, they found significantly higher levels of distress among patients treated with insulin (24.6%) compared with those taking tablets (17.8%) or diet alone (14.7%). The greater distress in patients on insulin was attributed to disease severity and the burdens of self-care.

● These two studies suggest a relationship between insulin therapy and increased anxiety. However, these findings should be taken seriously by doctors and nurses in view of the widespread pressure to introduce insulin therapy early in the course of Type 2 diabetes.

● A review of 18 studies from the US and Europe looked at 2584 patients with diabetes and showed that generalized anxiety disorder was present in 14% of those with diabetes compared with 3–4% of the general population. In this study, there were no differences between Type 1 and Type 2 diabetes.

schizophrenia, showed that the risk of having diabetes with complications was twice that of the population as a whole.

Schizophrenia

It has emerged that some of the newer antipsychotic drugs which are now used to treat conditions such as schizophrenia may actually cause diabetes. A recent survey of patients with schizophrenia in the US examined 15,767 patients, who had been treated for psychosis over several years with one of four drugs: olanzapine, risperidone, quetiapine, or haloperidol. Compared with the older drug haloperidol, all three newer agents increased the risk of diabetes by over 60%. The risk was higher in people over 50 years.

Research findings: depression and Type 2 diabetes

- A review of 42 studies showed that diabetes increased the odds of having depression by two to threefold. The wealth of data in this article makes it hard to single out a headline result. However, in controlled studies, the frequency of major depression was 9.0% in patients with diabetes compared with 5.0% in controls, while the risk of less severe depression using self-report scales was 26.1% in diabetes and 14.4% in controls. The increased risk of depression was identical in Type 1 and Type 2 diabetes (2.9 versus 2.9).

- A survey of 8 studies looking at the lifetime frequency of major depression found it to be significantly higher in those with diabetes than in control subjects: 17.5% versus 6.8% respectively.

- The increased chance of depression in adults with Type 2 diabetes was confirmed in a survey of 10 controlled studies, comprising 51,331 patients, which showed a frequency of 17.6% in people with Type 2 diabetes compared with 9.8% in control subjects.

- The 1999 National Health Interview Survey uncovered some interesting observations about the relationship between diabetes, depression and functional disability in a representative sample of the adult US population.

Over 30,000 individuals were interviewed to identify the presence of diabetes, depression and functional disability, which was defined as difficulty in performing activities of daily living and routine social activities. Depression without diabetes increased the risk of functional disability three-fold, while diabetes on its own increased the risk by 2½ times. The combination of depression and diabetes led to a sevenfold increase in the risk of disability.

- A recent study from Norway further examined the relationship between diabetes and depression. A huge population of 65,000 were included in the study, which came up with the following conclusions:

  (i) The presence of other conditions (mainly heart disease) was associated with depression in Type 2 diabetes but not in Type 1 diabetes.

  (ii) Individuals with Type 2 diabetes without other medical conditions had the same risk of depression as the healthy non-diabetic population.

  (iii) Depression itself appears to increase the risk of developing both Type 2 diabetes and heart disease. Factors normally associated with depression, namely low education and physical inactivity, have the same effect in people with diabetes.

Diabetes and severe psychosis

People with a psychosis that reduces their grasp of reality cannot make the connection between good blood glucose control and the risk of future complications and therefore have no motivation to maintain a disciplined way of life. Anecdotally, some of the most damaged and deformed feet are seen in patients with schizophrenia who have developed neuropathic sensory loss due to diabetes.

Type 2 diabetes and eating disorders

It would be easy to assume that the overweight, overeating person who develops Type 2 diabetes would be a likely candidate to have an eating disorder. The literature is ambivalent. A study from Italy compared three groups of patients: obese patients with Type 2 diabetes (n=156), obese non-diabetic individuals who were seeking treatment for weight loss (n=192) and a control sample of obese patients selected at random (n=48). Using a score to identify people with eating disorders, these turned out to be almost twice as common in the non-diabetic groups. Thus, in this population, the presence of diabetes did not lead to an increased risk of developing an eating disorder.

An Australian study found that in a group of 215 women with Type 2 diabetes, 22% had an eating disorder of some description. The problem was more common in those women who were diagnosed at a younger age and who were heavier. As a group, those with an eating disorder could not motivate themselves to control their food intake or to increase their exercise.

Can psychological interventions help?

The same Australian group went on to investigate whether psychological treatment could help patients who had Type 2 diabetes and an eating disorder. They found that CBT (cognitive behavioural therapy) and NPT (non-prescriptive therapy) were both helpful and also improved control of their diabetes.

A systematic review was carried out of randomized controlled trials comparing psychological interventions for improving control of diabetes with a control group receiving the usual care. In an analysis of 12 of these trials, psychological therapies resulted in significantly better glycaemic control, with a difference in HbA_{1c} of 0.76%. More intensive psychological therapies appeared to be even more effective, with a 1% reduction in HbA_{1c}. Psychological therapy, usually a variant of CBT, was associated with a reduction in psychological distress but did not appear to affect weight control.

Taking control

Emotional factors have a major influence on the way people cope with the demands of Type 2 diabetes. Clinicians should address the anxieties and guilt that many people experience and should try to help patients accept the diagnosis and clarify their treatment goals.

As a rule of thumb, anxiety and depression are twice as common in people with diabetes as those without, and the presence of cardiovascular complications magnifies the risk.

As time passes, most people are able to face up to the diagnosis of Type 2 diabetes and take control of their lives. It is worth trying to be positive about living with this intrusive condition.

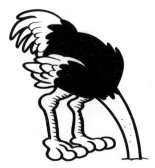

'Ostrich strategy', i.e. not caring about diabetes and not taking any responsibility for its management, is among the most dangerous things a person with diabetes can do. Your diabetes team can contribute with knowledge, tips and advice – but living with your diabetes is something only YOU can do.

Complications of the cardiovascular system

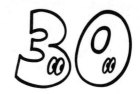

If you have Type 2 diabetes, much of the emphasis on good blood glucose control and many of the tablets you are prescribed will be designed to reduce the risk to your heart and blood vessels. These are known as macrovascular (i.e. large vessel) complications as opposed to microvascular (small vessel) complications, which are described in the next chapter.

What are macrovascular complications?

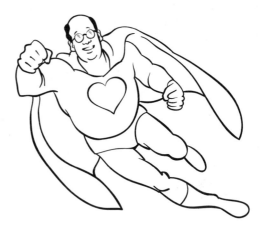

Macrovascular complications affect the large arteries in your body which supply blood to your heart, legs, kidneys and brain, among other parts of the body. If these become clogged up (the medical term is 'thrombosed'), you will be at risk of developing heart disease (often leading to heart attacks), kidney failure, foot ulcers and strokes. Unfortunately, heart attack and stroke represent the major cause of death (up to 75%) in patients with Type 2 diabetes. Thus, it is important to do everything possible to reduce your risk of large vessel complications.

Blood glucose levels

What is the evidence for a link between high blood glucose and macrovascular complications?

A number of studies have shown that the relationship between blood glucose and cardiovascular risk is a continuum. In other words, even before diabetes is diagnosed, while the blood sugar is slightly raised, there is a slightly increased risk of heart disease. As the sugar

becomes even higher and diabetes becomes apparent, so the risk becomes greater. Type 2 diabetes is also associated with a number of other risk factors for heart disease, such as hypertension, abnormal blood fats (cholesterol) and increased fat around the waist. The link between lowering blood sugar and reducing the rate of heart attack in diabetes has been shown in the UKPDS study (see Chapter 36 on Outcome studies). This study looked at the effect of reducing blood sugar and blood pressure on the rate of complications and found that, in the group who had intensive lowering of their blood sugar, there was a strong trend to a reduced risk of heart attack.

Other studies, such as the ORIGIN study which used insulin early after the diagnosis of diabetes, will help to further determine the link between reducing sugar and preventing heart disease. The PROactive study, which reported in 2005, was the first to suggest that a newer class of anti-diabetes drugs, the glitazones, might also reduce the risk of cardiovascular disease. That study looked at the effect of pioglitazone on a combined endpoint of all causes of death, heart

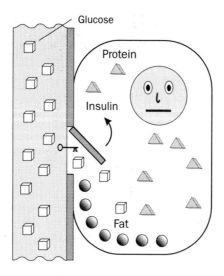

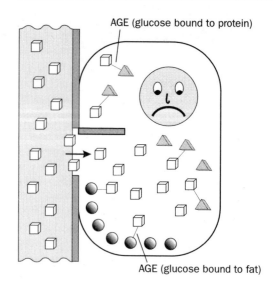

Even if the blood glucose is high, only a certain amount of glucose in the bloodstream will pass through into the cell as it is dependent on insulin to 'open the door'. Most cells in your body work this way.

Many important cells in your body can take in glucose without the help of insulin. In these cells, glucose will enter in direct proportion to the level in the blood. Such cells are found in the brain, nerves, retina, kidneys, adrenal glands, red blood cells and in the walls of the blood vessels. It may not seem logical that some cells can take in glucose without insulin, but in a situation where there is a lack of glucose in a healthy body (for example when starving) the production of insulin is stopped. This will lead to saving the available blood glucose for the organs in your body that are most vital. However, when a person has diabetes, this phenomenon will cause these cells to take in large amounts of glucose whenever the blood glucose is high. Glucose will bind within the cells to form so-called AGE (advanced glycation end products) that have the potential to damage the cells.

attack and stroke, and found that these events were reduced by a total of 16% over 3 years in patients taking pioglitazone compared with those taking a placebo.

What can I do about it?

The important message is that you should try to follow the advice you are given about your diet and anti-diabetic tablets. While controlling sugar is only part of the answer to reducing heart disease, strokes and other macrovascular complications, it does play an important role.

Blood pressure

What is the evidence for a link between higher blood pressure and macrovascular complications?

Raised blood pressure (hypertension) is very common in people who have diabetes. You have twice the risk of hypertension if you have Type 2 diabetes compared with a person of similar

age with no diabetes. The combination of uncontrolled blood pressure and diabetes doubles the risk of macrovascular complications. The best research evidence comes from the UKPDS (see Chapter 36 on Outcome studies). In this study, intensive, relatively small reductions in blood pressure of 10/5 mmHg caused a reduction in the risk of stroke by 44% and of heart attack by 21%. Larger trials, conducted across the whole population but including people with diabetes, also showed a reduction in a combined outcome of death, heart failure, stroke and heart attack if blood pressure was treated effectively. Medical societies now recommend a lower target for blood pressure in Type 2 diabetes of 140/80 mmHg. This is because the UKPDS showed that the lower the blood pressure, the lower the risk of these complications.

What can I do about it?

The key is to follow lifestyle advice and take the tablets your doctor prescribes for you. It goes against the grain for most people to take up to 10 different tablets a day, but each tablet will have a specific action either to improve blood glucose, reduce blood pressure or to control cholesterol. We know from the UKPDS that most people need three or more different tablets to achieve tight blood pressure control, especially now the target blood pressure is so stringent. The UKPDS also showed that the lower the blood pressure, the greater the protection, so the normal target is 140/80 mmHg. If there is any evidence of kidney damage, this target is lowered to 135/75 mmHg. Research studies have shown that a specific type of drug called an ACE (angiotensin-converting) inhibitor (drugs with names that end in '-pril', such as ramipril, enalapril, etc.) or an angiotensin II receptor blocker (with names that end in '-sartan', such as valsartan, losartan, etc.) may be particularly useful in diabetes because they protect the kidneys from the effects of diabetes and hypertension (see page 200). If you are not already taking this type of medication, perhaps you could ask your doctor about this. There are at least four different classes of drug which control blood pressure, and it is worth experimenting till you find a combination that controls your blood pressure without causing side effects.

Cholesterol levels

What is the evidence for a link between blood fats and macrovascular complications?

High blood fats (cholesterol) can lead to deposits being laid down within the blood vessels, particularly the arteries, causing them to become narrow and less efficient. This leads to a greater risk of heart attack or stroke than in someone whose arteries are normal.

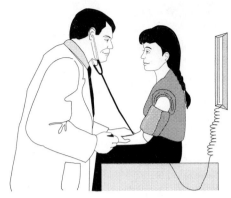

Control of blood pressure is very important in reducing your likelihood of developing complications of diabetes. Your blood pressure should be checked routinely at every clinic visit.

Until recently, all of the evidence for treating blood fats in patients with diabetes came from subsets of trials across the whole population. Several studies using drugs called statins which lower LDL or bad cholesterol, and one study using a drug called gemfibrozil, a fibrate which raises HDL or good cholesterol. All showed a substantial benefit for patients with diabetes who already have cardiovascular problems. The CARDS study used a statin (atorvastatin) to investigate its effect in preventing heart disease in people with diabetes who had not had previous heart problems. It showed a reduction of 37% in a combined outcome of stroke, acute coronary events, or the need for a coronary bypass operation. There is good evidence that people with Type 2 diabetes should take a statin to reduce their cholesterol level.

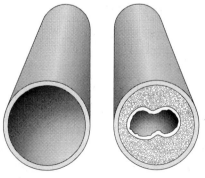

Build-up of fatty deposits in the arteries gradually blocks the flow of blood.

What can I do about it?

Unfortunately, dietary changes alone are not very effective in reducing your cholesterol in Type 2 diabetes, although of course you should try to reduce saturated fats and total calories. Based on the available evidence, medical scientific bodies such as the Joint British Societies (JBS) now recommend that all patients above the age of 40 years who have diabetes should take a statin. In addition, if you have microvascular complications, poor blood glucose control, a raised total cholesterol of more than 6.0 mmol/L, high blood pressure, low good cholesterol or high triglycerides (energy fats in the blood), they recommend that people with diabetes should start a statin any time above the age of 18 years. Of course, if you suffer any sort of cardiovascular event such as a stroke, TIA (ministroke), angina or heart attack and have diabetes, you should take lipid-lowering medication such as a statin without any question.

Insulin resistance

What is the evidence for a link between insulin resistance and macrovascular complications?

Insulin resistance is a condition where extra insulin is needed to maintain normal levels of blood glucose. Insulin resistance in fat cells leads to the breakdown of stored triglycerides to release fatty acids into the blood. Resistance to insulin means that higher levels of insulin are needed to bring about storage of glucose in muscle and liver, which both cause higher levels of glucose in the blood. Insulin resistance is the underlying cause of the metabolic syndrome (see Chapter 33 on Associated diseases). It is not easy to measure the degree of insulin resistance by means of a blood test. However, people with central obesity and a high waist circumference are likely to be resistant to insulin. In practice, the amount of insulin that people need to control their sugar levels is a good guide to the degree of insulin resistance.

> **Heart and large blood vessel diseases: Diagnosis**
>
> 1 Blood pressure measurements.
> 2 Examination of pulses in the feet and lower legs, with a Doppler device if necessary.
> 3 Analysis of cholesterol and triglycerides in the blood.
>
> **Treatment**
>
> 1 Stop smoking.
> 2 Increase the amount of physical exercise or physiotherapy.
> 3 Avoid putting on weight.
> 4 Avoid undue stress (see Chapter 20).
> 5 Don't drink too much alcohol.
> 6 Control high blood pressure.
> 7 Eat foods high in fibre and low in fat. Increase fruit and vegetable intake.

The problem is that insulin resistance occurs many years before diabetes is diagnosed and of course plays a major part in the causation of diabetes. In the time before diabetes comes to light, insulin resistance increases the risk of cardiovascular disease, which is why many people are diagnosed with diabetes at the time of a heart attack.

What can I do about it?

The most effective way of lowering insulin resistance is to lose weight and take exercise, which may be easier said than done! But even a small increase in your exercise regime will have a positive effect on your weight, blood pressure, blood glucose and blood fats. If you could lose 10% of your body weight, the effect on your level of insulin resistance (and hence your cardiac risk factors) would be substantial.

There is evidence from the UKPDS study (see above) that metformin, a drug which reduces insulin resistance and lowers blood glucose has positive effects on cardiovascular outcomes.

Metformin is therefore seen as the glucose-lowering therapy of choice for patients with Type 2 diabetes. There may be additional effects on cardiovascular risk factors of the glitazones (rosiglitazone and pioglitazone). Both drugs are potent reducers of insulin resistance and affect a range of cardiovascular risk factors such as blood pressure. In addition, a study with pioglitazone has actually shown an effect on the number of cardiovascular events in patients with diabetes at high risk over a period of around 3 years.

Rosiglitazone has been subject to some negative publicity regarding heart attacks. This came from an accumulation of several different studies, which appeared to show that the risk of heart attack was greater in patients taking this drug. However the manufacturers, who are understandably very sensitive to this sort of criticism, have responded by putting together *all* the available data on rosiglitazone and have shown that it does not appear to carry higher risk of heart attacks than other tablet treatments used in diabetes.

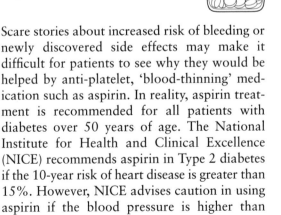

Who needs aspirin treatment?

Scare stories about increased risk of bleeding or newly discovered side effects may make it difficult for patients to see why they would be helped by anti-platelet, 'blood-thinning' medication such as aspirin. In reality, aspirin treatment is recommended for all patients with diabetes over 50 years of age. The National Institute for Health and Clinical Excellence (NICE) recommends aspirin in Type 2 diabetes if the 10-year risk of heart disease is greater than 15%. However, NICE advises caution in using aspirin if the blood pressure is higher than 145 mmHg. So control your blood pressure below this level before starting aspirin at a standard small dose of 75 mg daily. This is the equivalent of ¼ of a standard aspirin tablet, or one junior aspirin.

Your doctor will be able to identify conditions (mainly a history of bleeding stomach ulcers) which may preclude the use of aspirin. The take-home message is that, for the majority of patients, the advantages of using aspirin far outweigh the problems.

However, you should first consult your doctor to make sure there are no reasons for you not to take aspirin.

New cardiovascular risk markers

Scarcely a day goes by without a new marker for cardiovascular risk being reported in the tabloid press. Those in vogue recently include CRP (C-reactive protein – a marker of the amount of inflammation in your blood) and a number of other inflammatory chemicals in the blood, and homocysteine (an amino acid, one of the building blocks of proteins). There are good population studies which all support an association between these chemicals and increased cardiovascular risk. It is important to say though that there is no evidence that intervening in any of them has any effect at all in terms of reducing the risk of a cardiovascular event. While conventional drugs such as statins, metformin and glitazones have effects on some of these markers, these effects might have no connection at all with the reduction in heart attacks and strokes.

Helping yourself

In essence the message for reducing the risk of heart attacks, strokes or similar problems is simple. If you can lose weight and take regular exercise, anything at all you can manage will be helpful. In addition, your doctor may prescribe for you a large number of different medications, and you may feel it is too much. But you need to take them. A heart attack or a stroke is an all or nothing event, and there is good evidence that taking medication for high blood glucose, high blood pressure and high cholesterol can stave off the risk of a heart attack or a stroke.

Microvascular complications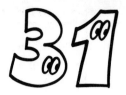

Microvascular complications are those which affect the small blood vessels of the body, specifically those in the eyes and the kidneys, and those affecting the supply of nutrients to the nerves. Damage to these small vessels can result in the following:

- Retinopathy, which may lead to blindness if left untreated;

- Kidney problems and sometimes kidney failure;

- Nerve damage – loss of sensation or problems with the functions of the body controlled by the internal nervous system. These include sexual problems (see Chapter 25).

In Type 1 diabetes, the risk of microvascular complications is largely governed by the degree of blood glucose control and the length of time the person has had diabetes. In Type 2 diabetes, the picture is a bit more complicated. The main explanation for the confusion is that some people with newly diagnosed Type 2 diabetes have actually had the condition for up to 10 years without it being discovered. During this time, a great deal of damage may have been done to small and large blood vessels. The UKPDS (see

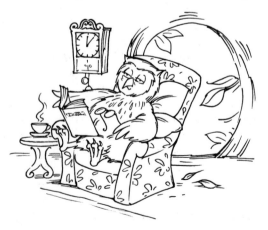

Chapter 36 on Outcome studies) found that over 25% of newly diagnosed patients already had some sign of retinopathy. We know that people with Type 2 diabetes are often diagnosed following a foot ulcer caused by nerve damage (neuropathy), and such people usually have some degree of retinopathy of which they have been unaware. If on the other hand, there are no signs of microvascular complications at diagnosis, the outlook is very good. Keeping the blood glucose and blood pressure under good control will minimize the risk of small vessel problems.

Complications affecting the eyes (retinopathy)

The risk of eye damage has decreased considerably with modern diabetes and eye care. However, a majority of people with 15–20 years of diabetes will have some degree of retinal changes, half of which need laser treatment. Of 1000 individuals with diabetes, one will sustain serious visual loss each year. But blindness due to diabetes is today very rare in countries where modern treatment methods are available.

High blood sugars and blood pressure can give rise to small swellings in capillaries called microaneurysms. These are described as 'background' problems that do not affect the sight. This type of early damage may sometimes get better if blood glucose control improves. On the other hand, continued high blood glucose and high blood pressure are likely to worsen the changes in the eyes until the threat of vision being affected becomes a real one. This is usually caused by fatty deposits at the macula, the central part of your retina, which is responsible for all detailed vision (reading, driving, recognizing people). In addition to these problems at the macula, the microaneuryms may develop to form new blood vessels at the back of the eye.

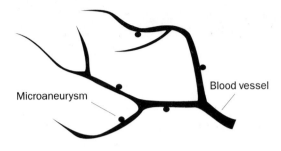

After many years of high blood glucose levels, the blood vessels of the retina will become brittle, and small bubbles (called microaneurysms) can form. They do not affect your vision, but can be seen on a photograph of the retina.

These new vessels are fragile and may rupture, leading to a bleed into the eye which will seriously affect vision.

Treatment

The most important treatment is good control of blood glucose and blood pressure.

If the changes reach the stage where they may lead to a reduction in vision, laser treatment is used. This effectively controls background problems and microaneurysms. Deposits (called exudates) in the region of the macula are usually treated by a small number of laser shots in the area. This is called 'focal' laser treatment and takes only a few minutes to perform. Laser treatment for new vessels is equally effective but requires many applications of laser over the back of the affected eye. This is a more arduous procedure and may take 20–30 minutes. Sometimes it takes more than one session with up to a thousand applications of laser at each sitting. Once the back of the eye (retina) has been widely treated with laser, the new vessels will recede and the risk of bleeding disappear. In order to detect eye problems at the earliest possible stage, everyone with diabetes should have a retinal photograph at diagnosis and then every subsequent year. This important screening service is now up and running in most areas in the UK. Drops are used to make the pupil open as wide as possible so that good quality photographs can be obtained.

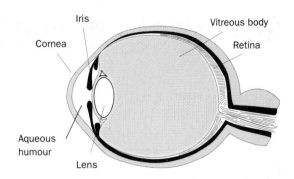

The eye seen in cross-section. Eye damage is first noted in the retina. At check-ups, the retina is photographed after dilatation of the pupil. An eye specialist will have a close look at the pictures.

Disturbed vision at unstable blood glucose levels

Blurred vision is a common symptom of unstable diabetes. This is due to the changes in glucose which affect the shape of the lens and hence make focusing difficult. It is not in any way dangerous for your vision, nor is it associated with future visual impairment.

Sometimes the disturbed vision can continue for several weeks and you may find that a pair of cheap reading glasses will resolve the problem. In any case, your vision will return to normal in time

Glasses

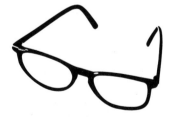

Your blood glucose levels should be stable when you are tested for new glasses. Otherwise, your vision will be affected by temporary changes in blood glucose. After the onset of diabetes, it may take 2–3 months of normal blood glucose levels before the lens returns to its usual shape, and you should obviously not be tested for new glasses during this time.

Contact lenses

People with diabetes can wear contact lenses. However, you should avoid long-term lenses (that are replaced every second or third week) as the protecting cell layer of the cornea tends to be more brittle if you have diabetes.

Complications affecting the kidneys (nephropathy)

The process of developing kidney failure is a gradual one. Only a small number of people with evidence of minor kidney damage go on to develop kidney failure. There are several distinct stages and each stage may last many years before progression to the next and there are well recognized ways of slowing down this process.

Stages of kidney damage

1 Microalbuminuria

The blood vessels of the kidneys are formed into small clusters where waste products in the blood are filtered into the urine. Damage to the walls of these blood vessels causes leakage of protein into the urine. Tiny amounts of protein (known as microalbuminuria) can be detected in the urine.

The structure of a kidney

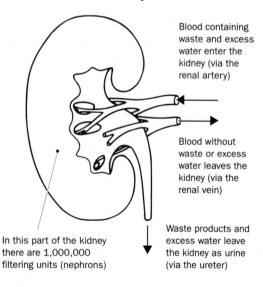

Blood containing waste and excess water enter the kidney (via the renal artery)

Blood without waste or excess water leaves the kidney (via the renal vein)

In this part of the kidney there are 1,000,000 filtering units (nephrons)

Waste products and excess water leave the kidney as urine (via the ureter)

The stages of kidney damage

1 Microalbuminuria.
2 Proteinuria.
3 Abnormal kidney function.
4 End stage kidney failure.

Treatment

1 Good glucose control (HbA$_{1c}$).
2 Stop smoking.
3 Microalbuminuria is treated with an ACE-inhibitor or angiotensin receptor blocker (ARB) to protect the kidneys.
4 Treatment of blood pressure (target less than 130/75).
5 Treatment of urinary tract infections.
6 Anaemia is treated with EPO injections.
7 Calcium abnormalities are treated with vitamin D.
8 Established kidney failure is postponed by the above.
9 When it occurs, treat with dialysis or transplant.

Microalbuminuria is measured on a small sample of urine and is expressed as a ratio of albumin to creatinine. The creatinine ratio corrects for the fact that the flow rate of urine varies greatly. The threshold for defining microalbuminuria is an albumin–creatinine ratio greater than 2.5 mg/mmol in men and 3.5 in women. It is a very sensitive test, and false positives can occur as a result of physical exercise, smoking and infection in the urine. If the test is positive, it should be repeated and a specimen of urine should be sent for testing to rule out an infection. Microalbuminuria is the first sign that there is a problem with the kidneys. However, it can be treated and often reversed by controlling blood glucose and blood pressure. There is also evidence that particular blood pressure tablets, called ACE inhibitors or angiotensin receptor blockers (ARBs, sometimes known as sartans) have a protective effect on kidneys at this early stage of damage.

2 Proteinuria

If the leakage progresses, there is a risk of high blood pressure, which leads to further leakage of protein into the urine (proteinuria). This can be detected by a simple urine testing strip (Albustix). The most basic protein in the blood is albumin, which is manufactured by the liver in response to the needs of the body. If the leakage of protein (albumin) becomes very severe (more than 5 g in 24 hours), it exceeds the amount that can be replaced by the liver even though it is working at full stretch. At this point, the level of albumin in the blood falls below normal, and this in turn leads to fluid retention. This condition is called the nephrotic syndrome, and once this has developed, it is difficult to reverse the leakage of protein. The fluid retention can only be treated by removing the excess fluid by diuretics – known as 'water tablets'. Its progression can be slowed by the usual measures of controlling blood glucose and blood pressure to tight targets. In the case of nephrotic syndrome, the fluid retention can be controlled with diuretics.

3 Abnormal kidney function

A number of people may drift quietly into kidney failure without feeling particularly unwell. Indeed, it is often picked up by chance on a random blood test. However, kidney failure does have a number of consequences, which affect the general working of the body. It is a slowly progressive process which takes place over years, but as the kidneys deteriorate, more metabolic problems arise and the person feels increasingly unwell. Because the body is unable to remove waste products, there is a build-up of acid in the blood. People with kidney failure also become anaemic and have problems with the calcium levels in their blood. This form of anaemia can be treated by injections and the calcium defect by vitamin D tablets.

4 Established (or end-stage) kidney failure

The kidneys can no longer remove waste products from the body, which puts the individual at risk of coma. The first line of treatment is dialysis, which normally takes place three times a week in a specialist centre. An alternative is peritoneal dialysis, which is usually done by the patient in his or her own home three times a day. This avoids the need for high-tech equipment and allows a little more independence. However, it is quite intrusive and interferes with normal daily activities. Most people who have dialysis are keen to receive a kidney transplant, which gives them back their freedom.

Complications affecting the nerves (neuropathy)

Nerve fibres are made of very long and thin cells, which can be affected after many years of diabetes. Damage to the blood vessels supplying the nerve fibres results in a decreased supply of oxygen. This causes injury to the insulating covering (myelin sheath) of the nerve and ultimately results in poorer nerve impulses. This can lead to loss of sensation and/or pain. The longest nerves are the most vulnerable, so problems arise primarily in the feet. Later on, this loss of sensation can progress up the legs. The fingers may eventually be affected by numbness, and people with this problem find difficulty in picking up small objects and doing up buttons.

Treatment: loss of sensation

This condition is painless and may only come to light when the feet are examined at the annual

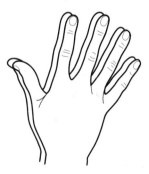

Mobility in the finger joints can be tested by the 'prayer sign'.

review. In other words, people usually are not aware that they have lost sensation. However, it is a potentially serious condition since it removes the warning that people receive when their feet are being damaged. People with loss of sensation in their feet must have regular foot checks and follow the specialist advice they are given regarding footwear.

Treatment: pain due to nerve damage

Unlike loss of sensation, this can be a very distressing condition. The type of pain people describe is very variable but tends to be like the effect of stinging nettles. It normally affects both feet or legs symmetrically and is typically worse when resting – especially when trying to get to sleep at night. There are a number of drugs which can ease neuropathic pain. The first tablet your doctor will probably try is amitriptyline, an anti-depressant, which often has a good effect on the pain and allows people to sleep undisturbed. If this fails or causes unacceptable side effects, try pregabalin. Pregabalin was designed to treat epilepsy, but it can often also relieve this irritating pain.

The autonomic nervous system

The autonomic nervous system controls those parts of the body which are not under our direct control and which tend to work automatically without us even being aware of them – until something goes wrong. The autonomic nerves control the digestive system, passing urine and emptying the bladder, sexual functions, the heart and blood vessels, the sweat glands and the eyes.

Because the autonomic nervous system normally does its work without us even being aware of it, it is usually very hard to cope when it fails to work normally. Any item on the above list may be present to a minor or severe degree, and sometimes the severity may vary from one day to the next. For instance, a mild degree of indigestion can be helped with an antacid purchased over the counter. However, if the nerves to the stomach are completely destroyed, the stomach becomes paralysed and behaves like a floppy

Problems with the autonomic nervous system

Organ	Problem
Digestive system	Indigestion, heartburn, feeling bloated.
	Food sits in the stomach undigested.
	Diarrhoea, constipation, loss of control of the bowels.
Urinary system	Having to pass urine little and often.
	Leaking urine.
	No urge to pass urine when the bladder is full.
Sexual function	Inability to maintain an erection (men).
	Vaginal dryness (women).
Heart and blood vessels	Feeling dizzy on suddenly standing up.
	Feeling faint on changing position.
	Heart beating rapidly at rest.
Sweat glands	Increased sweating, especially at night or when eating.
	Reduced sweating, even when hot.
	Dry skin on the feet.
Eyes	Hard to adjust when going from bright to dark.
	Difficulty night driving.

bag. This prevents the normal passage of food into the gut, causing a delay in absorption, which slows conversion of food to glucose. This condition (called gastroparesis) can make it impossible to control diabetes, especially in those who have an injection of insulin before each meal. Because the absorption of food is completely unpredictable, it is impossible to make the normal calculations about the type of food and the dose of insulin. Various forms of treatment, such as antibiotics, have been tried for gastroparesis, with variable results. In the last few years, specialist centres have treated this problem by injecting botulinum toxin into the muscles at the outlet of the stomach. Early results of this procedure are promising. If you have this rare complication, you may be advised to delay your mealtime insulin injection until 30–60 minutes after your meal.

Other consequences of autonomic neuropathy are listed in the box on the previous page. They are very rarely a problem in Type 2 diabetes, apart from sexual problems, which are discussed in Chapter 25.

Avoiding complications: the evidence

There is good evidence from the UKPDS study that controlling both blood pressure and blood glucose has profound effects on the risk of developing microvascular complications. This study showed that for every 1% reduction in HbA_{1c}, there was a 37% fall in the risk of microvascular complication. Blood pressure control also helped microvascular complications – with a 13% reduction for every 10 mmHg fall in blood pressure.

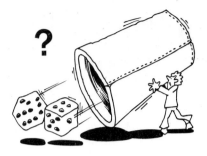

Many people believe that complications strike randomly among the population with diabetes. Others feel that it will not matter whether or not you 'manage well', complications will strike anyway. In fact, modern research has clearly shown that the degree of long-term complications depends directly upon the blood glucose levels over the course of the years that a person has diabetes.

The Steno-2 study from Denmark investigated the effect of controlling risk factors to the best possible extent in patients with Type 2 diabetes. By working hard to improve HbA_{1c}, blood pressure, cholesterol and lifestyle, patients in this study reduced their risk of microvascular complications by 60%.

A number of studies have shown that a particular class of drugs, the renin–angiotensin system drugs, ACE inhibitors and ARBs, are particularly valuable at protecting the kidneys from microvascular complications. Most clinicians now recommend ACE inhibitors or ARBs as the first-choice blood pressure-lowering drugs.

Problems with feet

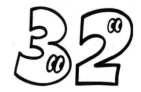

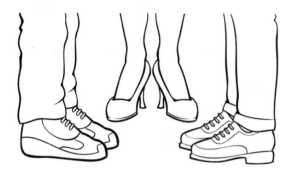

With the onset of Type 2 diabetes, you can no longer take your feet for granted. In the past, you could do whatever you wanted on or to your feet and be confident that they would recover with a bit of rest. Diabetes, however, may cause changes to your feet which put them at risk of permanent damage and, in particular, ulceration. It is effective, simple and cheap to check your feet every day, and to follow the advice laid out in this chapter.

Why do foot problems happen?

You need to be particularly careful if the sensation of your feet is reduced. Up to 80% of people with foot ulcers have a previous history of peripheral neuropathy. This causes loss of sensation, predominantly in the feet, due to damage to the nerve endings responsible for light touch, pain and other sensations. Autonomic neuropathy is a problem affecting nerves that operate automatically outside our direct control. This includes nerves that regulate the blood supply to the skin and control such functions as sweating. Damage to the autonomic nerves results in reduced sweating. This in turn can lead to dry and cracked skin, which may become an entry route for infection.

Nerves which control the way our muscles work (motor nerves) can also be affected by dia-betes, leading to motor neuropathy. This can lead to abnormalities in the shape of the feet, clawing of the toes and problems with callus formation. Ill-fitting shoes may then cause pressure areas, which are of course at risk of ulceration.

Foot problems in diabetes also result from poor blood supply to the feet, which is called peripheral vascular disease. Around 45% of patients with foot ulcers have problems with the arteries in their legs. This is why the blood supply to the feet should be assessed at the annual physical check for people with diabetes.

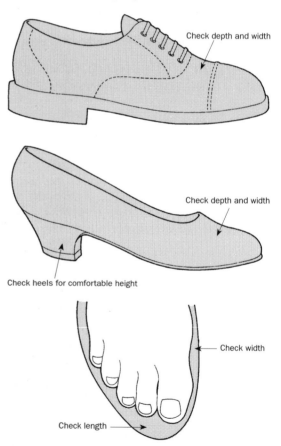

Always check the fitting of your shoes very carefully. Ill-fitting shoes can damage your feet.

Minimizing the risk of foot problems

Even if you have no nerve damage and a normal blood supply to the feet, you must take care of your feet. Neuropathy is related to poor control of blood glucose and blood pressure so by keeping these risk factors under good control, you can reduce the likelihood of developing it in the future. Vascular disease is related to the cluster of risk factors: insulin resistance, blood pressure, high cholesterol and to a lesser extent blood glucose. Smoking forms a deadly duo with diabetes to accelerate and accentuate the risk of a number of complications (see Chapter 23) so you must give this up. As usual, you should follow medical advice concerning treatment with a statin and for blood pressure.

If your doctor or diabetes nurse tells you that

The major complications of diabetes causing foot problems

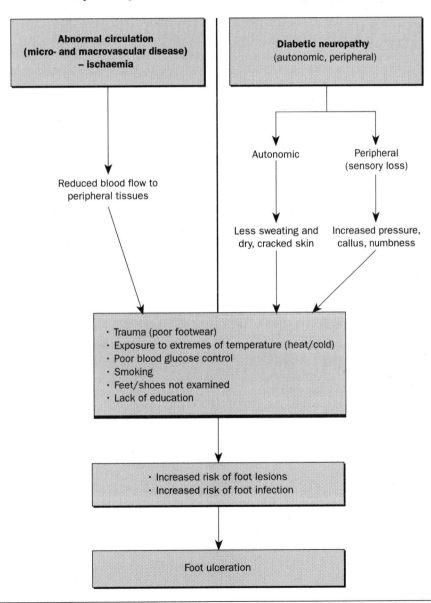

FOOT CARE RULES

DOs

- Do wash your feet daily with soap and warm water. Do not use hot water – check the temperature of the water with your elbow.

- Do dry your feet well with a soft towel; be especially gentle between your toes.

- Do apply a gentle skin cream, such as E45, if your skin is rough and dry.

- Do change your socks or stockings daily and keep them in good repair.

- Do wear well-fitting shoes. Make sure they are wider, deeper and longer than your foot, with a good firm fastening that you have to undo to get your foot in and out. This will prevent your foot from moving inside the shoe.

- Do run your hand around the inside of your shoes each day before putting them on to check that there is nothing that will rub your feet.

- Do 'wear in' new shoes for short periods of time and check your feet afterwards to see if the shoe has rubbed or pinched your feet.

- Do cut your toenails to follow the shape of the end of your toes, not deep into the corners. This is easier after a bath as your toenails will soften in the warm water.

- Do check your feet daily and see your podiatrist or doctor about any problems.

- Do see a registered podiatrist if in any doubt about foot care.

DON'Ts

- Do not soak your feet.

- Do not put your feet on hot-water bottles or sit too close to a fire or radiator, and avoid extremes of cold and heat.

- Do not use corn paints or plasters or attempt to cut your own corns with knives or razors in any circumstances.

- Do not neglect even slight injuries to your feet.

- Do not walk barefoot.

- Do not let your feet get dry and cracked. Use E45 or hand lotion to keep the skin soft. Avoid putting moisturiser between the toes.

- Do not cut your toenails too short or dig down the sides of your nails.

- Do not smoke.

Seek advice immediately if you notice any of the following:

* Any colour change in your legs or feet.

* Any discharge from a break or crack in the skin, from a corn or from beneath a toenail.

* Any swelling, throbbing or signs of inflammation (redness or heat) in any part of your foot.

---

your feet are at risk despite the fact that you have no signs of ulcers, what should you do? You should find out why your feet are at extra risk, which is likely to be either reduced sensation or poor blood supply. You must be under the care of a podiatrist, a foot specialist who can advise on care of nails, general foot hygiene and help with appropriate footwear. Your podiatrist should see you regularly, and you should follow his or her advice about footwear, foot inspection and general foot care. The podiatrist will probably give you a contact number so you can seek

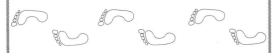

Looking after your feet: first aid measures

* Minor injuries can be treated at home provided that professional help is sought if the injury does not improve quickly.

* Minor cuts and abrasions should be cleaned gently with cotton wool or gauze and warm salt water. A clean dressing should be lightly bandaged in place.

* If blisters occur, do not prick them. If they burst, dress them as for minor cuts.

* Never use strong medicaments such as iodine.

* Never place adhesive strapping directly over a wound: always apply a dressing first.

advice if you have any worries, such as pain or discolouration in your feet.

Treating foot ulcers

If you develop a foot ulcer, no time should be wasted in starting treatment. A specialist podiatrist must examine your feet to assess the depth of the ulcer. You may need an X-ray of your foot to rule out any involvement of the bone. If there are signs of infection, a swab will be sent to identify the exact bacterium responsible. This will help with the choice of antibiotic. If there is a serious foot infection, you may need antibiotics given into a drip (intravenously), which is the most reliable way of getting antibiotics to the ulcer in the highest concentration. In the past, intravenous antibiotics could only be given in

hospital, but many areas employ specialist nurses who can visit people at home and administer antibiotics by this route. Any infection is likely to cause blood glucose levels to rise, and it is important to try and control them as high sugars will promote the infection. Swelling should be kept under control, usually by resting the foot and keeping it up as much as possible. Even when there is a serious foot infection involving the bone, there may be very little pain because of nerve damage.

Any dead tissue around the ulcer will interfere with the healing process, and the podiatrist will remove as much of this as possible – a process called debridement. Occasionally, an infection may be too deep and entrenched to be eradicated by antibiotic treatment and debridement. In such severe cases, some degree of amputation may be necessary and the surgeon will only remove areas of your foot if there is absolutely no hope of recovery. An amputation is a frightening experience. Your doctor or surgeon should discuss this with you honestly and supportively.

If the ulcer is partly or entirely due to poor circulation, you will have tests to identify the exact cause. The first test will be a colour Doppler, which will provide information about the site and degree of the narrowing of the blood vessels. If the results are positive, the next test will be an angiogram, where a small tube is threaded into the artery. Depending on the findings, it may be possible to reduce the block by mechanically widening the artery. This procedure is called an angioplasty. Alternatively, the surgeon may decide to carry out a bypass operation, using a graft to restore the blood supply to the foot.

Charcot foot

Charcot foot is a rare complication of Type 2 diabetes. It only occurs in people who already have a significant degree of nerve damage. The symptoms normally arise following minor trauma. The foot is often painful and is always swollen, warm and red. It is a serious condition,

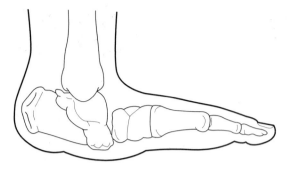

Deformity caused by Charcot's foot.

which if diagnosed late and not treated properly will lead to severe deformity of the foot. This in turn causes disability and the likelihood of future ulceration.

Because it is a rare condition, many doctors are unaware that this is the likely diagnosis if someone with diabetes comes to see them with a warm, swollen, red and painful foot. A podiatrist specialising in diabetes will be able to make the diagnosis and start the correct treatment.

First, there should be a careful examination of the foot, with measurement of the temperature difference between the feet. The Charcot process can only develop in the presence of a good blood supply and when there is already nerve damage. The foot should be X-rayed, which may reveal a fracture of one or more of the long bones in the foot.

Even without proper treatment, the warmth and redness of the foot will return to normal, but with continued walking, the arch will collapse and the foot take on a convex shape giving it a rocker-bottom appearance. This is unsightly and interferes with normal mobility.

Treatment consists of immobilisation of the foot with either a plaster cast or a special boot, designed to provide total support and maintain the normal shape of the foot. The active process lasts from 3 to 9 months, and throughout this period, it is important to rest as much as possible and to retain the normal shape of the foot by immobilization.

Associated diseases

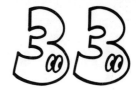

Type 2 diabetes has a different underlying cause from Type 1 diabetes and conditions associated with these two types of diabetes are also very different. Type 1 diabetes is an auto-immune disease, and thus people with this condition are at risk of other auto-immune conditions such as thyroid disease or coeliac disease. Type 2 diabetes is caused by insulin resistance, which is at the root of a number of other conditions all of which are related to Type 2 diabetes. In this chapter, we also discuss conditions similar to simple Type 2 diabetes, and diseases in which diabetes occurs as a secondary phenomenon.

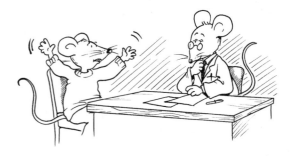

- Diseases associated with Type 2 diabetes are very different from those associated with Type 1 diabetes.

- Insulin resistance is associated with cardiovascular disease.

Insulin resistance

Insulin resistance occurs many years before the onset of Type 2 diabetes and indeed does not always progress to diabetes and raised blood sugars. We believe that insulin resistance is caused by increased storage of fat in the central portion of the body, particularly around the gut and the internal organs. This central fat is very poor at storing lipids called triglycerides, which are an energy source, so the level of triglycerides in the blood begins to rise. Central fat also produces a number of chemicals that promote a rise in the blood pressure. Thus, people who carry a lot of weight around their middle tend to have high blood pressure, high levels of triglyceride fats and low levels of good cholesterol or HDL. Chronic inflammation may occur inside the blood vessels, leading to atherosclerosis or narrowing of the arteries. Insulin resistance may

cause gout, which supports the view that gout is a 'disease of good living'. The high blood fats lead to insulin resistance, so that more insulin is needed to maintain the normal sugar levels in the body.

If, in addition to insulin resistance, there is failure of the pancreas to produce enough insulin, the sugar levels will drift upwards until diabetes develops. This combination of cardiac risk factors is known as 'the metabolic syndrome' (see box overleaf).

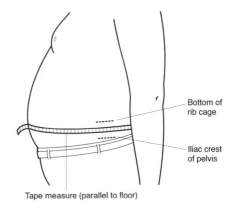

Tape measure (parallel to floor)

Bottom of rib cage

Iliac crest of pelvis

Carrying a lot of fat around your middle can put you at risk of developing the metabolic syndrome. The illustration shows you how to measure your waist. You are at risk of developing metabolic syndrome (and therefore Type 2 diabetes) if your waist is above 102 cm (40 inches) if you are a white man, 88 cm (35 inches) if you are an Asian man or a white woman, or 80 cm (32 inches) if you are an Asian woman.

> ### Features of the metabolic syndrome
>
> ⟹ Central obesity.
>
> ⟹ Raised triglycerides.
>
> ⟹ Raised LDL cholesterol.
>
> ⟹ Low HDL cholesterol (the protective form).
>
> ⟹ High blood pressure.
>
> ⟹ Insulin resistance.
>
> ⟹ Abnormal glucose metabolism/ Type 2 diabetes.

Problems associated with insulin resistance

In addition to the problems mentioned above, insulin resistance may be related to other important medical conditions, including polycystic ovarian syndrome (PCOS), non-alcoholic steatohepatitis (NASH) and acanthosis nigricans.

Polycystic ovarian syndrome

PCOS is a condition affecting women, which causes:

● Irregular periods;
● Reduced fertility;
● High testosterone levels;
● Excess body hair.

Most, but not all, patients with this condition are overweight with central obesity. Treatment with metformin, which is known to improve insulin resistance, may have a dramatic effect and lead to restoration of normal periods and often pregnancy. Metformin is not particularly effective at reducing body hair.

Non-alcoholic steatohepatitis

This is a potentially serious condition, in which excess fat is stored in the liver. This leads to enlargement of the liver and occasionally pain in the right side of the abdomen. Simple liver tests are raised and an ultrasound shows the typical appearance of fatty liver. However, the only way of proving the diagnosis is to do a liver biopsy.

NASH may progress to cause permanent liver damage (cirrhosis), although this process takes many years. People with NASH usually have central obesity and other markers of insulin resistance.

There is no proven treatment for NASH but a glitazone, which reduces insulin resistance, may be helpful.

Acanthosis nigricans

In this condition, the skin becomes thickened and dark with a velvety appearance. It is seen mainly at the back of the neck and in the skin folds – armpits and groin. It also affects pressure areas such as the elbows and knuckles. It is found in people with central obesity, and they carry a risk of diabetes. Skin tags are often found in the same patient.

The best way to reduce insulin resistance is to lose weight. The glitazone class of drugs lower blood sugar levels by reducing insulin resistance, but unfortunately these also lead to weight increase, which can be very dispiriting to people who are being encouraged to lose weight on medical grounds.

Maturity-onset diabetes of the young (MODY)

This condition was first described about 40 years ago and, more recently, has been the subject of research which has taught us a great deal about the causes of Type 2 diabetes. People with MODY develop Type 2 diabetes in their teens or 20s and are not usually overweight. It is a genetic disease and affects many people in the same family. There are at least six different types of MODY, but the most common variant can usually be controlled with sulphonylurea tablets. At the time of diagnosis, many people with MODY are assumed to have Type 1 diabetes

Consider MODY if you:

- Are thin;
- Are young;
- Have a strong family history;
- Present with Type 2 diabetes.

because they are young and not overweight. They are therefore started on insulin. Once the true diagnosis has been made, however, they can often be successfully switched to treatment with a sulphonylurea. (More information about MODY can be found in Chapter 22 on Type 2 diabetes and younger people.)

Causes of secondary diabetes

Hormonal causes

Several hormones oppose the action of insulin, and two of these may be produced in excess following other medical conditions.

Cushing's syndrome

This is a condition in which the body produces extra amounts of adrenal steroid hormones, which are known to have strong anti-insulin effect. In addition to diabetes, people with untreated Cushing's syndrome have high blood pressure and are overweight with a particular moon face.

Acromegaly

This is caused by overproduction of growth hormone due to a tumour in the pituitary gland, which lies at the base of the skull. This causes enlargement of the jaw, hands and feet and a number of other medical problems including high blood pressure and arthritis. Diabetes often seems to persist even when the underlying problem has been treated.

Pancreatic disease and pancreatitis

Any condition which causes damage to the pancreas may lead to diabetes. Pancreatitis is an inflammation of the pancreas which leads to a release of digestive juices into the abdomen. It is not easy to treat and often recurs. Each attack causes further permanent injury to the pancreas, and eventually it becomes so damaged that it can produce neither pancreatic juice nor the hormones insulin and glucagon. At this stage, the person will develop diabetes and, in addition to treatment with insulin, is likely to require replacement of pancreatic enzymes to allow the normal digestion of food.

Location of the pancreas

Any condition that damages your pancreas may lead to diabetes.

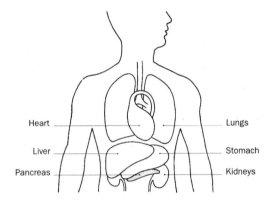

Heart — Lungs
Liver — Stomach
Pancreas — Kidneys

Haemachromatosis

This inherited condition also causes damage to the pancreas. In haemochromatosis, the body is unable to deal normally with iron, and there are high levels of iron in the blood. This is deposited in various parts of the body including the skin, joints and pancreas. After many years, the pancreas is destroyed by the iron and diabetes occurs. If diagnosed early, haemochromatosis can be treated simply by taking off a pint of blood every few weeks or months. The condition runs in families and, when detected, it is important to screen family members so those with the condition can be treated early and the unpleasant consequences avoided.

Type 2 diabetes in later life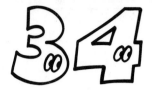

Management of Type 2 diabetes in later life needs to take into account the specific needs of the individuals concerned, with respect to health and wellbeing. If you are older and have Type 2 diabetes, drug side effects such as hypoglycaemia or gastrointestinal upset may take on more importance for you than aggressive targeting of your blood sugar to keep you healthy until the age of 110! Equally, staying free of cardiovascular problems or eye disease related to diabetes may be crucial to independent living, or helping you to deal with grandchildren or great-grandchildren. These considerations lead to competing pressures.

➡ On the one hand, do I really want to take 15 tablets and insulin and run the risk of hypoglycaemia, flatulence or diarrhoea?

➡ On the other hand, I have a real need to stay well for my grandchildren and to enjoy life as long as possible.

This chapter examines the treatment targets for an older population, specific drug side effects, and the needs of particular groups such as those older people who are living with special support in a nursing home.

Best possible blood glucose levels

If possible, you should still aim to get your average blood level, as measured by HbA_{1c}, down to around 7%. There is no evidence in an elderly population (above the age of 75 years of age) that the relationship between HbA_{1c} and complications of diabetes is any different from that found in younger people. So in general, older people should aim at the usual target for HbA_{1c}, namely 7%. However, the UKPDS (see Chapter 36) suggested that there was a delay between achieving good glucose control and seeing a

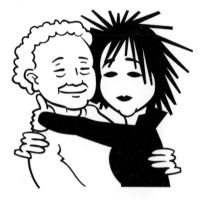

benefit in terms of reduced complications. Many older people find it very simple to achieve this degree of good control without any particular hardship, and there is some evidence from Australia that older people with diabetes tend to have lower HbA_{1c} results. However some people simply refuse to make the attempt at achieving good control, especially if this involves giving themselves insulin. Another group of people in this age group would like to have an HbA_{1c} of 7% but find this impossible, sometimes because of drug side effects and hypoglycaemia. Studies have shown that, in older people particularly, high blood sugars are associated with a worsening of memory problems. This is clearly an incentive to improve the HbA_{1c}.

There is, however, some flexibility in this target. If you have a lot of other medical problems, live alone, don't have easy access to help when needed, you might not want to run the risk of hypoglycaemia. This is perfectly understandable. It is also worth being honest with your doctor or diabetes nurse, so that you can discuss with them the fears and difficulties you face.

In addition, evidence is beginning to emerge that some people find their HbA_{1c} may increase a little as they get older. This is because, over time, the red blood cells may naturally attract more glucose than those of a younger person with the same level of blood glucose.

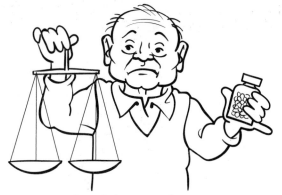

Most older patients find a compromise.

As a general rule, if your HbA_{1c} runs at a little above 7% and you feel well, you should not be coerced into reducing it further. Blood glucose targets in older people are a compromise between risks of hypoglycaemia, symptoms of allowing high blood glucose and benefit in terms of reduced complications.

Glucose-lowering drugs: which is best for you?

Metformin

As discussed in Chapter 13, metformin has good data to support a benefit in avoiding cardiovascular complications. It is now the first-choice drug for treating Type 2 diabetes. There are, however, some problems with metformin. It should not be used if there is a history of kidney failure, which is more likely in older people. It is also associated with stomach problems, particularly nausea, abdominal bloating, flatulence and diarrhoea. If you can take it, metformin is the best choice, but it may simply not be an option for significant numbers of older patients.

Sulphonylureas

The main difficulty with sulphonylureas is the risk of hypoglycaemia (low blood sugar). This is a particular worry when patients are taking a long-acting sulphonylurea such as glibenclamide or chlorpropamide. If you are taking one of these two older drugs, you should suggest to your GP that your prescription is changed to another class of anti-diabetes drug or a short-acting sulphonylurea. The likelihood of suffering a low blood sugar is increased if you have kidney failure, as sulphonylureas are eliminated from the body by the kidneys and this process is protracted if the kidneys are not working properly. If you have been found to have this problem, you may need to reduce your daily dose. Your risk of developing hypoglycaemia is increased if you miss a meal or work hard in your garden. In this case, you should take half the dose of sulphonylurea.

Rosiglitazone and pioglitazone

Glitazones are potentially useful in older people as they do not cause hypoglycaemia. While metformin is the automatic first-choice drug for patients who can take it, glitazones are challenging sulphonylureas for second place as the preferred treatment in Type 2 diabetes. Like all effective drugs, they cause side effects, and the main unwanted effect with glitazones is fluid retention. This can worsen or unmask problems of heart failure. For this reason, they must not be given to older patients if there is any suspicion of heart failure. Your GP will take a careful look at the condition of your heart before considering one of these two drugs. No one likes taking more tablets than necessary, and one of the advantages of both rosiglitazone and pioglitazone is that they are available as combined drugs with metformin. So anyone taking three metformin tablets a day can continue on the same number of tablets, but each one will contain both metformin and a glitazone.

There is a concern that rosiglitazone may carry an extra risk of heart attacks, and this has generated a heated debate. It appears that, putting together a number of studies, people taking rosiglitazone have a slightly higher risk of heart attacks, though the risks themselves are very small. The manufacturers have looked at all the research studies on rosiglitazone and have concluded that the risk for their drug is no higher than for patients taking metformin.

Insulins

Many older patients are scared of the idea of going on to insulin therapy, and no one enjoys the prospect of injecting themselves and doing regular blood tests. However, with modern blood testing devices and pens for injection, most people find this acceptable. The major concern with insulin in the older patient is hypoglycaemia. Severe hypoglycaemia, defined as needing help from a third party, occurs in less than 1% of patients per year, and a low blood glucose which the patient can correct on their own occurs in less than 5% per year. There is no doubt that these risks are higher in older people. Studies have shown that knowledge of the symptoms of hypoglycaemia is very poor in old people. There is also evidence that the symptoms of hypoglycaemia are different in the elderly. The usual complaint is lightheadedness and unsteadiness.

If you live alone and are becoming frail, hypoglycaemia can represent a real threat to your independence. It is worth talking to your GP or diabetes nurse about ways of avoiding the dangers of a low blood glucose, such as making sure a snack is near to hand, and identifying what support is available. Inevitably, to avoid the risk of low blood sugar, many patients allow their blood glucose targets to float upwards. Newer insulins may be used to reduce the risk of low blood sugars. In particular, the long-acting analogues (Lantus and Levemir) reduce the risk of night-time hypos.

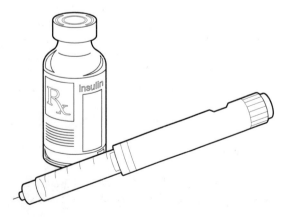

You should also talk to your diabetes nurse or doctor about the number of insulin injections that would be the best for you. As a rule, the more frequently you inject insulin, the easier it is to tailor the dose to your needs and adjust the dose in response to your blood glucose level, your food intake, your energy levels and the timing of meals. However, this makes your diabetes more intrusive, and it might be more attractive just to give a fixed dose of insulin once or twice a day and try to live your life round this. This is a decision you have to make yourself, and your diabetes nurse or doctor should be keen to have this debate with you.

Finally, you may be partially sighted, have arthritis, have had a previous stroke or have another disability which affects your ability to do glucose monitoring or manage the insulin injections. A number of aids do now exist, including a 'speaking' glucose monitor and devices which help you fix the pen or injector to a particular spot. A district nurse may be able to visit to give your insulin injections if you are unable to manage this yourself.

Management of other risk factors if you are older

Aspirin therapy

As discussed on page 197, there is good evidence for the use of aspirin treatment in older patients. A number of large studies have proven the benefit of using aspirin. These include the HOT study, the Early Treatment Diabetic Retinopathy study and a big meta-analysis (where researchers lump a number of trials together) called the Anti-Platelet Trialists Collaboration, all of which have shown positive benefits in the aspirin-treated group. There are of course risks of bleeding which may be higher in the older patient, so if you have uncontrolled high blood pressure or a history of stomach ulcers or persistent indigestion, you should discuss the question of aspirin with your doctor or diabetes nurse. In most cases, the benefits of aspirin in reducing cardiovascular events outweigh the risks.

Control of blood pressure

It used to be thought that controlling blood pressure aggressively in an older patient was positively dangerous and that more 'lax' limits could be allowed with increasing patient age. This is utterly untrue, and evidence from blood pressure-lowering studies in older patients has proved that blood pressure should be lowered to the same aggressive limits, 140/80 mmHg, without complications, and lower if you have complications from your diabetes. Evidence is accumulating that an ACE inhibitor such as ramipril or perindopril is an ideal initial choice in older people. Unfortunately, blood pressure is difficult to control in Type 2 diabetes, especially in the elderly, so you can expect to be taking a number of different tablets for your blood pressure. However, there is no doubt that reducing blood pressure can lessen the risk of stroke and heart attack, which are both more devastating in older people.

Control of blood fats (cholesterol)

We now have aggressive recommendations for statin use in people with Type 2 diabetes. Indeed, nearly everyone with Type 2 diabetes is encouraged to take them. But what is the evidence like for treating your blood fats if you are older, say 75 or more? There are a number of studies of using a statin which include elderly patients, up the age of 82. These show that statins have the same beneficial effect in older people and confirm that the danger of serious side effects is low. They reduce the risk of heart attacks by 20–40% but do not seem to protect people from strokes. People with Type 2 diabetes have high risks of heart disease, and it is reasonable to treat all risk factors aggressively, including the use of a statin.

Management of erectile dysfunction if you're older

Unfortunately, it seems that problems with maintaining an erection are associated with both Type 2 diabetes and increasing age. It's estimated that between 50 and 95% of men aged above the age of 60 years have some problems with their erections. Sex may well still be an important part of your life, and problems with performance can be distressing for you and your partner. Before your GP or health professional can arrange treatment for you though, it's important to assess any risk factors for vascular disease. Unfortunately, erectile dysfunction often goes hand in hand with cardiovascular problems, and angina or ischaemic heart disease can restrict access for you to tablet treatments for erection problems such as Viagra or Cialis.

The good news is that there are a number of possible treatments which may suit you; these include vacuum constriction devices to help you achieve erection, injections into the side of the penis and administering medication down the urethra to name a few options (see also Chapter 25). The difficult thing is talking about it, and once you've managed that, the rest is a great deal easier.

Diabetes foot care

Unfortunately, foot problems related to diabetes contribute significantly to the tribulations of older people with Type 2 diabetes. Old age is a risk factor for diabetic foot problems and also increases the risk of the main causes of foot ulcers, namely poor blood supply and nerve damage. Other risk factors include limited mobility, smoking, alcohol consumption and bony deformities. It is important that you educate yourself about the factors that lead to foot problems and act upon them. Your feet should be examined every time you consult for your diabetes. If you have any risk factors for diabetic foot problems, you should be looked after by a specialist foot team, either in the hospital clinic or in the community. More information about foot problems in diabetes can be found in Chapter 32.

Diabetes in a care home

Traditionally, people with Type 2 diabetes who live in a care home have less stringent diabetes

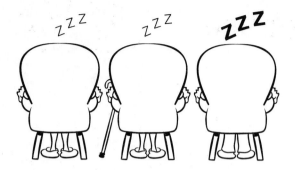

care than people in their own home. This may be due to a lack of knowledge on the part of staff, and studies have shown that intervention with a diabetes education programme for staff or affiliation to a university care of the elderly department for support improves the standard of care. If you live in a care home and have a number of other medical problems, you may wonder how important it is to control your diabetes well. However, a better control of blood glucose improves symptoms, such as thirst and urinary frequency, as has been shown to improve memory and other thought processes. In combination, these are likely to have a significant impact on your quality of life. Equally, if you have coexistent conditions like high blood pressure, managing them properly can significantly impact on the risk of further complications such as a stroke or a heart attack. Just because you live in a care home, it doesn't mean the care of your diabetes should be ignored. If you don't receive a regular diabetes review, ask to see your GP to discuss it.

Support and information

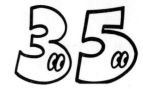

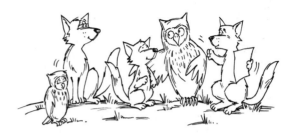

Once you have received your diagnosis of Type 2 diabetes, you will have diabetes as a companion for the rest of your life. There is plenty of support and information available to help you deal with this companion in a constructive way so that it does not disrupt your life or cause you distress. This chapter looks at what structures and organizations are in place to help you and how you can harness your time and energy in order to best help yourself. We begin by looking what sort of care and facilities you have a right to expect.

What should you be getting from your primary care team?

Once your diabetes has settled down, your primary care team are likely to be responsible for your regular care. You should not regard this care as in any way 'second class' as GPs and practice nurses have been specially trained to take on this role for over 20 years now. They are likely to know you, as an individual, better than a team in a hospital several miles away could hope to, and visiting them should be more convenient for you too.

Your GP and practice nurse will ensure that you go onto the practice's register of patients with diabetes. This will ensure that you are given regular appointments for the diabetes clinic and appropriate additional screening. Being on this register should also mean you receive reminders about immunizations such as the 'flu vaccination and other care such as eye tests.

The person with whom you have most contact will probably be a practice nurse with special training in diabetes care. This nurse will be your main point of contact should you have any worries about your diabetes or any related issues, so you may find you come to know him or her very well in time. Indeed, the practice nurse with a special knowledge of diabetes will have links with all the other professionals with whom you are likely to come into contact, and will be well placed to provide you with a great deal of support as well as information. You should also be referred to a dietitian, a podiatrist (chiropodist) and a pharmacist as appropriate.

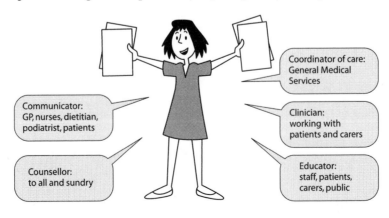

Coordinator of care:
General Medical
Services

Communicator:
GP, nurses, dietitian,
podiatrist, patients

Clinician:
working with
patients and carers

Counsellor:
to all and sundry

Educator:
staff, patients,
carers, public

National Service Frameworks

As part of the process of modernizing the National Health Service in the UK, the Department of Health began launching National Service Frameworks (NSFs) from April 1998. These NSFs are described as 'long-term strategies for improving specific areas of care' by setting measurable goals within specific time frames.

Each NSF is developed with the assistance of an external reference group (ERG) which brings together health professionals, service users and carers, health service managers, partner agencies and other advocates. ERGs adopt an inclusive process to engage the full range of views. The Department of Health supports the ERGs and manages the overall process.

**What do NSFs do?
(From the Department of Health website)**

⇒ They set national standards and identify key interventions for a defined service or care group.

⇒ They put in place strategies to support implementation.

⇒ They establish ways to ensure progress within an agreed timescale.

⇒ They form part of a range of measures to raise quality and decrease variations in service.

The NSF for diabetes

The 12 Standards of the Diabetes NSF cover all aspects of diabetes care and prevention and, together with the Delivery Strategy, set out a 10-year programme of change and improvement which will raise the quality of services and reduce unacceptable variations. Your local practice, and your primary health care team, have a duty to do everything possible to meet these standards of

---

The rolling programme of NSFs, launched in April 1998, covers:

● Coronary heart disease.

● Cancer.

● Paediatric intensive care.

● Mental health.

● Older people.

● Diabetes.

● Long-term conditions.

● Renal services.

● Children's and maternity services.

● Chronic obstructive pulmonary disease (COPD).

(From the Department of Health website)

---

care. The standards are listed here to let you know what sort of care you can expect from your primary care team. If you feel they are not being met in your case, you should ask to speak to the practice manager at your local surgery in the first instance. If you still feel you are not getting the care you should be getting, you should contact the Patient Advice and Liaison Service (PALS) for your local Primary Care Trust.

Structured patient education programmes

People living with diabetes have a crucial role in managing their condition on a day-to-day basis so supporting self-care should be an integral component of any local diabetes service.

Patient education is a vital part of this support package. There is a considerable amount of excellent work already being done to ensure that quality-assured training and education are available to all those who need it. For more information, consider contacting your local Diabetes UK group for advice on local courses available.

NSF for diabetes: standards

● **Standard 1**
Prevention of Type 2 diabetes.

● **Standard 2**
Identification of people with diabetes.

● **Standard 3**
Empowering people with diabetes.

● **Standard 4**
High-quality care of adults with diabetes.

● **Standard 5**
High-quality care of children and young people with diabetes.

● **Standard 6**
Smooth transition of young people from paediatric to adult care.

● **Standard 7**
Management of diabetic emergencies.

● **Standard 8**
Care of people with diabetes during admission to hospital.

● **Standard 9**
Diabetes and pregnancy.

● **Standard 10**
Surveillance for long-term complications.

● **Standard 11**
Timely and effective treatment of long-term complications and reduction of cardiovascular risk factors.

● **Standard 12**
Multi-agency integrated health care.

DESMOND

DESMOND is an acronym for Diabetes Education and Self Management for Ongoing and Newly Diagnosed. Still in development, this is a structured education programme based on recognized principles of adult learning and is promoted by the Department of Health. People are invited to DESMOND sessions in groups of eight, accompanied by partners if they wish. The sessions are run by two nurses or dietitians who have been specially trained to deliver patient education. Ideally, patients should have access to a DESMOND session within 4 weeks of their diagnosis. After this, they should be able to identify their own health risks and set their own specific goals.

To date, only sessions for people with newly diagnosed Type 2 diabetes are able to take part in DESMOND sessions, and a research project to test its effectiveness has recently reported. However, individuals who take part in these groups describe how their attitude towards diabetes has been altered completely by the programme. They have been able to tell their own story and listen to the accounts of diabetes from a peer group.

The results of the research study in 824 people showed a numerically greater reduction in HbA_{1c} for individuals enrolled in a DESMOND group versus those receiving normal care, but this wasn't statistically different from the normal care group. It is important to note though that the DESMOND group had significantly greater

DESMOND topics covered at the newly diagnosed patients' session with the time (in minutes) spent on each subject

DESMOND: newly-diagnosed curriculum	mins
Housekeeping	5
The patient story	10
What diabetes is	5
Main ways to manage diabetes	10
Diabetes consequences/ personal risk	15
Monitoring and taking action	10
Food choices	20
Physical activity	5
Stress and emotion	5
Screening and annual clinics	5

rates of smoking cessation and weight loss, and much stronger beliefs that they could have an impact on their own illness.

X-PERT

X-PERT is a 6-week structured patient education programme developed by Dr Trudi Deakin, which has been trialled initially in the North of England but is now being rolled out throughout the UK and Ireland. It consists of six sessions, leading to goal setting for a healthier lifestyle. An interactive CD-ROM and a DVD are being developed for those who cannot or prefer not to attend group sessions.

X-PERT programme: content

Week 1	What is diabetes?
Week 2	Weight management.
Week 3	Carbohydrate awareness.
Week 4	Supermarket tour.
Week 5	Complications of diabetes.
Week 6	Questions and evaluation.
Lifestyle experiment	Goal setting.

Diabetes UK

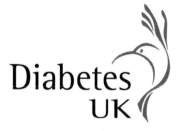

People react in different ways to the shock of diabetes: some try to become hermits and hide, while others set out to try to solve all the problems of mankind (including diabetes) in a few weeks. Whatever your reaction, you should make contact with your local Diabetes UK group. You will come across people who are living with diabetes and who have learnt to cope with many of the daily problems. These people should provide an extra dimension to the information that you have been given by doctors, nurses, dietitians and other professionals.

Diabetes UK (formerly the British Diabetic Association) was founded in 1935 by two people with diabetes, the author H.G. Wells, and Dr R.D. Lawrence, who worked at the diabetes clinic of King's College Hospital, London. In a letter to *The Times* dated January 1933, they announced their intention to set up an 'association open to all diabetics, rich or poor, for mutual aid and assistance, and to promote the study, the diffusion of knowledge, and the proper treatment of diabetes in this country'. They proposed that people with diabetes, members of the general public interested in diabetes, and doctors and nurses should be persuaded to join the projected association. Over 70 years later, Diabetes UK is a credit to its founders.

Diabetes UK now has more than 170,000 members and an income in 2005 of £23.7 million. In many countries, there are separate organizations for people with diabetes and for professionals, but Diabetes UK draws its strength from the fact that both interest groups are united in the same society.

Diabetes UK is the largest organization in the UK working for people with diabetes, funding research, campaigning and helping people to live with the condition. The Careline (020 7424 1030, Monday–Friday, 9am–5pm) offers confidential support and information on all aspects of diabetes. During 2006, the Careline handled an average of 200 calls each day. In order to make the Careline accessible to all, there is access to an interpreting service.

Diabetes UK

10 Parkway, London NW1 7AA
Helpline: **020 7424 1030/1000**
Careline: **0845 120 2960**
www.diabetes.org.uk

Publications

Up-to-date information and news is published in *Balance*, a magazine that appears every other month. *Diabetes for Beginners* is provided for newly diagnosed people, both Type 1 and Type 2 (insulin dependent and non-insulin dependent). Diabetes UK produces its own handbooks, leaflets and videotapes for teaching purposes and also sells those produced by other publishers. It constantly lobbies for high standards of care for those with diabetes. Diabetes UK has an excellent website.

Living with diabetes

Diabetes UK organizes 'living with diabetes' days. These are one-day conferences for people with diabetes, their carers, families and friends, giving an opportunity to talk to healthcare professionals and people living with diabetes and to discover more about Diabetes UK. For more information contact the conference team at Diabetes UK, telephone 020 7424 1000.

Diabetes UK holidays

The first diabetes holidays for children in the UK took place in 1935, and these have grown into a large enterprise. During the summer of 2006, at seven different sites throughout the UK, 250 children aged between 7 and 18 years enjoyed a week away with Diabetes UK. These educational holidays are organized by the care interventions team, and they give the opportunity for children to meet others with diabetes and to become more independent of their parents. They aim to give the children a good time and encourage them to try new activities, while teaching them more about their diabetes and providing a well-earned break for their parents.

Diabetes UK family weekends

The care intervention team also organizes family weekends to include the parents of children with diabetes. These cater for about 200 families each year. While parents have talks and discus-sions from specialist doctors, nurses and dietitians, there are activities for children throughout the weekend that are supervised by skilled and experienced helpers.

Local Diabetes UK groups – previously called branches

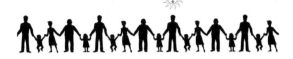

There are over 350 branches and parents' groups throughout the country. These are run entirely by volunteers, and because of their commitment large sums of money are raised for research into diabetes (£1.5 million being raised by groups in 2005). Diabetes UK groups also aim to increase public awareness of diabetes, and they arrange meetings for local people with diabetes and their families for support and information.

Parent support groups

The parents of children with diabetes often feel they have special needs – and that they can offer particular help to other parents in the same boat. Over 80 parent support groups exist throughout the UK, and these have added a sense of urgency to the main aim of Diabetes UK: to improve the lives of people with diabetes and to work towards a future without diabetes. In addition to self-help, the parents' groups also raise money for research.

The care intervention team now runs a 'Parent-link', which is a network support system for the parents of children with diabetes that aims to put parents in touch via a gradually expanding database. Parent-link sends out a newsletter called *Link-Up* four times a year.

Insurance

Many people with diabetes experience discrimination in terms of increased premiums or restricted terms, and even have policies refused when taking out insurance. Faced with the general lack of understanding within the insurance market, Diabetes UK has negotiated its own exclusive schemes to provide policies suited to the needs of people with diabetes and those living with them. Diabetes UK Services offers competitively priced home and motor, travel and personal finance products. For details of home, travel and motor insurance, as well as personal finance, telephone 0800 731 7431 (or e-mail diabetes@heathlambert.com).

Joining Diabetes UK

Diabetes UK works to influence the decisions made about living with diabetes, and the more members it has, the greater its influence can be. Diabetes UK cannot continue to provide its services and activities to all people with diabetes without your support. If you would like more information about joining Diabetes UK, contact the Supporter Development department on 0207 323 1531 or write to Diabetes UK at the address shown above.

Other useful organizations

International Society for Pediatric and Adolescent Diabetes

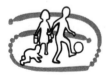

ISPAD is the only global (professional) advocate for children and adolescents with diabetes. It is an association for diabetes teams (doctors, nurses, dietitians, educators, psychologists and all others involved in the care of children with diabetes). The society is committed to promoting the best possible health, social welfare and quality of life for *all* children and adolescents with diabetes, anywhere in the world.

> **ISPAD**
> www.ispad.org

Juvenile Diabetes Research Foundation (JDRF)

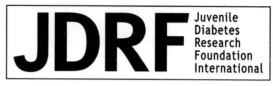

dedicated to finding a cure

This organization was founded in 1970 by a small group of parents of children with diabetes. The JDRF exists to find a cure for diabetes and its complications. It supports diabetes all over the world and provides research funds at a level comparable that provided by Diabetes UK.

> **JDRF**
> 19 Angel Gate, City Road,
> London EC1V 2PT
> Tel: **020 7713 2030**
> **www.jdrf.org.uk**

International Diabetes Federation (IDF)

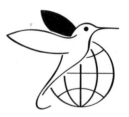

International Diabetes Federation

The IDF is open to members of all countries. It promotes diabetes interests in many different areas. An international conference is held every 3 years, with the two most recent being in Paris (2003) and South Africa (2006). The next conference is planned for Montreal in 2009.

You can obtain more information about the IDF from your local diabetes association, or from the website at www.idf.org

Diabetes Federation Ireland

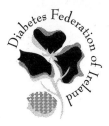

The aims of the Federation are:

- To represent people with diabetes.

- To help and provide information for people with diabetes, their families and the community.

- To create awareness and foster programmes for the early detection and prevention of diabetes.

- To support and encourage advances in diabetes care and research.

- To raise funds which will make the achievement of these aims possible.

The activities of the Federation include the dissemination of non-judgemental advice and information through meetings, its magazine (*Diabetes Ireland*) and by request. The Federation provides support through its telephone helpline and regular public meetings. It raises awareness of diabetes by running campaigns and actively lobbying on behalf of people with diabetes in areas where they are encountering discrimination, as well as for national service development. All the above activities are possible only through the close collaboration of all people concerned with diabetes, whether their interest arises through their work or through living with the condition.

Diabetes Federation Ireland
76 Lower Gardiner Street, Dublin 2
Republic of Ireland
Helpline: **1850 909 909**
www.diabetesireland.ie

Insulin-Pumpers
(insulin pump therapy group)

This group was formed to raise funds and provide information on insulin pumps. It will put users of insulin pumps in touch with each other if they wish, and also offers advice about obtaining funding for a pump if non are available on the NHS. Contact Insulin-Pumpers via their website: www.insulin-pumpers.org.uk

British Heart Foundation

This national charity funds research, promotes education and raises money to buy equipment to treat people with heart disease. Increasingly, it also provides information on preventing heart disease and heart attack, and staying as healthy as possible for as long as possible. The helpline, HeartstartUK, can arrange training in emergency life-saving techniques for lay people.

British Heart Foundation
14 Fitzhardinge Street, London W1H 6DH
Helpline: **0845 07 08 070**
www.bhf.org.uk

National Kidney Federation (NKF)

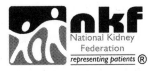

The NKF is a UK-wide charity run by kidney patients for kidney patients. While it used to be concerned almost solely with people with advanced or end-stage renal failure, there is now much more emphasis on people at earlier stages of kidney disease too. If you have even a

mild form of kidney disease, the NKF can help you find information and support to keep your kidneys as healthy as possible for as long as possible.

Given the high numbers of people with diabetes who go on to develop some degree of kidney damage, it is important to be aware of this organization and what it has to offer.

> **National Kidney Federation**
> The Point, Coach Road, Shireoaks,
> Worksop S81 8BW
> Helpline: **0845 601 02 09**
> **www.kidney.org.uk**

RNIB

 supporting blind and partially sighted people

If you have microvascular complications affecting your eyes, sooner or later you will want to be aware of this organization. The RNIB (founded as the Royal National Institute for the Blind) offers a range of information and advice on lifestyle changes and practical adaptations for people facing sight loss, and produces a mail order catalogue of useful aids. It also offers support and training in Braille.

> **RNIB**
> 105 Judd Street, London WC1H 9NE
> Helpline: **0845 766 99 99**
> **www.rnib.org.uk**

Stroke Association

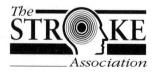

This UK-wide charity works to combat stroke in people of all ages, including people with diabetes. The Stroke Association funds research into prevention, treatment and better methods of rehabilitation. It also helps stroke patients and their families directly through its Rehabilitation and Support Services. These include Communication Support, Family and Carer Support, information services and welfare grants. The Association campaigns on behalf of people who are affected by stroke, and acts as a voice for its member.

The Stroke Association produces a number of publications including patient leaflets, *Stroke News* (a quarterly magazine) and information for health professionals.

> **The Stroke Association**
> 240 City Road, London EC1V 2PR
> Helpline: **0845 303 31 00**
> **www.stroke.org.uk**

Practical and financial support

Claiming benefits

Some people with diabetes may be eligible for disability benefits and incapacity benefits, depending on the effect that the condition has on their lives.

Disability Living Allowance (DLA) may be granted to you if you have a physical or mental disability, the disability is severe enough for you to have walking difficulties or problems looking

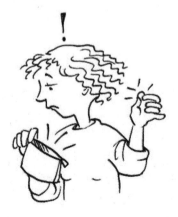

after yourself and you are under 65 years old when you claim. Both microvascular and macrovascular complications might lead to a situation where you need to claim disability living allowance. The amount you receive isn't normally affected by income.

Disability benefits are mainly for people who need help in their daily lives. They might pay for some of the extra transport costs involved in not being able to drive, a cleaner or home help for a few hours a week, or some aids to help you in activities around the home. Incapacity benefits are also available for people who are not fit to work.

You may also qualify for a type of disability benefit called Attendance Allowance. This is for people over 65 who are severely disabled and have needed attention or supervision during the day or night for at least 6 months. Carers may also be entitled to some benefit too depending on their involvement in caring for the person with diabetes. This may be useful if you are elderly and struggling with complications of your diabetes.

Your local Citizen's Advice Bureau can check whether you are getting all the benefits to which you are entitled. They, as well as your diabetes specialist team, should also be able to provide advice on filling in the forms. Information on the types of benefits available can also be obtained by calling your local benefits enquiry line or the Disability Benefits enquiry line on Freephone 0800 882 200.

It is very important to remember that you are not alone when it comes to applying for benefits, and these are not separate from your general care. If you are planning to apply for benefits, discuss this with your doctor or other healthcare professionals who look after you. They can often provide important supporting material about your diabetes, care of your condition and complications which may increase your chances of a successful application for financial support.

A number of benefits are also available for those affected by loss of vision. Details of these can be obtained from the RNIB. These may include qualification for disability living allowance or reduced price services such as your TV licence. The RNIB website also has contact numbers to talk to an adviser about what further help may be available.

Prescription advice

If you have Type 2 diabetes and are treated with tablets or insulin, you are entitled to free prescriptions. You do need to apply for an exemption certificate though; the nurse, doctor or pharmacist will have a leaflet with details of how to apply.

If you have diabetes, you are entitled to free eye tests. Unfortunately, however, you are not entitled to free dental care. If you are entitled to benefits such as Income Support, you may be able to claim some help with the cost of dental treatment.

Reimbursed accessories

In most countries, insulin is available free of charge for people who need it for their diabetes. Syringes, pen injectors and needles are often either free or reimbursed as well. Other accessories such as indwelling catheters are reimbursed in some countries, though not in all. Sometimes the person with diabetes has to pay for blood glucose meters, while the sticks for testing are free or reimbursed. In the UK, blood testing meters are usually available free, but you will need a prescription from your doctor for the testing strips. Sometimes the companies producing the meter will provide them free of charge at the onset of diabetes. Insulin pumps and accessories for these are often not reimbursed but

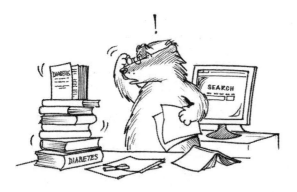

Diabetes and the Internet

There is a vast amount of diabetes information available on the Internet. You need to be aware that information on the Internet is often not reviewed by healthcare professionals and may only be the opinion of the person writing it. The associations listed below, however, can be trusted to produce reliable information.

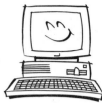

Associations:

Diabetes UK	www.diabetes.org.uk
Diabetes Federation of Ireland	www.diabetesireland.ie
American Diabetes Association (ADA)	www.diabetes.org
Diabetes Australia	www.diabetesaustralia.com.au
International Diabetes Federation (IDF)	www.idf.org
Juvenile Diabetes Research Federation (JDRF)	www.jdrf.org
Diabetes Exercise and Sports Association (DESA)	www.diabetes-exercise.org

Government departments:

Department of Health	www.dh.gov.uk
National Institute for Health and Clinical Excellence (NICE)	www.nice.org.uk

Since Internet pages are constantly being updated, and many change their addresses from time to time, we have chosen not to include more links in this book.

may be available through various insurance companies or under special conditions. In the UK, a recent report from the government organization NICE (the National Institute for Health and Clinical Excellence) has recommended that pumps be made available for those in special need, in particular people who have unstable diabetes. However, funding in the NHS remains a problem.

Using the Internet

An ever-increasing amount of information about diabetes is available on the Internet. Both medical companies and institutions have homepages displaying information and news. Use one of the search services to find the type of information you are looking for.

One thing is particularly important to remember when you are reading information on the Internet. Much of what you find will not have been reviewed by health professionals, and it may often be only the opinion of the person writing it. However, if you judge the information somewhat critically, you may find out a lot of interesting information about diabetes which you can then discuss with your diabetes nurse or doctor.

Over the past few years, there has also been an explosion in interactive sites such as chat rooms, and this may be a way to make new friends who share some of your experiences in adjusting to life with diabetes.

Outcome studies in Type 2 diabetes

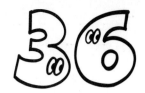

The world of Type 2 diabetes care has evolved rapidly. The main reason for this is that a large number of outcome studies have been completed over the past few years which have provided information about the best way of caring for people with Type 2 diabetes. This chapter looks at some of the key studies and what they tell us. It also looks forward to studies reporting in the near future.

UKPDS

The UKPDS study reported in 1998, and informed us about the importance of keeping both blood sugar and blood pressure under good control. It looked at 3867 patients with newly diagnosed Type 2 diabetes and measured the effects of tight control of blood glucose versus less tight control. It also looked at 1148 patients with newly diagnosed Type 2 diabetes and hypertension, again measuring the effects of tight versus less tight blood pressure control.

What did it show?

The 10-year follow-up from the study showed that for a difference of 0.9% in HbA_{1c} between the tight and the less tight groups for blood glucose control, there was a reduction in complications related to diabetes of 12%. Most of this was due to a 25% reduction in damage to the eyes and kidneys, known as microvascular events. The study also showed that the individuals taking metformin for lowering of blood glucose appeared to have fewer heart attacks and strokes than those taking other glucose-lowering treatments. The blood pressure study showed that a lowering of the blood pressure by 10/5 mmHg in the intensive blood pressure control group led to a 24% reduction in complications

More than 10,000 articles on diabetes research are produced every year. Many small advances have resulted, but so far no one has been able to solve the question of why a person develops diabetes or how to cure it. However, there is every reason to be optimistic about the future.

What is an 'outcome study'?

In any medical research project, it is important to define clearly what endpoints are being measured. In the UKPDS, hundreds of thousands of measurements were made during and after the study. Some of these looked at the effect of treatment on the blood glucose and the quality of life, but the most important findings were the actual medical problems (or outcomes) that affected patients in the study, such as heart attacks, laser therapy and, worst of all, death. Each endpoint was carefully checked independently by two separate adjudicators, and any disagreement was referred to a third arbitrator. So an outcome study examines what important events are prevented by a certain form of treatment, rather than just measuring differences in blood values, which do not affect people's lives in the same way.

related to diabetes. This included a 32% reduction in deaths and a 44% reduction in strokes, to name just a couple of the benefits.

What does all this mean?

The UKPDS study established the need for metformin to be used first for the treatment of raised blood glucose as, compared with other treatments used for lowering blood glucose, it showed positive benefits in reducing the risk of cardiovascular disease. The UKPDS also showed that reducing both the blood glucose and blood pressure has a large benefit in reducing complications related to diabetes.

Doctors have responded to the results of the UKPDS by trying to get as many people as possible below the recommended targets for blood glucose and blood pressure.

Over the past few years, the UKPDS has continued to provide a valuable resource to study a number of other risk factors related to Type 2 diabetes and will continue to give us useful insights for many years to come.

Heart Protection Study

The Heart Protection Study was one of the biggest studies of a cholesterol-lowering drug (simvastatin) and studied patients with and without diabetes.

What did it show?

There were 20,536 patients in the study, 5963 of whom had diabetes. These people were allocated randomly either to the group being given simvastatin 40 mg daily or to the group being given a placebo (dummy) tablet. Patients were followed up for a period of 5 years. Over that time, the simvastatin treatment group had cholesterol levels that were on average about 1 mmol/L less than those in the placebo group. In this study, the risk of major cardiovascular events such as stroke or heart attack was reduced by 33%. People with diabetes who had LDL (bad cholesterol; see page 210) levels lower than 3 mmol/L and

who would not have been treated in the past benefited with a 27% reduction in the risk of cardiovascular events.

This study also showed that simvastatin is an extremely safe drug with a low risk of side effects. There have been worries that simvastatin might cause liver problems, but less than 0.5% (five out of a thousand) of patients in this very large study had evidence of liver damage, and this risk was the same in both the simvastatin and the placebo group.

What does this mean?

If all the cholesterol-lowering studies with drugs of the statin family are taken together, there is now strong evidence that the vast majority of patients with Type 2 diabetes should be given a statin tablet to reduce their cholesterol and hence their cardiovascular risk. We know that Type 2 diabetes greatly increases the risk of cardiovascular events. So where we can demonstrate reductions in risk with a tried and tested drug, it is important to encourage their use.

CARDS

CARDS, the Collaborative Atorvastatin Diabetes Study, is the largest study of a statin (atorvastatin) to be carried out in people with Type 2 diabetes. The study involved an important collaboration between a number of key researchers in diabetes from across universities in the UK and Ireland.

What did it show?

A group of 2838 patients between the ages of 40 and 75 years with fairly average cholesterol levels (total cholesterol was 5.4 mmol/L and bad LDL level was 3.1 mmol/L) were randomized to receive the lowest dose of atorvastatin (10 mg) or a placebo tablet. As well as Type 2 diabetes, they also had to have another risk factor, such as cigarette smoking, high blood pressure, diabetic eye disease or proteinuria (indicative of diabetic kidney disease). These patients were followed up for about 4½ years. The number of patients who had at least one cardiovascular event such as a stroke or heart attack was reduced by 37%, and stroke reduction was greatest, at 48%. The people who joined this study would not have been considered a high-risk group, so the results are very impressive.

What does this mean?

Taken together with other studies looking at the use of statins in patients with Type 2 diabetes, this study has provided the final piece of the jigsaw to support the use of statin-type drugs in most patients with Type 2 diabetes. Since the publication of the CARDS study, an evidence review has taken place carried out by the joint British Societies (the specialist bodies for cardiovascular and diabetes care). These bodies now recommend statin treatment for almost all people with Type 2 diabetes over the age of 40, unless there is a contraindication which means they are unable to take them.

HOPE

The HOPE study examined the benefits of ramipril, an ACE inhibitor drug used for lowering blood pressure, in a mixed population of patients with and without Type 2 diabetes.

What did it show?

In total, 3577 people with diabetes were included in the study. They were randomized to ramipril 10 mg per day or placebo, and there was a 25% reduction in the risk of major cardiovascular events in the group taking ramipril. The study also showed that ramipril reduced the progression of albuminuria, effectively delaying the worsening of kidney disease due to diabetes.

What does this mean?

This study and a number of others using ACE inhibitors and the similar drugs called angiotensin-2 receptor blockers have shown

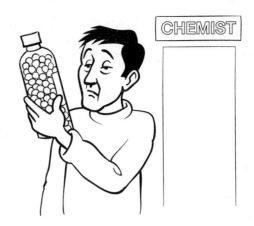

Statins have been found to be very effective in reducing the risk of strokes and heart attacks. If you have Type 2 diabetes, it is likely your doctor will put you on them at some stage.

positive effects on both cardiovascular events and a reduction in microalbuminuria – a marker of kidney disease. These drug classes now have a central place in the management of blood pressure and as part of a holistic strategy of managing Type 2 diabetes. As with statins, if you have diabetes you almost have to find a reason not to be taking one rather than look for a reason to start!

PROactive

The PROactive study was designed to look at the effects of pioglitazone, a glitazone drug used for reducing blood glucose, on cardiovascular events. The investigators wanted to test the hypothesis that, by reducing a number of cardiovascular risk factors apart from just blood sugar, pioglitazone might actually reduce the number of events suffered by patients in the study.

What did it show?

In total, 5238 patients at high risk of cardiovascular events were recruited into the study and followed up for an average of nearly 3 years. They were treated with 45 mg of pioglitazone added to their previous treatment. People with insulin-treated Type 2 diabetes patients took part in the study, in contrast to routine practice in Europe where pioglitazone is not licensed for use with insulin.

The main endpoint of the study was a combination of a number of unpleasant events including death, heart attack, stroke, amputation and also a number of active treatments for these conditions, such as coronary bypass surgery. There was no difference between the group receiving pioglitazone, compared with placebo, which was a disappointment to the study organisers. However, over the course of the study, which lasted over 2½ years, there was a 17% reduction in the risk of heart attack and a 23% reduction in strokes in the group taking pioglitazone. Thus, there were some important positive findings from the study. The downside is that the patients on pioglitazone put on an average of 3.6 kg (8 lb) in weight, some of which was due to fluid retention. The placebo group lost 0.4 kg (about 1 lb) in weight.

What does this mean?

While this study does show that pioglitazone impacts on cardiovascular risk in a high-risk population, excitement was tempered a little when the study was presented because of the increased fluid retention. Nevertheless, PROactive adds to the evidence that glitazones benefit people with Type 2 diabetes. However, they should be avoided when retention of extra fluid could be dangerous, such as in patients with heart failure.

ASCOT

ASCOT (the Anglo-Scandinavian Cardiac Outcomes Trial) was an international trial that recruited over 19,000 patients with high blood pressure but no previous heart disease. Approximately 4500 of these people had Type 2 diabetes. There were two 'arms' to the trial, one which confirmed the previous finding that lowering a slightly raised cholesterol level with a statin (this time atorvastatin) reduced the risk of

heart attack and stroke. The second arm compared the effects of two different regimes for reducing blood pressure.

What did it show?

The blood pressure-lowering arm reported in 2005. However, it had been stopped early because the benefits of treating patients with a combination of amlodipine (an ACE inhibitor drug) and perindopril (a calcium channel blocking drug), as opposed to a combination of atenolol (a beta-blocker) and bendrofluazide (a diuretic or 'water tablet'), were too clear to be ignored.

Combined results from both arms of the trial indicated the following:

⮕ The risk of heart attacks and strokes was lowered by approximately 46% for patients being treated with amlodipine, perindopril and atorvastatin.

⮕ Patients without diabetes who were being treated with amlodipine and perindopril appeared to be 29% less likely than those being treated with atenolol and bendrofluazide to develop Type 2 diabetes. This may be due in part to the withdrawal of bendrofluazide, to a protective effect of perindopril or to a combination of the two.

What does this mean?

The clear benefits enjoyed by those patients taking the combination of amlodipine and perindopril have prompted the British Hypertension Society to review its guidelines on prescribing. A combination of an ACE inhibitor drug with a calcium channel blocker is now the first treatment of choice for patients with heart disease.

Steno-2 study

For years, it was accepted that if you managed one risk factor aggressively, there would be little to be gained by managing other risk factors to

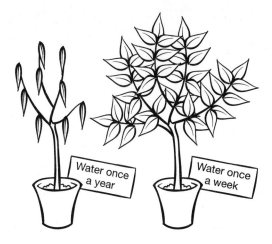

Sometimes the benefits of a particular treatment become evident during the course of a trial, so the trial is stopped early.

similar stringent targets. The Steno-2 study was designed to test the hypothesis that reducing all possible risk factors to tight targets would have a synergistic effect in reducing heart attacks, strokes and other cardiovascular problems.

What did it show?

The study looked at 160 people with diabetes who also had microalbuminuria, which put them at risk of heart disease. These were entered into either an intensive or a conventional management group. The conventional group were managed to standard Danish guidelines, whereas the intensive group were given very tight targets for glucose, blood pressure, lipids and microalbuminuria and treated with aggressive drug intervention and lifestyle advice. The greatest reductions were seen in blood pressure, lipids and microalbuminuria in the intensive group, with a much smaller fall in glucose, representing the fact that blood glucose targets are much harder to achieve. Over a period of 8 years, the group managed intensively were about half as likely to suffer cardiovascular problems. Now, 13 years after the study, the intensive therapy group still benefit from fewer cardiovascular events, and the death rate in this group is much reduced.

What does this mean?

The Steno-2 study reinforced the view that holistic management of Type 2 diabetes is the key and finally steered clinicians away from a view of the condition centering only on controlling sugar. It proved that treating to target is not just the preserve of randomized trials of new drugs, and that by adopting an aggressive approach to multiple targets, real benefits can be achieved.

DREAM

The main aim of the DREAM study was to establish whether rosiglitazone could prevent Type 2 diabetes in people with 'pre-diabetes' who were at high risk of developing the full condition. A total of 5269 people were studied for 3 years and tested for diabetes every year. The risk of diabetes was reduced from 26% in the control group and 11.6% in those receiving rosiglitazone, which represents a 62% reduction. However, because of the side effect of fluid retention, many more people in the rosiglitazone group developed heart failure – 14 compared with only two in the control group.

Although rosiglitazone has been shown to be effective in reducing the onset of diabetes in people at risk, it is not recommended for this by NICE, partly because of the unwanted side effects.

ADOPT

ADOPT is a study comparing the effectiveness of metformin, glibenclamide (a sulphonylurea) and rosiglitazone in reducing blood glucose levels in people with diabetes. Patients were asked to take one of the drugs under study and were followed for up to 6 years. If the fasting blood glucose rose above 10 mmol/L, this was regarded as the primary endpoint (i.e. the drug on its own was no longer holding the blood glucose) and a second drug was added. There were approximately 1450 patients in each group. At 5 years, there was a significant 32% reduction in relative risk of needing additional treatment in patients randomized to rosiglitazone compared with metformin, and a 63% reduction in those taking rosiglitazone compared with glibenclamide.

Thus roziglitazone on its own maintained good control of diabetes longer than the other two drugs.

Future outcome studies reporting in the next few years

NAVIGATOR

NAVIGATOR is similar in design to the DREAM study but uses valsartan (an angiotensin II receptor blocking drug) and nateglinide (a very short-acting drug which works like a sulphonylurea to increase insulin release from the pancreas). It is due to report imminently. The study is in people at high risk of developing diabetes and will tell us if these drugs can have a useful role in preventing diabetes and modifying cardiovascular risk in this group.

ORIGIN

ORIGIN looks at the use of insulin glargine in early diabetes or in patients who are yet to develop the disease but do have pre-diabetes (impaired glucose tolerance). It will tell us whether introducing insulin earlier has any effect on disease progression, from the point of view of worsening blood sugar levels and micro- and macrovascular complications. It should be completed in October 2009.

ACCORD and VADT

ACCORD and VADT are two studies being carried out by the National Institutes of Health (NIH), an American government medical research organization. They essentially look at whether an aggressive strategy to reduce blood sugar using modern combinations of glucose-lowering medicines will impact on complications.

BARI-2D

BARI-2D is another NIH study. This will look, in a similar way to PROactive did for pioglitazone, at whether rosiglitazone or pioglitazone given in addition to normal medication will reduce cardiovascular events after angioplasty for blocked blood vessels in the heart.

Outcome studies: what now?

The past few years have brought about a sea change in our level of knowledge about the best way to manage Type 2 diabetes. The studies described here are only a selection of key trials which have impacted on our clinical practice. The outcome trials due to report, and a raft of new medication classes, promise to inform us still further.

Outcome studies: key points

- Outcome evidence exists for aggressively treating a number of risk factors for diabetes complications.
- Individual studies show the importance of managing glucose, blood pressure and lipids to target and support using certain drug classes.
- There is also strong evidence that a holistic management of Type 2 diabetes brings additive benefits in reducing cardiovascular disease.
- We are due an explosion of new clinical trials over the next few years.

Outcome studies: useful websites

www.idf.org	Repository for the global guideline on Type 2 diabetes.
www.pubmed.com	Website used by medical researchers for medical evidence.
www.dtu.ox.ac.uk	Has links to the website with details about the UKPDS study that was run by Oxford University.
www.clinicaltrials.org	Site run by the NIH (the US government medical research organization) to give information on ongoing clinical studies.

Research and new developments

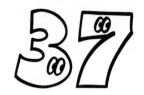

Huge efforts are put into diabetes research around the world, and more than 10,000 scientific studies are published every year. A large proportion of this is basic research, trying to throw light upon the causes of diabetes and the effects it may have on the body over the years. If you hear of a new treatment for diabetes from newspapers, television or the Internet, you must be aware that many of these reports are not based on scientific fact. In any case, it takes several years for a new exciting treatment becomes widely available. Unfortunately, many new 'wonder drugs' never become established treatments. There are, however, several lines of research that are looking promising.

Weight loss drugs

Everyone with a diagnosis of Type 2 diabetes tries their hardest to lose weight, and it can be a difficult task. It is natural to find it tough, and all healthcare professionals with an interest in diabetes are well aware of the problems you might have in getting rid of the excess kilos.

Unfortunately, neither of the present drug therapy options for treating excess weight is ideal. While orlistat and sibutramine are appropriate additions to diet and lifestyle advice for some, they don't suit everyone due to problems with diarrhoea (orlistat) or headaches and blood pressure (sibutramine). A new therapy, however, is about to be launched or may indeed have been launched worldwide by the time this book is published. Anyone who has used cannabis, or knows a friend who has, will be aware of the appetite stimulation which happens when people take it. Out of this observation comes the first of a new class of cannabis receptor blockers

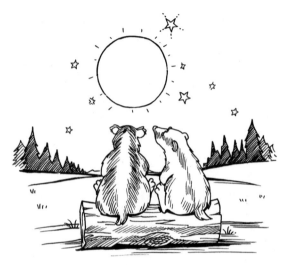

(cannabinoid antagonists) which block appetite and lead to weight loss.

Studies of rimonabant in obesity, the RIO studies have demonstrated significant reductions in weight, waist circumference, blood fats and blood glucose. This is extremely encouraging as these are the features most strongly associated with insulin resistance, the development of Type 2 diabetes and high cardiovascular risk. Compared with other treatments for obesity, the retention rate of patients continuing in these studies was higher than that for the orlistat or sibutramine trials, and weight loss was maintained out to 2 years. Although longer-term outcome studies are awaited, it finally seems that we have an effective option for weight loss. Rimonabant is the first in this new class of drugs and is an important development.

Unfortunately, rimonabant may lead to depression and should not be used in people with a history of depression or anxiety. For this reason, the manufacturers have withdrawn their application for this drug to be used in the US.

Newer glitazone-type drugs

When they were first launched in 1997, with troglitazone, the glitazones, or thiazolidine-diones, were heralded as the first treatment class to treat one of the underlying defects of Type 2 diabetes, insulin resistance. Unfortunately, this claim proved over optimistic as the drug was subsequently withdrawn due to unpredictable liver failure. The two currently marketed drugs, rosiglitazone and pioglitazone, offer advantages in sustained glycaemic control but are associated with weight gain and fluid retention. They only act on one class of receptor, the PPAR-gamma receptor, but two other types of PPAR receptor, alpha and delta, also exist. Drugs which act at receptors on the nucleus of the cell cause it to produce proteins and enzymes which change the way in which the cells of the body deal with chemicals such as fats and sugars.

Because of the problems with the current drugs, the pharmaceutical industry has worked hard to overcome the disadvantages of the present glitazones by producing drugs which act on more than one of the receptor sites. Drugs which act at the PPAR-alpha site include the fibrates, such as fenofibrate or bezafibrate. These have effects on lowering triglycerides (a form of bad cholesterol) and increasing HDL (good) cholesterol levels. Two drugs which act at PPAR-gamma and -alpha sites have reached the later stages of development, but these have both been abandoned because they cause severe fluid retention. A number of pharmaceutical companies are now trying to produce drugs which act at all three of the receptor sites. There is evidence that if the PPAR-delta receptor can also be stimulated, fluid retention can be ameliorated with potential for weight loss. In early animal studies, there is some evidence that exercise tolerance improves. Inevitably, the 'PPAR-pan' drugs which act at all three receptor sites are at an earlier stage of development, but preliminary studies look exciting.

With all drugs which act on the nucleus, the very heart of the cell, it is important to make sure that they don't cause harm. For this reason all of this class have to have at least 2 years of animal studies to prove that they don't increase the risk of cancer.

Incretins

When food passes from the stomach into the small bowel (the next part of the digestive tract), the distended part of the bowel produces very small chemicals called polypeptides. These signal to the brain to tell you that you are full and you don't need to eat any more, and signal to the beta cells of the pancreas, improving the release of insulin. They also have a local action in slowing the passage of food through the bowel. GLP-1 (glucagon-like peptide-1) is a polypeptide with these effects. However, it is broken down in the body so rapidly that if taken by injection, it only works for a few seconds. The Gila monster (an American desert lizard) produces in its saliva a substance that resembles GLP-1 but is not broken down so rapidly. This has been purified and is available as exenatide for injection. It has the benefit of improving blood glucose control and at the same time helping people lose weight. The drawback of exenatide is that it can make people feel sick, although this often wears off after a few weeks.

Another approach to harnessing the GLP-1 effect has been to develop a substance which slows down the rapid breakdown of GLP-1 in the body. These drugs are called DPP-4 inhibitors or gliptins. They are also available for

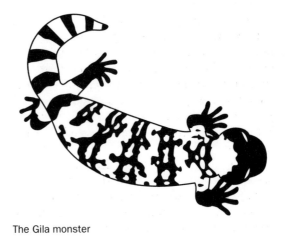

The Gila monster

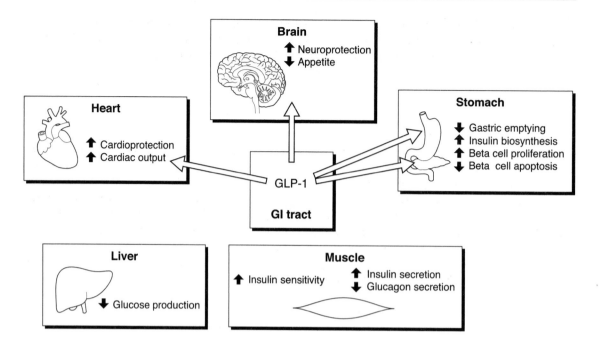

How GLP-1 affects the beta cells.

use and can be taken as tablets. They have proved to be effective but do not cause the weight reduction seen with exenatide.

Almost all the major multinational drug companies are currently investigating the incretin pathway for treating diabetes, and it seems likely that a number of drugs acting on this area will make it to the market over the next few years, for the benefit of large numbers of patients.

Drugs acting on glucose re-absorption in the kidney

Another way to reduce the amount of glucose in the body is to cause it to be excreted. Glucose is retained in the bloodstream by a complex system, using a chemical called an SGLT-2 transporter, which prevents glucose from passing into the urine via the kidney. A potential target is to block the SGLT-2 receptor, which would allow glucose to enter the urine, and which would have the added benefit of encouraging weight loss. At least two companies are at an advanced stage of research.

Other methods of insulin delivery

The holy grail of insulin delivery would be to give insulin in oral form, as either a liquid or tablets, but this has so far eluded the pharmaceutical industry. An insulin inhaler was available for a time for the delivery of short-acting insulin via the lungs (see pae 114), but the device was cumbersome and difficult to use. It has now been withdrawn.

A number of other firms are currently investigating different ways of delivering insulin. The lungs lend themselves well to the delivery of drugs as the border between the external environment and the bloodstream is very thin at the level of the alveoli where oxygen exchange occurs. Other delivery devices under investigation include nasal and oral sprays; the latter would deliver insulin through the mucous membrane inside the mouth. There are also attempts to coat insulin and thus protect it from the digestive enzymes in the digestive tract so that it can be delivered orally. These developments look quite promising.

The problem of just delivering insulin to your body if you have Type 2 diabetes is that this has no effect on obesity and insulin resistance, primary defects which contribute greatly to poor diabetic control associated with the disease.

Pancreas transplants

Although pancreatic transplants have received a great deal of publicity, they are not the answer for Type 2 diabetes. They deal solely with the relative deficiency of insulin rather than effecting the obesity and insulin resistance associated with the condition. In addition, even when islet cells which produce insulin are the only thing transplanted, anti-rejection therapy needs to be taken, and this may be associated with long-term complications such as a low blood count or

even some forms of cancer. Stem cell technology may offer the best alternative to pancreas transplants from the deceased, but this is still very much at the research stage

Looking ahead

When your diabetes was diagnosed and while you were settling into a treatment pattern, it was difficult to view the future with optimism. Reading this book, you must be aware of a wide range of treatment that is available, and there is a promise of more effective medications in the future. In time, we can be sure that more effective and convenient forms of treatment will be developed.

Well-known people with diabetes

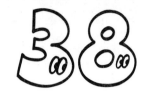

Brian Cox

The first actor to play the fearsome Hannibal Lecter (in the 1986 film *Manhunter*), Brian Cox has performed in numerous roles on the large and small screens (including recent success as Daphne's father in the popular comedy series *Frasier*). He started his career on the stage, and early – with the Dundee Repertory Company at the age of 14, then with the acclaimed Birmingham Rep and the Royal Shakespeare Company.

Brian, who never watches his own work, often plays villains. Some notable performances include Agamemnon in *Troy*, a devious CIA official in the *Bourne Supremacy* and Hermann Göering in a television miniseries about the Nuremberg trials. He has gained awards and accolades for his work, including an Emmy award for his complex portrayal of a paedophile in *L.I.E.* in 2001. He has also used his voice to great effect in the videogame industry.

Brian manages his diabetes so it rarely affects his work. A notable exception, however, occurred during the filming of *Super Troopers*, in which he played a senior police officer. Once scene called for this character to eat a bar of 'soap' – which the props staff had arranged to be made out of white chocolate. But because of his diabetes, production had to be halted until a sugar-free substitute could be found.

Brian is a native of Dundee and has been a leading figure in a campaign to raise millions of pounds for the Sir James Black Centre at the University of Dundee, described as 'a world-class global diseases research facility'. Type 2 diabetes is one of the conditions that will benefit from research at this centre, which was opened in 2006. The new building includes a Brian Cox Seminar Room in recognition of the actor's enthusiastic support. Professor Sir Philip Cohen, Research Dean in the College of Life Sciences, says: 'We are delighted to continue our association with Brian and it is entirely fitting that his efforts are recognized in this way.'

Steve Redgrave

Sir Steve Redgrave won gold medals for rowing at five consecutive Olympics. He was diagnosed with Type 2 diabetes at the age of 35 and started on insulin treatment immediately.

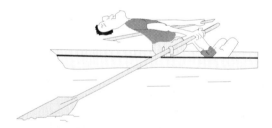

Sir Steve admits that he had considered giving up competing after being told that he had diabetes in 1997. 'My first thought was that my rowing career was at an end. I spoke to my GP and my specialist, and both said that I should be aware that the path to success was not going to be easy. However, very little is known about endurance sports and diabetes, so it has been a steep learning curve for all of us.' With the support of his doctors and his family, he thought again about competing in the Sydney Olympics and decided, 'I felt I had to give it a go.'

'But let's not be blasé about it', he continues. 'At first I went into a denial phase – you do not want to know that this thing is happening to you – and took as little insulin as possible. But after some months, I ended up taking as much as I could, always keeping in mind the maximum permitted doseage. It isn't rocket science – frankly it's pretty straightforward.'

Although he no longer takes part in competitive rowing, Sir Steve remains a strong and positive role model with a high profile as an inspirational speaker and campaigner. He is also an honorary Vice President of Diabetes UK. He explains how coping with diabetes is as much about controlling your lifestyle as it is about health. 'As an athlete you have to be tremendously disciplined, and I test six or seven times a day. I'll help spread the message on a national and international basis, stressing that regular testing is vital for people with the condition. This is an area where I can use my status as a sportsman to project a positive message and get people to think about the issues associated with testing.'

Sue Townsend

The creator of Adrian Mole has written her way from rags to riches, thanks to her acute powers of social observation, her gift for storytelling and her ready wit. She has written 14 novels, which have sold tens of millions of copies and been translated into 42 languages, as well as eight plays and four screenplays.

For her work Sue has received two Honorary Doctorates, one from the University of Leicester and one from Loughborough University in July 2007, along with the James Joyce Award of the Literary and Historical Society of University College Dublin.

Sue was diagnosed with Type 2 diabetes in the mid 1980s, when she was 38 years old. She admits she was 'cavalier' about looking after her health, and in an interview with *The Scotsman* in November 2006 she said: 'I used to keep my blood sugar deliberately high so that when I was working in the rehearsal room, say, on one of my plays, I didn't disturb anyone at quiet moments by unwrapping a Mars bar if I felt I was about to slip into a coma.' One has the impression of a life of creativity, colour and not a little chaos: 'And I was always in a hurry, leaping on to trains as they moved out of the station, running, running everywhere, forever rushing around from one place to another, and that made it difficult to stick to the diabetic routine.'

Sue has suffered considerably from complications of her diabetes. She has been registered blind for some years – although she can see a little with help. The creativity, colour and chaos haven't gone though. She dictates her work now to her husband Colin, and her youngest daughter helps her maintain a zany dress sense, with raffish pirate patches to shield her weaker eye. One of her much quoted sayings is 'Live with all of your senses.' She does that.

There are many other successful people in the world who live with Type 2 diabetes. They include sportsmen and women, actors, writers, professors, captains of industry and health professionals. All of them how you can live with diabetes successfully with courage and motivation.

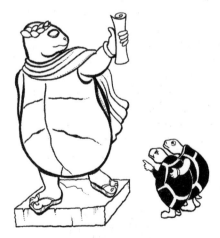

Glossary

Terms in *italics* in these definitions refer to other terms in the glossary.

acarbose A drug that slows the digestion and absorption of complex carbohydrates.

Acesulfame-K A low-calorie intense sweetener.

acetone One of the chemicals called *ketones* formed when the body uses up fat for energy. The presence of acetone in the urine usually means that more insulin is needed.

adrenaline A hormone produced by the adrenal glands, which prepares the body for action (the 'flight or fight' reaction) and also increases the level of blood glucose. Produced by the body in response to many stimuli, including a low blood glucose.

AGE Abbreviation for advanced glycation end products, the name given to glucose bound to fat which causes damage to certain cells in the body.

albumin A protein present in most animal tissues. The presence of albumin in the urine may denote kidney damage or be simply due to a urinary infection.

alpha cell The cell that produces *glucagon* – found in the *islets of Langerhans* in the *pancreas*.

alpha-glucosidase inhibitor A tablet that slows the digestion of carbohydrates in the intestine (acarbose).

analogue insulin Insulin that has the molecular structure changed to alter its action.

angiography A special type of X-ray where dye is injected into an artery to detect narrowing.

angioplasty A technique which uses an inflatable balloon to widen narrowed arteries.

antigens Proteins, which the body recognizes as 'foreign' and which trigger an immune response.

arteriosclerosis or **arterial sclerosis** or **arterial disease** Hardening of the arteries. Loss of elasticity in the walls of the arteries from thickening and calcification. Occurs with advancing years in those with or without diabetes. May affect the heart (causing thrombosis), the brain (a stroke) or the circulation to the legs and feet.

aspartame A low-calorie intense sweetener. Brand name NutraSweet.

autonomic neuropathy Damage to the system of nerves that regulate many automatic functions of the body such as stomach emptying, sexual function (potency) and blood pressure control.

bacteria A type of germ.

balanitis Inflammation of the end of the penis, usually caused by yeast infections as a result of sugar in the urine.

beta-blockers Drugs that block the effect of stress hormones on the cardiovascular system. Often used to treat angina and to lower blood pressure. May change the warning signs of *hypoglycaemia*.

beta cell The cell that produces insulin – found in the *islets of Langerhans* in the *pancreas*.

biguanides A group of anti-diabetes tablets that lower blood glucose levels. Their mode of action is not well understood, but they work in part by increasing the body's sensivity to insulin. Metformin is the only preparation in this group.

blood glucose monitoring System of measuring blood glucose levels at home using a portable meter and reagent sticks.

bran Indigestible husk of the wheat grain. A type of *dietary fibre*.

brittle diabetes Refers to diabetes that is very unstable with swings from very low to very high blood glucose levels and often involves frequent admissions to hospital.

calories Units in which energy or heat are measured. The energy value of food is measured in calories.

carbohydrates A class of food that comprises starches and sugars and is most readily available to the body for energy. Found mainly in plant foods. Examples are rice, bread, potatoes, pasta, beans.

cataract Opacity of the lens of the eye, which obscures vision. It may be removed surgically.

Charcot foot Swelling of the foot, sometimes leading to deformity, as a result of lack of sensation (neuropathy).

clear insulin This term used to refer to short-acting insulins. However, the two long-acting *analogue insulins* (Lantus and Levemir) are also clear so the term must be used with caution.

cloudy insulin Longer-acting insulin with fine particles of insulin bound to protamine or zinc.

coma A form of unconsciousness from which people can only be roused with difficulty. If caused by diabetes, may be a *diabetic coma* or an *insulin coma*.

complications Long-term consequences of imperfectly controlled diabetes. For details, see Chapters 30, 31 and 32.

control Usually refers to blood glucose control. The aim of good control is to achieve normal blood glucose levels (4–10 mmol/L) and *HbA$_{1c}$* less than 7%.

coronary heart disease Disease of the blood vessels supplying the heart.

cystitis Inflammation of the bladder, which usually causes frequent passing of urine, accompanied by a burning pain.

DESMOND Diabetes Education and Self Management for Ongoing and Newly Diagnosed. An education programme for people with Type 2 diabetes.

detemir A new insulin analogue designed to last for 24 hours and act as basal insulin. Also called Levemir.

diabetes insipidus A disorder of the pituitary gland accompanied by excessive urination and thirst. Nothing to do with *diabetes mellitus*.

diabetes mellitus A disorder of the *pancreas* characterized by a high blood glucose level. This book is about diabetes mellitus.

diabetic amyotrophy Rare condition causing pain in and/or weakness of the legs from the damage to certain nerves.

diabetic coma Extreme form of *hyperglycaemia*, usually with *ketoacidosis*, causing unconsciousness.

diabetic diarrhoea A form of diabetic *autonomic neuropathy* leading to diarrhoea.

diabetic foods Food products targeted at people with diabetes, in which ordinary sugar (*sucrose*) is replaced with substitutes such as *fructose* or *sorbitol*. These foods are not recommended as part of your food plan.

diabetic nephropathy Type of kidney damage that may occur in diabetes. See Chapter 31.

diabetic neuropathy Type of nerve damage that may occur in diabetes. See Chapters 31 and 32.

diabetic retinopathy Type of eye disease that may occur in diabetes. See Chapter 31.

dietary fibre Part of the plant material that resists digestion and gives bulk to the diet. Also called fibre or roughage.

diuretics Agents that increase the flow of urine, commonly known as water tablets.

DPP-4 inhibitors. New generation of agents to treat Type 2 diabetes. DPP-4 inhibitors (gliptins) can be taken in tablet form and work by slowing the breakdown of *GLP-1* (see below). Sitagliptin is now available and may be joined soon by vildagliptin.

erectile dysfunction Inability to achieve or maintain an erection (impotence).

fibre Another name for *dietary fibre*.

fructosamine Measurement of diabetes *control* that reflects the average blood glucose level over the previous 2–3 weeks. Similar to *haemoglobin A$_{1c}$* which averages the blood glucose over the longer period of 2–3 months.

fructose Type of sugar found naturally in fruit and honey. Since it does not require insulin for its *metabolism*, it is often used as a sweetener in *diabetic foods*.

gangrene Death of a part of the body due to a very poor blood supply. A combination of *neuropathy* and *arteriosclerosis* may result in infection of unrecognized injuries to the feet. If neglected, this infection may spread, causing further destruction.

gastroparesis Delayed emptying of the stomach as a result of *autonomic neuropathy*. Can lead to erratic food absorption and vomiting.

gestational diabetes Diabetes which is diagnosed during pregnancy.

glargine A new insulin analogue designed to last for 24 hours to act as basal (background) insulin. Also called Lantus.

glaucoma Disease of the eye causing increased pressure inside the eyeball.

glitazones A group of drugs that reduce insulin resistance – see *thiazolidinedione*.

GLP-1 Glucagon-like peptide-1 – a hormone which increases the production of insulin in response to food and reduces the production of glucagon. Two GLP-1 agents (exenatide and liraglutide) are soon to arrive in the UK.

glucagon A *hormone* produced by the *alpha cells* in the *pancreas* which causes a rise in blood glucose by freeing *glycogen* from the liver. Available in injection form for use in treating a severe *hypo*.

glucose Form of sugar made by digestion of *carbohydrates*. Absorbed into the bloodstream where it circulates and is used as a source of energy.

glucose tolerance test Test used in the diagnosis of *diabetes mellitus*. The *glucose* in the blood is measured at intervals before and after the person has drunk a large amount of glucose while fasting.

glycaemic index (GI) A way of describing how a *carbohydrate*-containing food affects blood *glucose* levels.

glycogen The form in which *carbohydrate* is stored in the liver and muscles. It is often known as animal starch.

glycosuria Presence of *glucose* in the urine.

glycosylated haemoglobin Another name for *haemoglobin A$_{1c}$*.

haemoglobin A$_{1c}$ The part of the haemoglobin or colouring matter of the red blood cell which has *glucose* attached to it. A test of diabetes *control*. The amount of haemoglobin A$_{1c}$ in the blood depends on the average blood glucose level over the previous 2–3 months.

HbA$_{1c}$ See *haemoglobin A$_{1c}$*.

hormone Substance generated in one gland or organ which is carried by the blood to another part of the body to control another organ. *Insulin* and *glucagon* are both hormones.

human insulin Insulin that has been manufactured to be identical to that produced in the human *pancreas*. Differs slightly from older insulins, which were extracted from cows or pigs.

hydramnios An excessive amount of amniotic fluid, i.e. the fluid surrounding the baby before birth.

hyperglycaemia High blood glucose (above 10 mmol/L).

hypo Abbreviation for *hypoglycaemia*.

hypoglycaemia (also known as a hypo or an insulin reaction) Low blood glucose (below 3.5 mmol/L).

impotence Failure of erection of the penis.

injector Device to aid injections.

Innolet A simple injector for insulin designed for people with poor vision or problems with their hands such as arthritis.

insulin A *hormone* produced by the *beta cells* of the *pancreas* and responsible for control of blood glucose. Insulin can only be given by injection because digestive juices destroy its action if it is taken by mouth.

insulin coma Extreme form of *hypoglycaemia* associated with unconsciousness and sometimes convulsions.

insulin-dependent diabetes (abbreviation IDD) Former name for *Type 1 diabetes*.

insulin pen Device that resembles a large fountain pen that takes a cartridge of *insulin*. The injection of insulin is given after dialling the dose and pressing a button that releases the insulin.

insulin reaction Another name for *hypoglycaemia* or a hypo. In America it is called an insulin shock.

insulin resistance A condition where the normal amount of insulin is not able to keep the blood glucose level down to normal. Seen particularly in patients with Type 2 diabetes. Such people need large doses of insulin to control their diabetes. The glitazone group of tablets is designed to reduce insulin resistance.

intermediate-acting insulin Insulin preparations with an action lasting 12–18 hours.

intradermal Meaning 'into the skin'. Usually refers to an injection given into the most superficial layer of the skin. *Insulin* must not be given in this way as it is painful and will not be absorbed properly.

intramuscular A deep injection into the muscle.

islets of Langerhans Specialized cells within the *pancreas* that produce *insulin* and *glucagon*.

isophane A form of *intermediate-acting insulin* that has protamine added to slow its absorption.

joule Unit of work or energy used in the metric system. There are about 4.18 joules in each calorie. Some dietitians calculate food energy in joules.

juvenile-onset diabetes Outdated name for *Type 1 diabetes*, so called because most patients receiving insulin develop diabetes under the age of 40. The term is no longer used because Type 1 diabetes can occur at any age, although it is more common in young people.

ketoacidosis A serious condition due to lack of insulin which results in body fat being used up to form *ketones* and acids. Characterized by high blood glucose levels, ketones in the urine, vomiting, drowsiness, heavy laboured breathing and a smell of *acetone* on the breath.

ketones Acid substances (including *acetone*) formed when body fat is used up to provide energy.

ketonuria The presence of *acetone* and other *ketones* in the urine. Detected by testing with a special testing stick (Ketostix, Ketur Test). Presence of ketones in the urine is due to lack of *insulin* or periods of starvation.

laser treatment Process in which laser beams are used to treat a damaged *retina* (back of the eye). Used in *photocoagulation*.

lente insulin A form of *intermediate-acting insulin* that has zinc added to slow its absorption.

lipoatrophy Loss of fat from injection sites. It used to occur before the use of highly purified insulins.

lipohypertrophy Fatty swelling usually caused by repeated injections of insulin into the same site.

maturity-onset diabetes Another term for *Type 2 diabetes*, most commonly occurring in people who are middle-aged and overweight.

metabolic rate Rate of oxygen consumption by the body; the rate at which you 'burn up' the food you eat.

metabolism Process by which the body turns food into energy.

metformin A *biguanide* tablet that works by reducing the release of *glucose* from the liver and increasing the uptake of glucose into the muscle.

microalbuminuria Small amounts of protein in the urine, not detectable by dipstick for albumin (*proteinuria*). Raised levels indicate early kidney damage.

microaneurysms Small red dots on the *retina* at the back of the eye which are one of the earliest signs of diabetic *retinopathy*. Represent areas of weakness of the very small blood vessels in the eye. Microaneurysms do not affect the eyesight in any way.

micromole One thousandth (1/1000) of a millimole.

millimole Unit for measuring the concentration of glucose and other substances in the blood. Blood glucose is measured in millimoles per litre (mmol/L). It has replaced milligrammes per decilitre (mg/dl or mg%) as a unit of measurement, although this is still used in some other countries. 1 mmol/L = 18 mg/dl.

MODY Maturity-onset diabetes of the young: a form of Type 2 diabetes that affects young people and runs in families. See Chapter 22.

nateglinide A prandial glucose regulator.

nephropathy Kidney damage. In the first instance, this makes the kidney more leaky so that *albumin* appears in the urine. At a later stage, it may affect the function of the kidney, and in severe cases, it leads to kidney failure.

neuropathy Damage to the nerves, which may be *peripheral neuropathy* or *autonomic neuropathy*. It can occur with diabetes especially when poorly controlled, but also has other causes.

NICE National Institute for Health and Clinical Excellence. An independent organization to provide national guidance to promote good health. It provides guidelines for the use of new and existing drugs in the NHS.

non-insulin dependent diabetes (abbreviation NIDD) Former name for *Type 2 diabetes*.

orlistat A tablet that blocks the digestion of fat. Brand name Xenical. Used to help people lose weight, which in turn may improve control of diabetes.

pancreas Gland lying behind the stomach, which as well as secreting a digestive fluid (pancreatic juice) also produces the *hormones insulin* and *glucagon*. Contains the *islets of Langerhans*.

peripheral neuropathy Damage to the nerves supplying the muscles and skin. This can result in diminished sensation, particularly in the feet and legs, and in muscle weakness. May also cause pain in the feet or legs.

phimosis Inflammation and narrowing of the foreskin of the penis.

photocoagulation Process of treating diabetic *retinopathy* with light beams, either laser beams or a xenon arc. This technique focuses a beam of light on a very tiny area of the *retina*. This beam is so intense that it causes a very small burn, which may close off a leaking blood vessel or destroy weak blood vessels that are at risk of bleeding.

pioglitazone A glitazone tablet that targets insulin resistance. Trade name Actos.

PKC inhibitors (protein kinase C inhibitors). Developed to try and reverse the changes in small blood vessels which cause diabetic eye disease (*retinopathy*). Though they seem to help in isolated cases, the overall results have been disappointing.

polydipsia Being excessively thirsty and drinking too much. It is a symptom of untreated diabetes.

polyuria The passing of large quantities of urine due to excess *glucose* in the bloodstream. It is a symptom of untreated diabetes.

pork insulin Insulin extracted from the *pancreas* of pigs.

prandial glucose regulators Tablets taken before meals that stimulate the release of *insulin* from the *pancreas* (repaglinide and nateglinide). Only used in *Type 2 diabetes*.

pre-eclampsia A condition which occurs towards the end of pregnancy and leads to high blood pressure, protein in the urine and, in severe cases, convulsions. Pre-eclampsia normally resolves soon after delivery.

protein One of the classes of food that is necessary for the growth and repair of tissues. Found in fish, meat, eggs, milk and pulses. Can also refer to *albumin* when found in the urine.

proteinuria *Protein* or *albumin* in the urine.

pruritus vulvae Irritation of the vulva (the genital area in women). Caused by an infection that occurs because of an excess of sugar in the urine and is often an early sign of diabetes in the older person. It clears up when the blood glucose levels return to normal and the sugar disappears from the urine.

pyelonephritis Inflammation and infection of the kidney.

renal threshold The level of *glucose* in the blood above which it will begin to spill into the urine. The usual renal threshold for glucose in the blood is about 10 mmol/L; i.e. when the blood glucose rises above 10 mmol/L, glucose appears in the urine.

repaglinide A *prandial glucose regulator*.

retina Light-sensitive coat at the back of the eye.

retinal screening Photograph of the *retina* to identify changes due to diabetes at a stage at which they can be treated to prevent loss of vision. Usually carried out once a year.

retinopathy Damage to the *retina*.

rimonabant New drug designed to help obese patients by reducing appetite. May also help people give up smoking, though it is not licensed for this. It is not yet available in the NHS and is being evaluated by *NICE*. Also named Acomplia.

rosiglitazone A glitazone tablet that targets *insulin resistance*. Trade names Avandia and Avandamet (in combination with metformin).

roughage Another name for *dietary fibre*.

saccharin A synthetic sweetener that is *calorie* free.

short-acting insulin Insulin preparations with an action lasting 6–8 hours.

sitaglitpin (Januvia) A DPP-4 inhibitor tablet that increases levels of GLP-1, now available in the US and Europe.

Snellen chart Chart showing rows of letters in decreasing sizes. Used for measuring *visual acuity*.

sorbitol A chemical related to sugar and alcohol that is used as a sweetening agent in foods as a substitute for ordinary sugar. It has no significant effect upon the blood *glucose* level but has the same number of *calories* as ordinary sugar so should not be used by those who need to lose weight. Poorly absorbed and may have a laxative effect.

steroids *Hormones* produced by the adrenal glands, testes and ovaries. Also available in synthetic form. Tend to increase the blood *glucose* level and make diabetes worse.

subcutaneous injection An injection beneath the skin into the layer of fat that lies between the skin and muscle. The normal way of giving *insulin*.

sucrose A sugar (containing *glucose* and *fructose* in combination) derived from sugar cane or sugar beet (i.e. ordinary table sugar). It is a pure *carbohydrate*.

sulphonylureas Anti-diabetes tablets that lower the blood *glucose* by stimulating the *pancreas* to produce more insulin. Commonly used sulphonylureas are gliclazide and glibenclamide.

thiazolidenedione Generic name for the group of tablets that target *insulin resistance* and improve diabetes in *Type 2 diabetes*. Pharmaceutical names are rosiglitazone and pioglitazone, brand names are Avandia and Actos.

thrombosis Clot forming in a blood vessel.

tissue markers *Proteins* on the outside of cells in the body that are genetically determined.

toxaemia Poisoning of the blood by the absorption of toxins. Usually refers to the toxaemia of pregnancy, which is characterized by high blood pressure, *proteinuria* and ankle swelling.

Type 1 diabetes Name for insulin-dependent diabetes which cannot be treated by diet and tablets alone. Outdated name is juvenile-onset diabetes. Age of onset is usually below the age of 40 years.

Type 2 diabetes Name for non-insulin-dependent diabetes. Age of onset is usually above the age of 40 years, often in people who are overweight, which contributes to insulin resistance. These people do not need insulin treatment immediately and can usually be successfully controlled with diet alone or diet and tablets for a period of time. Formerly known as maturity-onset diabetes.

U-40 insulin The old weaker strength of *insulin*, no longer available in the UK. It is still available in Eastern Europe and in some countries in the Far East, such as Vietnam and Indonesia.

U-100 insulin The standard strength of *insulin* in the UK, USA, Canada, Australia, New Zealand, South Africa, the Middle East and the Far East.

U-500 insulin A stronger strength of insulin used for patients who are particularly insulin resistant.

urine testing The detection of abnormal amounts of *glucose*, *ketones*, *protein* or blood in the urine, usually by means of urine testing sticks.

vildagliptin (trade name Galvus) A DPP-4 inhibitor tablet, that is likely to be vailable soon.

virus A very small organism capable of causing disease.

viscous fibre A type of *dietary fibre* found in pulses (peas, beans and lentils) and some fruit and vegetables.

visual acuity Acuteness of vision. Measured by reading letters on a sight testing chart (a *Snellen chart*).

water tablets The common name for *diuretics*.

Xenical The brand name for *orlistat*.

References and additional reading

2 Getting to grips with diabetes

Fox, C. and Kilvert, A. *Type 2 Diabetes: Answers at your fingertips.* London: Class Publishing, 2007

Rodgers, J. and Walker, R. *Type 2 Diabetes: Answers at your fingertips.* London: Dorling Kindersley, 2006

3 Caring for your own diabetes

Department of Health: *National Service Framework for Diabetes: Standards.* London: DH, 2001

Department of Health: *National Service Framework for Diabetes: Delivery Strategy.* London: DH, 2002

Fox, C. and Kilvert, A. *Type 2 Diabetes: Answers at your fingertips.* London: Class Publishing, 2007

4 Diabetes: some background

Bonora, E., Kiechl, S., Willeit, J. *et al.* Population-based incidence rates and risk factors for type 2 diabetes in white individuals. The Bruneck Study. *Diabetes,* 53 (July): 1782–9, 2004

Botazzo, G.F. On the honey disease. *Diabetes,* 42: 778–800, 1993

Ettisham, S., Barrett, T.G. and Shaw, N.J. Type 2 diabetes in children: an emerging problem. *Diabetic Medicine,* 17: 867–71, 2000

Rosenbloom, A.L. The cause of the epidemic of Type 2 diabetes in children. *Current Opinion in Endocrinology and Diabetes,* 7: 191–6, 2000

Willi, S.M. Type 2 diabetes mellitus in adolescents. *Current Opinion in Endocrinology and Diabetes,* 7: 71–6, 2000

5 How your body works

Amiel, S. and Gale, E. Physiological responses to hypoglycaemia: counterregulation and cognitive function. *Diabetes Care,* 16 (suppl 3): 48–55, 1993

Escalante, D., Davidson, J. and Garber, A. Maximizing glycemic control. How to achieve normal glycemia while minimizing hyperinsulinemia in insulin-requiring patients

with diabetes mellitus. *Clinical Diabetes,* Jan/Feb: 3–6, 1993

Malherbe, C., de Gasparo, M., de Hertogh, R. and Hoet, J. Circadian variations of blood sugar and plasma insulin. *Diabetologia,* 5: 397–404, 1969

6 Regulation of blood glucose

Franz, M.J., Bantle, J.P., Beebe, C.A. *et al.* Evidence-based nutrition principles and recommendations for the treatment and prevention of diabetes and related complications. *Diabetes Care,* 25: 148–98, 2002

Johnston, D.G. and Alberti, K.G.M.M. Hormonal control of ketone body metabolism in the normal and diabetic state. *Clinics in Endocrine Medicine,* 11: 329–61, 1982

Hirsch, I.B. and Polonsky, W.H. Hypoglycemia and its prevention. In Fredrickson, I. (ed.) *The Insulin Pump Therapy Book.* Los Angeles: MiniMed, 1995

McIntosh, A., Hutchinson, A., Home, P.D. *et al.* Clinical guidelines and evidence review for Type 2 diabetes: management of blood glucose. Sheffield: ScHARR, University of Sheffield, 2001. Available at www.nice.org.uk/pdf/NICE_full_blood_glucose.pdf

Nathan, D.M., Buse, J.B., Davidson, M.B. *et al.* Management of hyperglycaemia in Type 2 diabetes: a consensus algorithm for the initiation and adjustment of therapy: a consensus statement from the American Diabetes Association and the European Association for the Study of Diabetes. *Diabetologia,* 49: 1711–21, 2006

7 High blood glucose levels

Chang, F.Y., Shaio, M.F. Decreased cell-mediated immunity in patients with non-insulin-dependent diabetes mellitus. *Diabetes Research in Clinical Practice,* 28 (2): 137–46, 1995

Draelos, M.T., Jacobson, A.M., Weinger, K. *et al.* Cognitive function in patients with insulin-dependent diabetes mellitus during hyperglycaemia and hypoglycaemia. *American Journal of Medicine,* 98: 135–44, 1995

International Diabetes Federation (2005) *Global Guideline for Type 2 Diabetes*, especially Section 06, Glucose control levels. Available at www.idf.org

Manley, S.M., Meyer, L.C., Neil, H.A.W. *et al.* Complications in newly diagnosed Type 2 diabetic patients and their association with different clinical and biochemical risk factors. UKPDS 6. *Diabetes Research,* 13: 1–11, 1990

Robins, M. Short-term complications of diabetes. In Dunning, T. (ed.) *Nursing Care of Older People with Diabetes.* Oxford: Blackwell, 2005

8 Nutrition

Anderssen, H., Asp, N.G. and Hallmans, G. Diet and diabetes. *Scandinavian Journal of Nutrition,* 30: 78–90, 1986

Bowling, S. *The Everyday Diabetic Cookbook.* London: Grub Street Publishing, 1993.

Department of Health (last modified, 2007) Five a day. Available at www.dh.gov.uk/policyandguidance/healthandsocialcaretopics/FiveADay/

Foster-Powell, K., Holt, S.H. and Brand-Miller, J.C. International table of glycemic index and glycemic load values. *American Journal of Clinical Nutrition,* 76: 5–56, 2002

Govindji, A. *The Good Housekeeping Diabetic Cookbook.* London: Collins & Brown, 2005.

Holzmeister, L.A. *The Diabetes Carbohydrate and Fat Gram Guide.* Alexandria, Virgina: American Diabetes Association, 2000

Jenkins, D.J., Kendall, C.W., Marchie, A. *et al.* Type 2 diabetes and the vegetarian diet. *American Journal of Clinical Nutrition,* 78 (suppl): 610S–16S, 2003.

Truby, H., Baic, S., de Looy, A. *et al.* Randomised controlled trial of four commercial weight loss programmes in the UK: initial findings from the BBC "diet trials". *British Medical Journal,* 332: 13091–314, 2006

Waldron, S. Childhood diabetes: current dietary managment. *Current Pediatrics,* 3: 138–41, 1993

9 Weight control

Brinkworth, G.D., Noakes, M., Keogh, J.B. *et al.* Long-term effects of a high-protein, low-carbohydrate diet on weight control and cardiovascular risk markers in obese hyperinsulinemic subjects. *International Journal of Obesity,* 28: 661–70, 2004

Dietitians Working in Obesity Managment UK. *Position Statement on Meal Replacement Approaches in the Management of Overweight and Obesity.* Essex: British Dietetic Association, 2005

Dujovne, C.A., Zavoral, J.H., Rowe, E. and Mendel, C.M. (Sibutramine Study Group). Effects of sibutramine on body weight and serum lipids: a double-blind, randomized, placebo-controlled study in 322 overweight and obese patients with dyslipidemia. *American Heart Journal,* 142 (3): 489–97, 2001. Summary for patients in *Current Atherosclerosis Reports,* 4 (1): 51, 2002

Heymsfield, S.B., van Mierlo C.A.J., van der Knaap, H.C.M., Heo, M. and Frier, H.I. Weight management using a meal replacement strategy: meta and pooling analysis from six studies. *International Journal of Obesity,* 27 (5): 536–49, 2003

Hsieh, C., Wang, P., Liu, R. *et al.* Orlistat for obesity: benefits beyond weight loss. *Diabetes Research and Clinical Practice,* 67 (1): 78S–83S, 2003

Jarvi, A.E., Karlstrom, B.E., Granfelt, Y.E. *et al.* Improved glycemic control and lipid profile and normalized fibrinolytic activity on a low–glycemic index diet in Type 2 diabetic patients. *Diabetes Care,* 22: 10–18, 1999

Roberts, M. Obesity and diabetes. *Nutrition Review,* March 2004

10 Exercise

American Diabetes Association. Physical Activity/Exercise and Type 2 Diabetes: a consensus statement. *Diabetes Care,* 29 (6): 1433–38, 2006

Boulé, N.G., Haddad, E., Kenny, G.P., Wells, G.A. and Sigal, R.J. Effects of exercise on glycemic control and body mass in Type 2 diabetes mellitus: a meta-analysis of controlled clinical trials. *Journal of the American Medical Association,* 268 (15): 1218–27, 2001

Cicerone, K.D., Dahlberg, C., Malec, J.F. *et al.* Evidence-based cognitive rehabilitation: updated review of the literature from 1998 through 2002. *Archives of Physical Medicine and Rehabilitation,* 86 (8): 1681–92, 2005

Diabetes Prevention Program Research Group. Reduction in the incidence of Type 2 diabetes with lifestyle intervention or metformin. *New England Journal of Medicine,* 346: 393–403, 2002

Hu, F.B., Sigal, R.J., Rich-Edwards, J.W. *et al.*

Walking compared with vigorous physical activity and risk of Type 2 diabetes in women. *Journal of the American Medical Association*, 282 (15): 1433–39, 2006

Thomas, D.E., Elliott, E.J. and Naughton, G.A. Exercise for Type 2 diabetes mellitus. *Cochrane Database of Systematic Reviews*, 1, 2007

11 Monitoring

Ellison, J.M., Stegmann, J.M., Colner, S.L. *et al.* Rapid changes in post-prandial blood glucose produce concentration differences at finger, forearm, and thigh sampling sites. *Diabetes Care*, 25: 961–4, 2002

Farmer, A., Wade, A., Goyder, E. *et al.* Impact of self monitoring of blood glucose in the management of patients with non-insulin treated diabetes: open parallel group randomised trial. *British Medical Journal*, 335: 132, 2007

Fogh-Andersen, N. and D'Orazio, P. Proposals for standardizing direct reading biosensors for blood glucose. *Clinical Chemistry*, 44: 655–9, 1998

Franciosis, M., Pellegrini, F., De Berardis, G. *et al.* Self-monitoring of blood glucose in non-insulin-treated diabetic patients: a longitudinal evaluation of its impact on metabolic control. *Diabetic Medicine*, 22: 900–6, 2005

International Diabetes Federation (2005) Global Guideline for Type 2 Diabetes, Section 08, Self-monitoring. Available at www.idf.org

Jungheim, K. and Koschinsky, T. Glucose monitoring at the arm: risky delays of hypoglycemia and hyperglycemia detection. *Diabetes Care*, 25: 956–60, 2002

Reynolds, R.M. and Strachan, M.W. Home blood glucose monitoring in Type 2 diabetes. *British Medical Journal*, 329: 754–5, 2004

Welschen, L.M., Bloemendal, E. Nijpels, G. *et al.* Self-monitoring of blood glucose in patients with Type 2 diabetes who are not using insulin: a systematic review. *Diabetes Care*, 28: 1510–17, 2005

12 Glycosylated haemoglobin (HbA$_{1c}$)

American Diabetes Association. Tests of glycemia in diabetes: clinical practice recommendations 2003. *Diabetes Care*, 26 (Suppl 1): S106–8, 2003

DCCT Research Group. The relationship of glycemic exposure (HbA$_{1c}$) to the risk of development and progression of retinopathy in the Diabetes Control and Complications Trial. *Diabetes*, 44: 968–83, 1995

Little, R.R. and Goldstein, D.E. Measurements of glycated haemoglobin and other circulating glycated proteins. In de Greyter, W. (ed.) *Research Methodologies in Human Diabetes.* Berlins, 1994

Reichard, P. Are there any glycemic thresholds for the serious microvascular diabetic complications? *Journal of Diabetes Complications*, 9: 25–30, 1995

Rohlfing, C.L., Wiedmeyer, H-M.,Little, R.R., England, J.D., Tennill, A. and Goldstein, D.E. Defining the relationship between plasma glucose and HbA$_{1c}$. *Diabetes Care*, 25: 275–8, 2002

Tahara, Y. and Shima, K. Kinetics of HbA$_{1c}$, glycated albumin and fructosamine and analysis of their weight functions against preceding plasma glucose levels. *Diabetes Care*, 18: 440–47, 1995

13 Tablets for lowering blood sugar

American Diabetes Association (ADA) Abstracts for vildagliptin, sitagliptin, exanetide, 2007. Available at www.ada.org

Bailey, C.J. and Feher, M.D. *Therapies for Diabetes, Including Oral Agents and Insulins*. Birmingham: Sherborne Gibbs, 2005

Calabrese, A.T., Coley, K.C., Swanson, D. and Rao, R.H. Risk of lactic acidosis with metformin therapy. *Archives of Internal Medicine*, 162: 434–7, 2002

European Association for the Study of Diabetes. Abstracted presentations for sitagliptin, 2007. Available at www.easd.org

Summary of product characteristics for rosiglitazone, pioglitazone, sitagliptin, metformin, acarbose, exenatide and sulphonylureas. Available at emc.medicines.org.uk

Turner, H. and Wass, J.A.H. *Oxford Handbook of Endocrinology and Diabetes*. Oxford: Oxford University Press, 2002

14 Insulin treatment

Hordern, S.V., Wright, J.E., Umpleby, A.M., Shojaee-Moradie, F., Amiss, J. and Russell-Jones, D.L. Comparison of the effects on glucose and lipid metabolism of equipotent doses of insulin detemir and NPH insulin with a 16-h euglycaemic clamp. *Diabetologia*, 48: 420–6, 2005

International Diabetes Federation (2005) *Global Guideline for Type 2 Diabetes*, Section 10, Glucose control: insulin therapy. Available at www.idf.org

Larger, E. Weight gain and insulin treatment. Diabetes Metabolism, 31: 4S51–4S56, 2005

National Institute for Health and Clinical Excellence. *Guidance on the Use of Long-acting Insulin Analogues for the Treatment of Diabetes: Insulin Glargine.* NICE Technology Appraisal Guidance No. 53. London: NICE, 2005

Plank, J., Bodenlenz, M., Sinner, F. *et al.* A double-blind, randomized, doseresponse study investigating the pharmacodynamic and pharmacokinetic properties of the long-acting insulin analog detemir. *Diabetes Care*, 28: 1107–12, 2005

Raskin, P., Allen. E., Hollander, P. *et al.* Initiating insulin therapy in Type 2 diabetes: a comparison of biphasic and basal insulin analogues. *Diabetes Care*, 28: 260–65, 2005

Raskin, P., Bode, B.W., Marks, J.B. *et al.* Continuous subcutaneous insulin therapy and multiple daily injection therapy are equally effective in Type 2 diabetes. *Diabetes Care*, 26: 2598–603, 2003

Siebenhofer, A., Plank, J., Berghold, A. *et al.* Short-acting insulin analogues versus regular human insulin in patients with diabetes mellitus. *Cochrane Database of Systematic Reviews*, 4, CD003287.pub3, 2004

15 Administering insulin

Frid, A. and Linde, B. Intraregional differences in the absorption of unmodified insulin from the abdominal wall. *Diabetic Medicine*, 9: 236–9, 1992

Herman, W.H., Ilag, L.L., Johnson, S.L. *et al.* A clinical trial of continuous subcutaneous insulin infusion versus multiple daily injections in older adults with Type 2 diabetes. *Diabetes Care*, 28: 1568–1573, 2005

Thow, J. and Home, P. Insulin injection technique. *British Medical Journal*, 301: 3–4, 1990

Wittlin, S. Treating the spectrum of Type 2 diabetes: emphasis on insulin pump therapy. *Diabetes Education*, 32(1 suppl): 39S–46S, 2006

16 Changing insulin requirements

Douek, I.F., Allen, S.E., Ewings, P. *et al.* Continuing metformin when starting insulin in patients with

Type 2 diabetes: a double-blind randomized placebo-controlled trial. *Diabetic Medicine*, 22 (5): 634–40, 2005

International Diabetes Federation (2005) *Global Guideline for Type 2 Diabetes*, especially Section 09, Glucose control: oral therapy, and Section 10, Glucose control: insulin therapy. Available at www.idf.org

Royal College of Physicians/British Diabetic Association. *Good Practice in the Diagnosis and Treatment of NIDDM.* London: RCP/BDA, 1993

Turner, R.C., Cull, C.A., Frighi, V. and Holman, R.R. (1999) Glycaemic control with diet, sulphonylurea, metformin and insulin therapy in patients with Type 2 diabetes: progressive requirement for multiple therapies. *Journal of the American Medical Association*, 281: 2005–12, 1999

17 Side effects and problems with insulin treatment

Chawdhury, T.A. and Escudier, V. Poor glycaemic control caused by insulin induced lipohypertrophy. *British Medical Journal,* 327: 383–4, 2003

Donnelly, L.A., Morris, A.D., Frier, B.M. *et al.* Frequency and predictors of hypoglycaemia in Type 1 and insulin-treated Type 2 diabetes: a population-based study *Diabetic Medicine*, 22, 749–55, 2005

Rosenstock, J., Dailey, G., Massi-Benedetti, M. *et al.* Reduced hypoglycemia risk with insulin glargine. A meta-analysis comparing insulin glargine with human NPH insulin in Type 2 diabetes. *Diabetes Care,* 28: 950–55, 2005

18 Hypoglycaemia

Amiel, S.A. Cognitive function testing in studies of acute hypoglycaemia: rights and wrongs? *Diabetologia*, 41: 713–19, 1998

Amiel, S.A. and Gale, E. Physiological responses to hypoglycaemia: counterregulation and cognitive function. *Diabetes Care*, 16 (suppl 3): 48–55, 1993

Cerosimo, E., Garlick, P. and Ferretti, J. Renal glucose production during insulin-induced hypoglycemia in humans. *Diabetes*, 48: 261–6, 1999

Eckert, B., Riding, E. and Agardh, C.D. The cerebral vascular response to a rapid decrease in blood glucose to values above normal in poorly controlled (insulin-dependent) diabetes mellitus.

Diabetes Research in Clinical Practice, 27 (3): 221–7, 1995

Hirsch, I.B. and Polonsky, W.H. Hypoglycemia and its prevention. In Fredrickson. I. (ed.) *The Insulin Pump Therapy Book*. Los Angeles: MiniMed, 1995

19 Treating hypoglycaemia

Amiel, S.A., Pottinger, R.C., Archibald, H.R. and Chusney, G. Effect of antecedent glucose control on cerebral function during hypoglycaemia. *Diabetes Care*, 14: 109–18, 1991

Brodows, G., Williams, C. and Amatruda, J. Treatment of insulin reactions in diabetics. *Journal of the American Medical Association*, 24 (252): 3378–81, 1984

Cox, D.J., Gonder-Frederick, L., Polonsky, W., Schlunt, D., Julian, D. and Clarke, W. A multicenter evaluation of blood glucose awareness training, II. *Diabetes Care*, 18: 523–8, 1995

Cryer, P., Fisher, J. and Shamoon, H. Hypoglycemia. *Diabetes Care*, 17: 734–55, 1994

Eckert, B., Rosen, I., Stenberg, G. and Agardh, C.D. The recovery of brain function after hypoglycemia in normal man. *Diabetologia*, 35 (suppl 1): abstract 161, 1992

Felig, P. and Bergman, M. Integrated physiology of carbohydrate metabolism. In Rifkin, H. and Porter, D. (eds) *Diabetes Mellitus: Theory and Practice*. Oxford: Elsevier, 1990

King, P., Kong, M.F., Parkin, H., Macdonald, R.A. and Tattersall, R.B. wellbeing, cerebral function and physical fatigue after nocturnal hypoglycemia in IDDM. *Diabetes Care*, 21: 341–45, 1998

20 Stress

Inul, A., Kitaoka, H., Majima, M. *et al.* Effect of the Kobe earthquake on stress and glycemic control in patients with diabetes mellitus. *Archives of Internal Medicine*, 158: 274–8, 1998

Lustman, P.J., Anderson, R.J., Freedland, K.E. *et al.* Depression and poor glycemic control. A meta-analytic review of the literature. *Diabetes Care*, 23: 934–42, 2000

Mazze, R.S., Lucido, D. and Shamoon, H. Psychological and social correlates of glycemic control. *Diabetes Care*, 7: 360–66, 1984

Moberg, E., Kollind, M., Lins, P.E. and Adamsson, U. Acute mental stress impairs insulin sensitivity in IDDM patients. *Diabetologia*, 37: 247–51, 1994

Peyrot, M.F. and Pichert, J.W. Stress buffering and glycemic control. *Diabetes Care*, 7: 842–46, 1992

21 Coping with sickness

Fox, C. and Kilvert, A. Emergencies. In *Type 2 Diabetes: Answers at your fingertips*. London: Class Publishing, 2007

Silink, M. Sick day rules. In Baba, S. and Kaneko, T. (eds), *Diabetes*, Elsevier Science, 1995

Tenovuo, J., Alanen, P., Lajava, H, Vilkari, J. and Lehtonen, O.P. Oral health of patients with insulin dependent diabetes mellitus. *Scandinavian Journal of Dental Research*, 94: 33–46, 1986

Tesfaye, S., Cullen, D.R., Wilson, R.M. and Wooley, P.D. Diabetic ketoacidosis precipitated by genital herpes infection. *Diabetes Research and Clinical Practice*, 13: 83–4, 1991

22 Type 2 diabetes and younger people

Ettisham, S., Barrett, T.G. and Shaw, N.J. Type 2 diabetes in children: an emerging problem. *Diabetic Medicine*, 17: 867–71, 2000

Rosenbloom, A.L. The cause of the epidemic of Type 2 diabetes in children. *Current Opinion in Endocrinology and Diabetes*, 7: 191–6, 2000

Rosenbloom, A.L., Silverstein, J.H., Shin, A., Zeitler, P. and Klingensmith, G.J. Type 2 diabetes in the child and adolescent. *Pediatric Diabetes* 2008 (in press)

Velho, G. and Froguel, P. Genetic, metabolic and clinical aspects of maturity-onset diabetes in the young. *European Journal of Endocrinology*, 138: 233–9, 1998

Willi, S.M. Type 2 diabetes mellitus in adolescents. *Current Opinion in Endocrinology and Diabetes*, 7: 71–6, 2000

23 Smoking

Bupropion summary of product characteristics. Available at www.medicines.org.uk

Rimm, E.B., Chan, J., Stampfer, M.J., Colditz, G.A.and Willett, W.C. Prospective study of cigarette smoking, alcohol use, and the risk of diabetes in men. *British Medical Journal*, 310: 555–9, 1995

Woolacott, N.F., Jones, L., Forbes, C.A. *et al.* The clinical effectiveness and cost-effectiveness of

bupropion and nicotine replacement therapy for
smoking cessation: a systematic review and
economic evaluation. *Health Technology
Assessment*, 6 (16): 1–245, 2002

24 Alcohol and other substances

Advisory Council on the Misuse of Drugs. *Further
Consideration of the Classification of Cannabis
under the Misuse of Drugs Act 1971*. London:
Home Office, 2005

Brand-Miller, J.C., Fatima, K., Middlemiss, C. *et al.*
Effect of alcoholic beverages on post-prandial
glycemia and insulinemia in lean, young, healthy
adults. *American Journal of Clinical Nutrition*,
85 (6): 1545–51, 2007.

Johnson, K.H., Bazargan, M., and Cherpitel, C.J.
Alcohol, tobacco, and drug use and the onset of
Type 2 diabetes among inner-city minority
patients. *Journal of the American Board of
Family Medicine*, 14 (6): 430–36, 2001

Kolvisto, V.A., Haapa, E., Tulokas, S., Pelkonen, R.
and Tolvenen, M. Alcohol with a meal has no
adverse effect on post-prandial glucose
homeostasis in diabetic patients. *Diabetes Care*,
12 (16): 1612–14, 1993

Rimm, E.B., Chan, J., Stampfer, M.J., Colditz, G.A.
and Willett, W.C. Prospective study of cigarette
smoking, alcohol use, and the risk of diabetes in
men. *British Medical Journal*, 310: 555–9, 1995

25 Sexual issues

Berardis, G., Pellegrini, F., Franciosi, M. *et al.*
Longitudinal assessment of quality of life in
patients with Type 2 diabetes and self-reported
erectile dysfunction. *Diabetes Care*, 28: 2637–43,
2005

Currie, H. *Menopause: Answers at your fingertips*.
London, Class Publishing, 2006

Vinik, A. and Richardson, D. Erectile dysfunction.
In Sinclair, A.J. and Finucane, P. (eds) *Diabetes in
Old Age*, 2nd edn. Chichester: John Wiley, 2001

26 Pregnancy and diabetes

American College of Obstetricians and
Gynecologists. Practice Bulletin: Clinical
Management Guidelines for
Obstetrician-Gynecologists. Number 60, March
2005. Pregestational diabetes mellitus. *Obstetrics
and Gynecology*, 105 (3): 675–85, 2005

International Diabetes Federation (2005) *Global

Guideline for Type 2 Diabetes*, Section 17,
Pregnancy. Available at www.idf.org

Lauenborg, J., Hansen, T., Moller Jensen, D. *et al.*
Increasing incidence of diabetes after gestational
diabetes. *Diabetes Care*, 27: 1194–9, 2004

Linné, Y., Barkeling, B. and Rössner, S. Natural
course of gestational diabetes mellitus: long term
follow up of women in the SPAWN study. *British
Journal of Obstetrics and Gynaecology*, 109 (11):
1227–31, 2002

27 Social and employment issues

Department of Transport. *Think! Advice for older
drivers*. Available at www.thinkroadsafety.gov.uk/
advice

Diabetes UK. *Driving and diabetes: What you need
to know*. Available at www.diabetes.org.uk/
guide-to-diabetes/living_with_diabetes/everyday_life/

Fox, C. and Kilvert, A. Life with diabetes. In *Type 2
Diabetes: Answers at your fingertips*. London:
Class Publishing, 2007

28 Travelling with diabetes

Fit For Travel (NHS Scotland) Diabetes mellitus
and travel. Available at www.fitfortravel.scot.nhs.uk/
advice/travellers/diabetes.htm

Kassianos, G. Some aspects of diabetes and travel.
Diabetes Reviews International 2, 3: 11–13,
1992

Travel Medicine Handbook. Available on
www.travelmedicine.dk

29 Psychological aspects of Type 2 diabetes

Ali, S., Stone, M.A., Peters, J.L., Davies, M.J., and
Khunti, K. Prevalence of co-morbid depression in
adults with Type 2 diabetes: a systematic review
and meta-analysis. *Diabetic Medicine*, 23:
1165–73, 2006

Cembrowicz, S. and Kingham, D. *Beating
Depression: A Question and Answer Guide to
Symptoms, Causes and Treatment*, 2nd edn.
London: Class Publishing, 2006

Delahanty, L.M., Grant, R.W., Wittenberg, E. *et al.*
Association of diabetes-related emotional distress
with diabetes treatment in primary care patients
with Type 2 diabetes. *Diabetic Medicine*, 24:
48–54, 2007

Grigsby, A.B., Anderson, R.J., Freedland, K.E.,
Clouse, R.E. and Lustman, P.J. Prevalence of
anxiety in adults with diabetes: a systematic

review. *Journal of Psychosomatic Research,* 53: 1053–60, 2002

Hermanns, N., Kulzer, B., Krichbaum, M., Kubiak, T. and Haak, T. Affective and anxiety disorders in a German sample of diabetic patients: prevalence, comorbidity and risk factors. *Diabetic Medicine,* 22: 293–300, 2005

Ismail, K., Winkley, K. and Rabe-Hesketh, S. Systematic review and meta-analysis of randomised controlled trials of psychological interventions to improve glycaemic control in patients with Type 2 diabetes. *Lancet,* 363: 1589–97, 2004

Kenardy, J., Mensch, M., Bowen, K. *et al.* Disordered eating behaviours in women with Type 2 diabetes mellitus. *Eating Behaviours,* 2: 183–192, 2001

Mannucci, E., Tesi, F., Ricca, V. *et al.* Eating behavior in obese patients with and without Type 2 diabetes mellitus. *International Journal of Obesity,* 26: 848–53, 2002

Van Winkel, R., De Hert, M., Van Eyck, D. *et al.* Screening for diabetes and other metabolic abnormalities in patients with schizophrenia and schizoaffective disorder: evaluation of incidence and screening methods. *Journal of Clinical Psychiatry,* 67: 1493–1500, 2006

30 Complications of the cardiovascular system

Bonora, E., Kiechl, S., Willeit, J. *et al.* Population-based incidence rates and risk factors for Type 2 diabetes in white individuals. The Bruneck Study. *Diabetes,* 53 (July): 1782 –9, 2004

Selvin, E., Marinopoulos, S. Berkenblit, G. *et al.* Meta-analysis: glycosylated hemoglobin and cardiovascular disease in diabetes mellitus. *Annals of Internal Medicine,* 141: 421–31, 2004

United Kingdom Prospective Diabetes Study (UKPDS) Group. Intensive blood-glucose control with sulphonylureas or insulin compared with conventional treatment and risk of complications in patients with Type 2 diabetes (UKPDS 33). *Lancet,* 352: 837–53, 1998

United Kingdom Prospective Diabetes Study (UKPDS) Group. Tight blood pressure control and risk of macrovascular and microvascular complications in Type 2 diabetes (UKPDS 38). *British Medical Journal,* 317: 703–13, 1998

31 Microvascular complications

Ohkubo, Y., Kishikawa, H., Araki, E. *et al.* Intensive insulin therapy prevents the progression of diabetic microvascular complications in Japanese patients with non-insulin dependent diabetes mellitus: a randomized prospective 6-year study. *Diabetes Research and Clinical Practice,* 28: 103–17, 1995

Stein, A. and Wild, J. *Kidney Failure Explained,* 3rd edn. London: Class Publishing, 2007

Stratton, I.M., Adler, A.I., Neil, H.A. *et al.* Association of glycaemia with macrovascular and microvascular complications of Type 2 diabetes (UKPDS 35): a prospective observational study. *British Medical Journal,* 321: 405–12, 2000

Vinik, A.I., Maser, R.E., Mitchell, B.D. and Freeman, R. Diabetic autonomic neuropathy. *Diabetes Care,* 26: 1553–79, 2003

32 Problems with the feet

Campbell, L., Colagiuri, S., O'Rourke, S, Chen, M. and Colagiuri, R. *Evidence-based Guidelines for Type 2 Diabetes. Detection and Prevention of Foot Problems.* Canberra: Diabetes Australia and NHMRC, 2005

Frykberg, R. Diabetic foot ulcers, pathogenesis and management. *The American Family Physician,* 66 (9), 1: 1655–62, 2002

National Institute for Health and Clinical Excellence. *Type 2 Diabetes: Footcare.* London: NICE, 2004

Pitocco, D., Ruotolo, V., Caputo, S. *et al.* Six-month treatment with alendronate in acute Charcot neuroarthropathy. *Diabetes Care,* 28: 1214–15, 2005

Singh, N., Armstrong, D.G. and Lipsky, B.A. Preventing foot ulcers in patients with diabetes. *Journal of the American Medical Association,* 293: 217–28, 2005

33 Associated diseases

Ganda, O.P. Prevalence and incidence of secondary diabetes. In Harris, M.J., Cowie, C.C., Stern, M.P., Boyko, E.J., Reiber, G.E. and Bennett, P.H. (eds) *Diabetes in America,* 2nd edn. Available at diabetes.niddk.nih.gov/dm/pubs/america/pdf/chapter5.pdf

Sattar, N., Gaw, A., Scherbakova, O. *et al.* Metabolic syndrome with and without C-reactive protein as a predictor of coronary heart disease and diabetes in the West of Scotland Coronary Prevention Study. *Circulation*, 108: 414–19, 2003

34 Diabetes in later life

Colhoun, H.M., Betteridge, D.J., Durrington, P.N. *et al.* Primary prevention of cardiovascular disease with atorvastatin in Type 2 diabetes in the Collaborative Atorvastatin Diabetes Study (CARDS): multicentre randomised placebo-controlled trial. *Lancet,* 364: 685–96, 2004

Dunning, T. *Nursing Care of Older People with Diabetes.* Oxford: Blackwell, 2005

European Diabetes Working Party for Older People. Clinical Guidelines for management of Type 2 diabetes mellitus 2001–2004. Available at www.eugms.org

Hansson, L., Zanchetti, A., Carruthers, S.G. *et al.* Effects of intensive blood-pressure lowering and low-dose aspirin in patients with hypertension: principal results of the Hypertension Optimal Treatment (HOT). Collaborative overview of randomised trials of antiplatelet therapy, I, Prevention of death, myocardial infarction, and stroke by prolonged antiplatelet therapy in various categories of patients. Antiplatelet Trialists. Collaboration. *British Medical Journal,* 8: 308(6921): 81–106, 1994

Sinclair, A.J. and Finucane, P. *Diabetes in Old Age,* 2nd edn. Chichester: John Wiley, 2001

34 Support and information

Davies, M.J., Heller, S., Skinner, T.C. *et al.* Effectiveness of the diabetes education and self management for ongoing and newly diagnosed (DESMOND) programme for people with newly diagnosed Type 2 diabetes: cluster randomised controlled trial. *British Medical Journal,* 336 (7642): 491–5, 2008

36 Outcome studies in Type 2 diabetes

Colhoun, H.M., Betteridge, D.J., Durrington, P.N. *et al.* Primary prevention of cardiovascular disease with atorvastatin in Type 2 diabetes in the Collaborative Atorvastatin Diabetes Study (CARDS): multicentre randomised placebo-controlled trial. *Lancet* 2004; 364: 685–96, 2004

Collins, R., Armitage, J., Parish, S. *et al.* MRC/BHF Heart Protection Study of cholesterol-lowering with simvastatin in 5963 people with diabetes: a randomised placebo controlled trial. *Lancet,* 361: 2005–16, 2003

Dormandy, J.A., Charbonnel, B., Eckland, D.J., *et al.* Secondary prevention of macrovascular events in patients with type 2 diabetes in the PROactive Study (PROspective pioglitAzone Clinical Trial In macroVascular Events): a randomised controlled trial. *Lancet,* 366: 1279–89, 2005

Effects of ramipril on cardiovascular and microvascular outcomes in people with diabetes mellitus: results of the HOPE study and MICRO-HOPE substudy *Lancet,* 355: 253–59, 2000

Intensive blood-glucose control with sulphonylureas or insulin compared with conventional treatment and risk of complications in patients with Type 2 diabetes (UKPDS 33). *Lancet,* 352: 837–53, 1998

Tight blood pressure control and risk of macrovascular and microvascular complications in Type 2 diabetes (UKPDS 38). *British Medical Journal,* 317: 703–13, 1998

van Haehling, S. and Anker, S.D. Statins are being hailed as the new aspirin – but are they beneficial for patients with heart failure? *Heart,* 91: 1–52, 2005

Index

Page numbers followed by an italic *g* refer to glossary entries.

hypoglycaemia (hypos) *cont'd*
  and meals 94, 96, 101, 138
  and menstruation 168
  neuroglycopenic symptoms 126, 127, 128
  night-time 43, 45, 69, 93, 97, 98, 119,
    132–4, 214
    causes and symptoms 133
  and older people 212, 213, 214
  pregnancy and baby 173, 174
  rebound phenomenon 132
  recognizing symptoms 141
  recovery from 141
  and recreational drugs 163, 164
  relationship between blood sugar and
    hypoglycaemia 135
  risks associated with 134
  severe 75–6, 77, 127, 129, 131
  and smoking 158
  and stress 144
  and surgery 149
  symptoms 13, 31, 32, 33, 43, 66, 67, 68, 69,
    77, 126, 129, 134, 141
  testing 64, 65, 66
  timing and hypoglycaemia 137–9
  travel 183, 186
  treating hypoglycaemia 136–41
  warning signs 119, 126, 130, 134
  work related aspects 177, 178–9, 180

I

IDD insulin dependent diabetes *see* Type 1
    diabetes
illness while abroad 185
impaired glucose tolerance (pre-diabetes) 59,
    83, 232
  monitoring 126
  symptoms 126
impotence 242*g*
incapacity benefits 224, 225
Income Support 225
incretins 235, 236
influenza 150
information on diabetes, need for 188
injection sites, problems affecting 121, 125
injector 111–12, 242*g*
Innolet 242*g*

Insuflon 112, 113
insulin pen 94, 98, 100, 104, 105, 107–10,
    133, 176, 186, 225, 242
  and air travel 184–5
insulin pumps 35, 91, 103, 105–6, 108,
    112–14, 225–6
insulin sensitizers *see* glitazones
insulin 7, 12, 17–19, 21, 242*g*
  'insulin analogue' 124, 240*g*
  absorption of 98–9
  administering insulin 102–15
    injection techniques 102–6
    disinfecting skin 104, 105
    risk of intramuscular injection 105
  basal bolus insulin regime 72, 122, 176, 179,
    184
  basal insulin 19, 21, 22, 33, 90, 91,92, 93,
    97, 101
  bedtime insulin 97, 106, 133
  beef insulin 90, 124, 125, 131
  bolus secretion and injection 90, 94–5
  changing insulin requirements 116–20
  and changing sleep patterns 101
  clear insulin 108, 117, 240*g*
  cloudy insulin 90–1, 108, 109, 240*g*
  animal and human insulin 90, 124
  combining insulin and tablets 116
  complications of insulin therapy 40, 124,
    125, 190
  depot effect 98
  and diabetes 190
  effects of 26
  effects of insufficient insulin 31
  and exercise 59, 60
  factors influencing effect of insulin 98, 100
  forgetting to take insulin 99
  guidelines 117
  and high blood sugar 33
  history of discovery 12
  how insulin works 17–19, 22, 102
  human insulin production 90
  human insulin 90, 107, 124, 125, 131, 242*g*
  and hypoglycaemia 35, 136–7
  importance of 18
  injection patterns 94–7, 100–1
  injections 4
  injection and disinfection 105–6
  injection sites 98–9, 100, 102–3

2 | Treatment without insulin

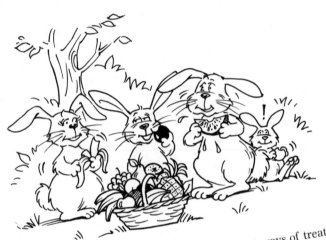

In this chapter and the next we describe different ways of treating diabetes. Most people diagnosed with Type 2 diabetes respond at first to changes in their diet. This alone may have a dramatic effect on their condition, especially in people who are overweight and manage to get their weight down. If changes in diet fail to control diabetes, tablets will be needed, but these will not work indefinitely and once they fail, insulin is the only alternative. A small number of people with Type 2 diabetes, who feel very unwell at the time of diagnosis, may need insulin immediately. Treatment with insulin is discussed in Chapter 3.

The most important thing for anyone with newly-diagnosed diabetes is to access good diabetes education. In the past, people were often given instructions about what to eat and which tablets to take without any explanation as to why it was important. Not surprisingly,

[Pages are shown smaller than actual size]

For details on how to order *Type 2 Diabetes: Answers at your fingertips*, please see our order form at the back of this book.

they did not always follow the advice. The importance of structured education has been recognised in the national frameworks for diabetes (see p. 140), and education programmes have been developed for both Type 1 and Type 2 diabetes. The DAFNE programme was introduced for Type 1 diabetes in 2002, and following its success, a group of people interested in diabetes education started to develop a course for people with Type 2 diabetes. They devised the DESMOND programme – Diabetes Education Self Management Ongoing and Newly Diagnosed. DESMOND is still being developed and the plan is to make it available nationally. Eventually everyone with Type 2 diabetes should have access to a standardised education programme, which will help them to understand diabetes and make important decisions about lifestyle changes.

DIABETES EDUCATION

My doctor has just told me that I have diabetes and I am feeling very shocked and confused as I don't know much about it but I know it can be serious. My doctor has given me the telephone number of Diabetes UK so I can get more information but I would really like to talk to someone with diabetes. Can you help me?

Most people who are told they have diabetes feel very upset at the news. One of the problems is the uncertainty about exactly how diabetes will impinge on their life. We agree that a phone call to Diabetes UK helpline is a good idea; it has gone to a lot of trouble to produce useful information for people with newly diagnosed diabetes. However, the most important thing they can do is put you in touch with the local branch of Diabetes UK. Naturally these vary in their level of activity, but in some areas the local branch is very well organised to provide support and information to new members. This will give you the opportunity to speak to other people who are in the same boat.

Have you found **Type 2 Diabetes in Adults of All Ages** *useful and practical? If so, you may be interested in titles from our award-winning 'Answers at your fingertips' series.*

Answers at your fingertips

'Woe betide any clinicians or nurses whose patients have read this invaluable source of down-to-earth information when they have not.' – The Lancet

Our best selling series, *Answers at your fingertips*, seeks to help those who, having been diagnosed with a condition, have countless questions that need answering. These essential handbooks answer all the questions that patients want to know about their health and condition. The formula for the series follows a question-and-answer format, with real questions from sufferers and their families answered by medical experts at the top of their fields, without the jargon of medical texts. All these books are packed full of practical information for patients and their families.

Each title is only £14.99 plus £3.00 p&p. Topics covered range from diagnosis to treatment, and from relationships to welfare entitlements.

'Contains the answers the doctor wishes he had given if only he'd had the time.' – Dr Thomas Stuttaford, *The Times*

Titles currently available (or coming soon*):

Acne • Allergies • Asthma • Autism • Breast Cancer*
COPD • Alzheimer's & other dementias • Diabetes • Epilepsy
Eczema • Gout • Heart Health • High Blood Pressure
Kidney Dialysis & Transplants • Motor Neurone Disease
Multiple Sclerosis • Osteoporosis • Parkinson's • Psoriasis
Sexual Health for Men • Stroke

For current availability of the *Answers at your fingertips* range, please contact us using our Freepost address:

Class Publishing Priority Service,
FREEPOST,
London W6 7BR

The *Class Health* Feedback Form

We hope that you found this *Class Health* book helpful. We always appreciate readers' opinions and would be grateful if you could take a few minutes to complete this form for us.

❶ How did you acquire your copy of this book?

From my local library ☐

Read an article in a newspaper/magazine ☐

Found it by chance ☐

Recommended by a friend ☐

Recommended by a patient organisation/charity ☐

Recommended by a doctor/nurse/adviser ☐

Saw an advertisement ☐

❷ How much of the book have you read?

All of it ☐

More than half of it ☐

Less than half of it ☐

❸ Which copies/chapters have been most helpful?

....

....

....

....

❹ Overall, how useful to you was this *Class Health* book?

Extremely useful ☐

Very useful ☐

Useful ☐

❺ What did you find most helpful?

....

....

....

....

6 **What did you find least helpful?**

....

....

....

....

7 **Have you read any other health books?**

Yes ☐   No ☐

If yes, which subjects did they cover?

....

....

....

....

How did this *Class Health* book compare?

Much better   ☐

Better   ☐

About the same   ☐

Not as good   ☐

8 **Would you recommend this book to a friend?**

Yes ☐   No ☐

Thank you for your help. Please send your completed form to:

Class Publishing, FREEPOST, London W6 7BR

Surname   First name
_____

Title Prof/Dr/Mr/Mrs/Ms
_____

Address
_____

Town   Postcode   Country
_____

☐ Please add my name and address to receive details of related books

[Please note, we will not pass on your details to any other company]

Have you found *Type 2 Diabetes in Adults of all Ages* useful and practical? If so, you may be interested in these other books from Class Publishing.

Type 1 Diabetes in Children, Adolescents and Young Adults £19.99
Dr Ragnar Hanas

If you have diabetes, you need to become better informed than the average doctor. Dr Hanas's book tells you everything you need to know to take good care of your condition, live a full, healthy and happy life, and control your diabetes rather than being controlled by it.

'This extraordinary book . . . will help you to understand diabetes better'
DR PETER SWIFT, Consultant Paediatrician, Leicester Royal Infirmary.

Dump Your Toxic Waist! £14.99
Dr Derrick Cutting

The easy, drug-free and medically accurate way to lose inches, beat diabetes and stop that heart attack.

'. . . an excellent book for those who are interested in unclogging their arteries, or getting down to their ideal weight for good, or controlling their blood pressure, or discovering a new vitality.'
The Family Heart Digest

Kidney Failure Explained £17.99
Dr Andy Stein and Janet Wild

Written by two experienced medical authors, this practical handbook covers every aspect of living with kidney disease – from diagnosis, drugs and treatment, to diet, relationships and sex.

'. . . without doubt, the best resource currently available for kidney patients and those who care for them.'

VAL SAID, kidney transplant patient

Beating Depression £17.99
Dr Stefan Cembrowicz and Dr Dorcas Kingham

Depression is one of most common illnesses in the world – affecting up to one in four people at some time in their lives. This book offers tried and tested techniques for overcoming depression.

'All you need to know about depression, presented in a clear, concise and readable way.'

ANN DAWSON, World Health Organization

Type 2 Diabetes: Answers at your fingertips £14.99
Dr Charles Fox and Dr Anne Kilvert

The latest edition of our bestselling reference guide on diabetes has now been split into two books covering the two distinct forms of the disease. These books maintain the popular question-and-answer format to provide practical advice for patients on every aspect of living with the condition.

'I have no hesitation in commending this book.'
SIR STEVE REDGRAVE, Vice President, Diabetes UK

Irritable Bowel Syndrome: Answers at your fingertips £17.99
Dr Udi Shmueli

IBS is a trying problem that can affect confidence and lifestyles. This practical and reassuring book looks at the science behind the symptoms, examines possible ways of finding relief, and gives advice about taking control of your condition.

'. . . an ideal first step in achieving better bowel health.'
KATHLEEN MCGRATH, Director of Medical Services, Medical Advisory Service

Heart Health: Answers at your fingertips £14.99
Dr Graham Jackson

This practical handbook, written by a leading cardiologist, answers all your questions about heart conditions. It tells you how to keep your heart healthy or, if it has been affected by heart disease, how to make it as strong as possible.

'Those readers who want to know more about the various treatments for heart disease will be much enlightened.'
DR JAMES LE FANU, The Daily Telegraph

Stroke: Answers at your fingertips £17.99
Dr Anthony Rudd, Penny Irwin and Bridget Penhale

This essential guidebook tells you all about strokes – most importantly how to recover from them. Full of practical advice, including recuperation plans. You will find it inspiring.

'If you only buy one book about stroke, it should be Stroke: Answers at your fingertips'
JON BARRICK, Chief Executive, the Stroke Association

PRIORITY ORDER FORM

Cut out or photocopy this form and send it (post free in the UK) to:

Class Publishing
FREEPOST 16705
Macmillan Distribution
Basingstoke RG21 6ZZ

Tel: 01256 302 699
Fax: 01256 812 558

Please send me urgently
(tick below)

Post included
price per copy (UK only)

☐ **Type 2 Diabetes in Adults of All Ages** (ISBN 978 1 85959 166 6) £23.99

☐ **Type 1 Diabetes in Children, Adolescents and Young Adults** (ISBN 978 1 85959 153 6) £23.99

☐ **Type 2 Diabetes – Answers at your fingertips** (ISBN 978 1 85959 176 5) £17.99

☐ **Dump Your Toxic Waist!** (ISBN 978 1 85959 191 8) £17.99

☐ **Kidney Failure Explained** (ISBN 978 1 85959 145 1) £20.99

☐ **Beating Depression** (ISBN 978 1 85959 150 5) £20.99

☐ **IBS: Answers at your fingertips** (ISBN 978 1 85959 156 7) £20.99

☐ **Heart Health: Answers at your fingertips** (ISBN 978 1 85959 097 3) £17.99

☐ **Stroke: Answers at your fingertips** (ISBN 978 1 85959 113 0) £20.99

TOTAL _____

Easy ways to pay

Cheque: I enclose a cheque payable to Class Publishing for £ _____

Credit card: Please debit my ☐ Mastercard ☐ Visa ☐ Amex

Number _____ Expiry date _____

Name _____

My address for delivery is _____

_____

Town _____ County _____ Postcode _____

Telephone number (*in case of query*) _____

Credit card billing address if different from above _____

_____

Town _____ County _____ Postcode _____

Class Publishing's guarantee: remember that if, for any reason, you are not satisfied with these books, we will refund all your money, without any questions asked. Prices and VAT rates may be altered for reasons beyond our control.